Health

—— AND ——

Numbers

Health

—— AND ——

Numbers

A Problems-Based Introduction to Biostatistics, Third Edition

Chap T. Le, Ph.D.

Distinguished Professor of Biostatistics,
School of Public Health
Director of Biostatistics & Informatics,
Comprehensive Masonic Cancer Center
University of Minnesota, Twin Cities

WILEY

A John Wiley & Sons, Inc., Publication

Published by John Wiley & Sons, Inc., Hoboken, New Jersey
Published simultaneously in Canada

For general information on our other products and services or for technical support, please contact our Customer Care Department within the United States at (800) 762-2974, outside the United States at (317) 572-3993 or fax (317) 572-4002.

Wiley also publishes its books in a variety of electronic formats. Some content that appears in print may not be available in electronic formats. For more information about Wiley products, visit our web site at www.wiley.com.

Library of Congress Cataloging-in-Publication Data:

ISBN 978-0470-18589-6

Printed in the United States of America

10 9 8 7 6 5 4 3 2 1

To my wife, Minh-Ha,
& my daughters, Mina and Jenna
with deepest love and appreciation

Contents

Preface

A course in introductory biostatistics is often required for professional students in public health, dentistry, nursing, and medicine, and graduate students in nursing and other biomedical sciences. It is only a course or two, but the requirement is often considered as a roadblock causing anxiety in many quarters. The feelings are expressed in many ways and in many different settings but all leading to the same conclusion that simply surviving the endurance is the only practical goal. And students need help, in the form of a user-friendly text, in order to do just that, surviving. In the early 1990s, we decided it's time to write our own text, and *Health and Numbers: Basic Biostatistical Methods* was published in 1995 reflecting our experience after teaching introductory biostatistics courses for many years to students from various human health disciplines. The second edition, *Health and Numbers: A Problems-based Introduction to Biostatistics* was also aimed to the same audience for whom the first edition was written: professional and beginning graduate students in human health disciplines who need help to successfully pass and to benefit from the basic biostatistics course requirement. Our main objective was not only to avoid the perception that statistics is just a number of formulas that students need to get over with, but to present it as a way of thinking, thinking about ways to gather and analyze data so as to benefit from taking the required course. And there is no better way to do that than making our book problem-based: many problems with real data in various fields are provided at the end of all eight chapters as aids to learning how to use statistical procedures, still the nuts and bolts of elementary applied statistics. The most appealing feature of Health & Numbers, through the first two editions, has been that it is based on the most popular, most available, cheapest computer package, the Microsoft Excel. The second edition was successful; however: (1) there are not enough details in the use of Excel, and (2) the book covers many topics — some are difficult for beginners. Therefore, in this third edition, Health and Numbers: A Problems-Based Introduction to Biostatistics, I try to overcome those weaknesses by cutting out a few advanced topics and adding many more hints and examples on the use of Excel in every chapter.

The "way of thinking" called statistics has become important to all professionals who not only are scientific or business-like but also caring people who want to help and make the world a better place. But what is it? What is biostatistics and what can it do? There are popular definitions and perceptions of statistics. For this book and its readers, we don't emphasize the definition of "statistics as things", but instead offer an active concept of "doing statistics". The doing of statistics is a way of thinking about numbers, with emphasis on relating their interpretation and meaning to the manner in which they are collected. Our working definition of statistics, as an activity, is that it is a way of thinking about data, its collection, its analysis, and its presentation. Formulas are needed but not as the only things you need to know.

To illustrate statistics as a way of thinking, let's start with a familiar scenario of our criminal court procedures. A crime has been discovered and a suspect has been identified. After a police investigation to collect evidence against the suspect, a prosecutor presents summarized evidence to a jury. The jurors learn about the rules and debate the rule about convicting beyond a reasonable doubt and the rule about unanimous decision. After the debate, the jurors vote and a verdict is reached: guilty or not guilty. Why do we need this time-consuming, cost-consuming process called trial by jury? Well, the truth is often unknown, at least uncertain. It is uncertain because of variability (every case is different) and because of incomplete information (missing key evidence?). Trial by jury is the way our society deals with uncertainties; its goal is to minimize mistakes.

How does society deal with uncertainties? We go through a process called trial by jury, consisting of these steps: (1) we form assumption or hypothesis (that every person is innocent until proven guilty), (2) we gather data (evidence supporting the charge), and (3) we decide whether the hypothesis should be rejected (guilty) or should not be rejected (not guilty). Basically, a successful trial should consist of these elements: (1) a probable cause (with a crime and a suspect), (2) a thorough investigation by police, (3) an efficient presentation by the prosecutor, and (4) a fair and impartial jury.

In the above-described context of a trial by jury, let us consider a few specific examples: (1) the *crime* is lung cancer and the *suspect* is cigarette smoking, or (2) the *crime* is leukemia and the *suspect* is pesticides, or (3) the *crime* is breast cancer and the *suspect* is a defective gene. The process is now called *research*, and the tool to carry out that research is biostatistics. In a simple way, biostatistics serves as the biomedical version of the trial by jury process. It is the *science* of dealing with uncertainties using incomplete information. Yes, even science is uncertain; scientists arrive at different conclusions in many different areas at different times; many studies are inconclusive. The reasons for uncertainties remain the same. Nature is complex and full of unexplained biological variability. But, most important of all, we always have to deal with incomplete information. It is often not practical to study the entire population; we have to rely on information gained from *samples.*

How does science deal with uncertainties? We learn from how society deals with uncertainties; we go through a process called biostatistics, consisting of these steps: (1) we form assumption or hypothesis (from the research question), (2) we gather data (from clinical trials, surveys, medical records abstractions), and (3) we make decision(s) (by doing statistical analysis/inference, a guilty verdict is referred to as *statistical significance*). Basically, a successful research should consist of these elements: (1) a good research question (with well-defined objectives and endpoints), (2) a thorough investigation (by experiments or surveys), (3) an efficient presentation of data (organizing data, summarizing, and presenting data; an area called *descriptive statistics*), and (4) proper *statistical inference*. This book is a problems-based introduction to the last three elements; together they form a field called *biostatistics*. The coverage is rather brief on data collection, but very extensive on descriptive statistics (Chapters 1 and 2), and on methods of statistical inference (Chapters 4, 5, 6, 7 and 8). Chapter 3, on probability and probability models, serves as the link between descriptive and inferential parts.

The author would like to express his sincere appreciation to colleagues for feedback, to teaching assistants who helped with examples and exercises, and to students for feedbacks. Finally, my family bore patiently the pressures caused by my long-term commitment to write books; to my wife and daughters, I am always most grateful.

CHAP T. LE
Edina, Minnesota

Introduction from the First Edition

We have taught introductory biostatistics courses for many years to students from various human health disciplines, and decided it's time to write our own book. We as teachers are very familiar with students who enter such courses with an enormous sense of dread, based on a combination of low self-confidence in their mathematical ability and a perception that they would never need to use statistics in their future work, even if they did learn the subject, especially those students who enter health fields that emphasize caring, human contact view statistics as the antithesis of interpersonal warmth. We are sympathetic to the plight of students taking statistics courses simply because it is a requirement, and consequently we have tried to write a friendly text. By friendly we mean *fairly thin book* and *emphasizing a few basic principles* rather than a jumble of isolated facts. The perception that statistics is just a bunch of formulas and long columns of numbers is the main misunderstanding of the field. Statistics is a way of thinking, thinking about ways to gather and analyze data. The formulas are tools of statistics, just like stethoscopes are tools for doctors and wrenches are tools for auto mechanics. The first thing a good statistician does when faced with data is to learn how the data were collected; the last thing is to apply formulas and do calculations. It's amazing how many times statistical formulas are misused by a well-intentioned researcher simply because the data wasn't collected correctly. Start to pay attention to the number of times the media will announce that studies have been done that lead to such-and-such a conclusion, but never tell you how the study was done or the data collected. Most of the time the reporters don't even know that the methods of the study or the method of data collection is crucial to the study's validity; their job is to seek out newsworthy findings and dramatize the implications.

Almost all of the formal statistical procedures performed fall into two categories: testing and estimation. This book covers the most commonly used, elementary procedures in both categories: the z-test, the t-test, the chi-square test, point estimation, confidence interval estimation, and correlation and regression. These are the nuts and bolts of elementary applied statistics. We also throw in some basic ideas of standardization of rates and graphical techniques that are easy to learn and incredibly useful. Exercises are added as aid to learning how to use statistical procedures. Learning to use statistics takes practice. It's not an easy subject, but it's worth learning. Let us know how we can improve the book.

Recently, we met Carmen, a middle-aged woman. During social chit-chat, she told us that she is a nurse in a cancer ward. When we announced that we are statistics professors, she said she was planning on getting her master's degree in nursing and that we might be interested in some advice she heard from other nurses who get master's degrees. "If you get only one chance for a pass-fail option, use it on the stat course," they counseled. They made it clear that the statistics course required of graduate students in nursing is really hard and that simply surviving it is the only practical goal.

We neither had problem believing Carmen nor did we question the sincerity of the students' recommendation. Many times this sentiment is expressed: Statistics courses are experiences to be endured and even honest people are tempted to cheat to pass. Survival skills are in order: "Do anything, including neglecting the other courses for one quarter, to get it behind you. Use flash cards, buy other books, and make friends with nerds if you must, but get through the requirement."

These feelings are expressed in many ways and in many different settings by those who have taken required statistics courses. In the social setting of a party, the revelation that we teach statistics usually provokes such comments from a course survivor or one who is dreading the experience. Indeed, the required statistics course may well be described as a hostage situation, with the students as prisoners and the teacher as torturer.

The drama of the required statistics course is re-enacted year after year throughout the country. Students from a wide variety of helping professions take statistics courses as they prepare for a career. This book is written especially for those who feel inadequate with statistics in any form but are forced by journal editors, government funding agencies, and degree requirements to deal with it. If you are one of those people, this book is for you.

Statistics is a hard subject; many people, however, realize that it is essential not only in science and government but also in the human services fields. As the federal budget problems continue, both the Pentagon and the Department of Health and Human Services cite statistics to help their cases. Applicants for increased government funding for worthy causes can no longer claim only their good intentions as the sole reason for a bigger chunk of the pie. They have to present numbers to show that funding their cause is a better bargain "for the people" than funding a competing worthy cause. This creates a demand for an objective way of thinking and an art of communication, called *statistics*.

The "way of thinking" called statistics has become important to all professionals who are not only scientific or business-like but also caring people who want to help and make the world a better place. Such people have big hearts, high ideals, and a concern for humanity. They are good people who work hard and expect only a modest income. They become teachers or nurses or clergy or social workers, the kind of people inclined to join the Peace Corps. They even do volunteer work in a wide variety of human services. Such people are the special audience of this book. Due to funding pressures and self-imposed requirements that their field be more research-based, those who seek higher degrees are forced to take statistics courses, read journal articles, and write reports using numbers and statistical formulas. They and their administrators must defend their work by counting and measuring, and defend against those who attack their counting and measuring methodology.

This book is written for helpers who are *forced* to deal with the world of statistics but feel inadequate because of low mathematical ability, lack of self-confidence, and the perception that they will never need to use statistical concepts and techniques in their future work.

WHAT IS STATISTICS?

There are several popular public definitions and perceptions of statistics. We see "vital statistics" in the newspaper, announcements of life events such as births, marriages, and deaths. Motorists are warned to drive carefully, to avoid "becoming a statistic." The public use of the word is widely varied, most often indicating lists of numbers or data. We have also heard people use the word *data* to describe a verbal report, a believable anecdote. Statisticians define statistics to be summarizing numbers, like averages; for example, the average age of all mothers on AFDC is a statistic because it is a (partial) summary of a list of numbers too long and too varied to describe individually. The average is a useful partial summary and thus a statistic.

For this book and its readers, we don't emphasize the definition of "statistics as things," but offer instead an active concept of "doing Statistics." The doing of statistics is a way of thinking about numbers, with emphasis on relating their interpretation and meaning to the manner in which they are collected. The relation of method of collection to technique of analysis, by the way, is absolutely central to the understanding of statistical thought. Anyone who claims facility with statistical formulas but is oblivious to the method of collection of the data to be analyzed must not portray him/herself as a statistician. Failing to see the important relationship of collection with analysis is the root cause of mindless throwing of statistical formulas at data.

Our working definition of statistics, as an activity, is that it is a way of thinking about data, about their collection, about their analysis, and about their presentation to an audience. Formulas are only a part of that thinking, simply tools of the trade.

To illustrate statistics as a way of thinking, we notice that our local radio station has a practice of conducting radio polls and announcing their results during the morning rush hour. One question was whether an old baseball player (who was personally popular among the locals and had a high batting average) should be recruited to play for the Minnesota Twins again. Of the people who called in their answer, 74% said "yes" and 26% said "no." As the people who are well-groomed into statistical thinking, we wondered whether the 74% meant that 74% of the people in the city want him back or 74% of baseball fans want him back or what? In trying to figure out whether the 74% meant anything, we listened to the method by which the data were collected. The announcer said that only people who had touch-tone phones could vote because only such phones would work for their voting system. So now the poll was limited to people with touch-tone phones, who aren't too busy at 8:30 a.m. Of those who had the phones and the time, what kind of people cared enough to vote? Thinking through this maze of selections is doing statistics. All this kind of thinking must be done before applying any statistical formula makes sense. There are many people who don't know statistical formulas but naturally think statistically. Someone who throws statistical formulas at data but doesn't appreciate the subtleties of data collection is dangerous.

WHAT CAN STATISTICS DO?

There is a broad spectrum of beliefs among nonstatisticians about what the field of statistics can actually do. At one extreme are the cynical disbelievers who think the only contribution of statisticians was the discovery that, at cocktail parties, 2% of the people eat 90% of the nuts. At the other extreme are the blind believers who envision statistics as a crime lab going over the murder room with a fine-tooth comb. They also think of statisticians as archaeologists digging gingerly into mounds of data, extracting from them every bit of truth.

WHY IS STATISTICS SO HARD TO LEARN?

Statistical formulas commonly result in numbers that have no intuitive meaning. They do not relate to any ordinary experience. At the end of the calculations for a *t*-test, the number one is considered very small but the number three is very large. This defies intuition. The person performing a *t*-test looks in t-tables at the back of a statistics book to find that the probability associated with 1 is .32. Next, the reader of the table is told that .32 is too large to be called significant. It is *not* significant. You might well think that .32 is not a significant number in some ordinary sense but because it is too small. The t-table tells you it's *too large* to be significant. If, after calculating the *t*-test, you get the "large" number 3 and then look in the t-table to find the probability associated with it is .005, you are told that .005 is small enough to be highly significant. What is this, anyway? How does a 1 get you a .32 while a 3 leads to a .005? What's going on when little numbers like .005 are highly significant? Any logical person thinks big numbers are significant, not small ones. This turning upside down of brand new meanings assigned to small numbers and large ones is a major adjustment for the student of statistics. Anyone who gets confused converting inches to centimeters or Celsius to Fahrenheit is in for hard work learning to use statistical formulas.

One class of volunteers who want to learn statistics are the graduate students seeking a master's or doctoral degree in biostatistics, a specialization of statistics. These students study full-time for at least a year before starting to get an integrated notion of statistics, and many of them come to our program already having earned a bachelor's degree in mathematics.

The nonvolunteers have an even worse time. The ones we see are the graduate students in fields such as nursing or environmental sanitation who are required to take one or two statistics courses for their masters or doctoral degrees. When we teach them, we do what we can to minimize their frustration with the material. Some of them seem to learn the formulas fairly easily, but few of them can get a good handle on the concepts. A good number of those students spend an inordinate amount of time on the course, neglecting their other courses, to pass statistics and get beyond the hurdle. Several students try hard to find a statistics course taught by an easy grader. They dread the statistics requirement.

REASONS FOR THE DIFFICULTY

There are two kinds of reasons for statistics being a difficult subject to learn: intellectual and emotional.

Intellectual Reasons

There are concepts in statistics that are difficult to understand. For one thing, although statistics is definitely not the same as mathematics, it *uses* mathematics. Anyone who has trouble with arithmetic and algebra has trouble with statistics, and there are lots of people with excellent communication skills (reading, writing, and speaking) who have trouble with arithmetic and algebra. The Graduate Record Exam, as well as other standard examinations such as the Scholastic Aptitude Test taken by high school students, has the separate categories of verbal and quantitative; they are different. To attain the master's degree, knowledge of statistics requires a good knowledge of calculus and some facility with a topic called "matrices" or linear algebra. A doctoral degree requires, in addition to the knowledge of statistics, advanced calculus and something called "measure theory" as a basis for understanding probability. In other words, getting deeply into statistical theory requires the knowledge of mathematics that is attained by very few people. The mathematics of advanced statistics is approximately the level of the mathematics of theoretical physics.

In addition to the mathematics of statistics, there are other difficult concepts. The main difficulty is in visualizing the distribution of numbers you cannot see. Many students have a hard time getting straight the sampling distribution of the sample means when the end point of the study is only one sample mean. That is, they have to be able to visualize infinitely many numbers, of which they see only one, and think about what the other numbers might have been.

Emotional Reasons

There are aspects other than statistics being intellectually difficult that act as barriers to learning. For one thing, statistics does not benefit from a glamorous image that motivates students to persist through tedious and frustrating lessons. A premedical or prelaw student is commonly sustained through long discouraging times in school by dreams of wealth and high social status, heroism in the not-too-distant future. However, there are no TV dramas with a good-looking statistician playing the lead, and few mothers' chests swell with pride as they introduce their son or daughter as "the statistician."

The public images of statisticians leave much to be desired as sources of recruitment. *How to Lie with Statistics* (by Darrell Huff) is the statistics book whose title is most often quoted by nonstatisticians. One image of statisticians is that of sports nuts who are fascinated by numerical trivia of games. Another image is of the librarian, the solemn keeper of dry details, of "more than you'd ever want to know about . . ." Yet another is the role of the manipulator of numbers, the crook who can make numbers say anything he or she wants them to. Presidential campaigns in which both incumbent and challenger cite "statistics" showing why they should be elected don't give statistics a good name.

Have you ever heard of a child who answered the question, "What are you going to be when you grow up?" with "I'm going to be a statistician!"?

Another emotional barrier to the learning of statistics is the one related to the difficulty of learning mathematics. The intellectual difficulty of learning mathematics not infrequently creates a phobia currently labeled "math anxiety," a feeling of inadequacy in doing anything mathematical. Such people who dread having to do mathematical work are particularly uncomfortable in the "required" statistics course. We have had many students in our elementary courses who contacted us early in the quarter tell us how nervous they are about passing the course. Many of them tell their history of math anxiety. Some describe their childhood math teachers as particularly stern and unforgiving.

One reason for math anxiety, leading to stat anxiety, is the fact that mathematics is an especially unforgiving *field*. The typical student of arithmetic or elementary algebra doesn't see the beauty and artistry of higher mathematics. Such students see that there is only one correct answer and that no credit is given for approximately correct, or not exactly right but useful. Two plus two equals four, not 4.001. It's either all right or all wrong. In most other subjects, there is a little give: answers are not so "right" or "wrong."

Those people very facile with numbers can easily intimidate the innumerate. The expert who spews forth a barrage of numerical facts is one up; numerical facts seem more precise and more correct, and the speaker of the facts thus seems more in charge. Robert McNamara, at one time the president of Ford Motor and later the Secretary of Defense under Lyndon Johnson, used to explain the Vietnam War on live television. His command of facts and confidence with which he spewed forth a barrage of war data gave the impression that he was on top of every detail. He was very impressive, due partly to his command of numbers.

THE THREE LEVELS OF STATISTICAL KNOWLEDGE

Level One

The first level of knowledge is that of familiarity with some of the statistical formulas. These formulas, like the formulas for the *t*-test or the Chi-square test, are gadgets. They are analogous to the stethoscopes used by physicians, wrenches used by auto mechanics, or desk calculators used by accountants. The formulas of statistics are as important to the field of statistics as the stethoscope, wrench, and desk calculator are for the aforementioned occupations. It's appropriate and natural when learning a new field to play with and get used to its gadgets. It's also a good way to see if you have a chance of liking the field and could be happy working in it. If you can't use a stethoscope, don't consider becoming a physician. If you can't use a wrench, cancel any plans to be an auto mechanic.

The formulas of statistics are qualitatively different from stethoscopes and wrenches. To use a stethoscope requires the ability to find the key spots on the human body, a good ear for subtle sounds, and willingness to tolerate the discomfort of the little black knobs that stick in your ears. Using a wrench requires a good sense of selecting the appropriate size and type of wrench, sufficient arm and shoulder strength to loosen tight nuts, and a light enough touch to avoid ruining a nut. Using statistical formulas requires good facility with algebra at the "college algebra" level, real skill and comfort with mathematical calculations, and a low rate of mistakes in arithmetic.

The skill in using the gadgets of a profession is obviously necessary for its practice. A candidate for the profession is well advised to test the waters by trying to attain at least minimal skill with its gadgets. After attaining minimal skill, the candidate can go on to learn to use them in context.

Level Two

The second level of knowledge of statistics is that of knowing how and when to use what gadgets for standard problems. Just as every physician must know what to do for a patient who is in every way healthy but has cracked a rib, or every auto mechanic knows how to install a new gas tank, the Level Two statistician knows how to analyze the data from a well-designed household survey when the households are selected using a random number table and every household has an adult respondent at home when the interviewer arrives. The Level Two statistician also knows how to work with a cooperative laboratory researcher who wants to design an experiment to allocate different chemotherapy doses to mice with cancer.

Level Three

The Level Three statistician is one who is perfectly familiar with the formulas and can handle difficult messy problems. A Level Three statistician can assess the possibility of making sense out of large data sets with many missing observations and chaotic methods of collection.

Setting Your Own Goal Level

The skill essential to learning statistical formulas is that of working with algebra. In other words, you need to be fairly good with abstract symbols and arithmetic. Being solid in the four basic operations of arithmetic (addition, subtraction, multiplication, and division) and taking square roots is absolutely essential for mastery of statistical formulas. Also, being good at looking up numbers in tables is required. There are inexpensive pocket calculators that will do the calculations of statistical formulas, but anyone shaky at arithmetic is in deep statistical water even with calculators. Without the ability to do the calculations by hand, there is great danger of pushing the wrong buttons or pushing the right buttons in the wrong order and not realizing that something is wrong. Another skill essential to the use of statistical formulas is a sense of magnitude, to know when the calculations result in a number that is way too large or too small, or negative when it should be positive. People who confuse debits with credits in their checkbooks have a very hard time with statistical formulas. If you are shaky at arithmetic, don't expect success with even Level One knowledge of statistics.

If you are good at arithmetic and algebra, you should be ready to learn statistical formulas. You would then be ready to follow the instructions of formulas (which you may think of as recipes) and thus correctly perform the calculations.

Learning Level Two requires an additional talent, that of understanding analogies. The ability to see that choosing households for a survey is mathematically equivalent to pulling names out of a hat is essential. Level Two also requires a good memory to keep in mind the many situations and where to find the formulas to fit them.

Level-Three knowledge of statistics requires, in addition to mastery of the first two levels, the ability and nerve to deal with problems for which there is no standard solution. Working at Level Three requires either finding new solutions or using an old technique that works imperfectly but will do the job. It requires cleverness and adaptability.

Time Required for Learning Statistics

For someone good at arithmetic and the symbol manipulations used in algebra, a few of the most popular formulas can be learned in a one-quarter or one-semester elementary course. In a course lasting one academic year, you can cover quite a few of the well-used formulas; you can also start to learn some of the concepts of statistics, although that is a much harder task than learning the formulas.

Learning Level Two takes two years of full-time study, assuming that you have had a year of calculus (with at least a B grade) and are an advanced undergraduate or graduate student. Level Two is essentially a master's degree in statistics and attaining it is a major effort. Level Three is acquired only after a good four years of full-time effort in the field of statistics. It can be obtained by a master's degree plus two years full-time experience. Some statisticians attain Level Three by the time they graduate with a doctorate in statistics. Attaining a very advanced Level Three requires natural statistical talent and many years of experience.

DEALING WITH FORMULAS

People who tend to grimace and flinch at the thought of statistics tend to be most repelled by statistical formulas. We have seen a number of them gingerly open a new statistics book, whose cover beckons the reader with come-ons such as "statistics made easy" or "statistics for the layman." The Introduction assures the reader that he or she need have no background in anything whatsoever and should simply relax and read on. The scarred veteran of previous statistics books doesn't believe it, however, and flips through the book to check for the presence of "formulas." Upon finding them, like bones in a fish, the reader snaps the book shut, defeated once again.

Statistical formulas are frightening to anyone suffering from math anxiety. They remind one of the worst days of the old algebra classes. Some even have Greek letters in them. This book is intended to be light on formulas, but we want to walk the reader through one of the most common ones, just to show how statisticians think about formulas.

There are a couple of well-worn formulas that are used frequently even by nonstatisticians. They are the formulas for the two-sample t-test and the Chi-square, the latter represented symbolically by the Greek letter "chi" with a 2 in the upper right corner: ξ^2. By purely arbitrary choice, we'll introduce the former, the two-sample t-test:

A statistics text will typically present the two-sample t-test as follows: To test

$$H_0 : \mu_1 = \mu_2$$

versus

$$H_A : \mu_1 \neq \mu_2$$

At the α-level, the process is to form

$$t = \frac{\bar{x}_2 - \bar{x}_1}{\text{SE}(\bar{x}_2 - \bar{x}_1)}$$

where

$$\text{SE}(\bar{x}_2 - \bar{x}_1) = s_p \sqrt{\frac{1}{n_1} + \frac{1}{n_2}}$$

$$s_p^2 = \frac{(n_1 - 1)s_1^2 + (n_2 - 1)s_2^2}{n_1 + n_2 - 2}$$

Then to "reject" H_0 if and only if t exceeds a certain cut-point obtained from some table (at the back of the book) or with the help of some computer software.

How are you doing? Had enough? That formula, one of the two most used, is full of frightening symbols and jargon. It contains the Greek letters α, μ, and σ. It has subscripts, indices, and may include absolute value symbol.

A statistician can dive right in, plugging in numbers for the xs, and get the job done. To the uninitiated, however, the formula is overwhelming. Students in statistics courses need days, sometimes weeks, to get used to it and working with it. Many keep forgetting what α, μ, and σ are. It seems very artificial, without intuitive appeal. It's intuitively natural to subtract one sample mean from another, but the whole denominator seems weird; it doesn't make any intuitive sense. Students have a hard time keeping standard deviation separate from standard error, forgetting to take square roots, putting the ns in the wrong place. When they should be getting a $+3$, they're getting a -3, and have no instinct that the -3 is wrong. We don't blame them; it is difficult and confusing.

Using statistical formulas is like cooking from recipes or putting together lawn furniture from a set of cut-away drawings. Just as the recipe is a kind of shorthand that could be written in prose form, and the drawings for the swing set could be eliminated by substituting a few paragraphs of English, a statistical formula *could* be expressed in words. A statistician reading the formula does just that, translating the formula into English, seeing it as a set of directions as to what to do with two sets of numbers. It is no surprise, of course, that statisticians write the statistics books in their own language, using formulas instead of English prose because they themselves are so comfortable reading formulas. Formulas, although in principle are similar to recipes, are more abstract. A recipe that says "Break two eggs into a cup of milk" is referring to objects and actions more common than μ, the population mean. Eggs, cups, and milk can be felt and tasted; α, μ, and σ are abstract concepts. Most people are so used to the small counting numbers, that is, 1, 2, 3, ... that they forget how abstract numbers themselves come about. Even the number "1" is a figment of the imagination; it cannot be touched or tasted. It has no volume or weight and is not on display in some museum. It is a property that an apple, a truck, and an ocean have in common, namely their oneness.

In summary, formulas are fine for those very comfortable with algebra and good at following a long list of complicated instructions. If you're weak in either of those areas, don't expect statistical formulas to be easy. But the computer can sure help. And that is why we introduce Excel.

1

Proportions, Rates, and Ratios

Most introductory textbooks in statistics and biostatistics start with methods for organizing, summarizing, and presenting continuous data–numbers measured on a continuous scale; for example, measurements of height, weight, blood pressure, or cholesterol level. We have decided, however, to adopt a different starting point because our focused areas are research in biomedical sciences, and health decisions are more frequently based on proportions, ratios, or rates. In addition, it is easier to learn methods for categorical data and, therefore, to build knowledge and confidence. In this first chapter we will see how the concepts of proportion, rate, and ratios appeal to common sense, and learn their meaning and uses. You will be able to apply what you learn quickly to tackle real-life data, concepts, and applications—concepts such as case–control study, measures of morbidity, and mortality—before moving on to more complicated methods for continuous data in Chapter 2.

1.1. PROPORTIONS

Many outcomes can be classified as belonging to one of two possible categories: Presence and Absence, Nonwhite and White, Male and Female, Improved and Not-improved. The resulting data are called "binary data" or "dichotomous data." Of course, one of these two categories is usually identified as of primary interest; for example, Presence in the Presence-and-Absence classification, Nonwhite in the White-and-Nonwhite classification. We can always, in general, relabel the two outcome categories as positive $(+)$ and negative $(-)$. An outcome is positive if the primary category is observed and is negative if the other category is observed.

It is obvious that, in the summary to characterize observations made on a group of individuals, the number "x" of positive outcomes is not sufficient; the group size "n", or total number of observations, should also be recorded and used. The number "x" tells us very little and only becomes meaningful after adjusting for the size "n" of the group; in other words, the two figures "*x*" and "*n*" are often combined into a *statistic*, called *proportion*:

$$p = \frac{x}{n}$$

The term "statistic" means a summarized figure from observed data; a summary, some calculated number. It can be easily seen that $0 \leq p \leq 1$ because the number "*x*" of positive outcomes cannot be negative and, as the size of a subgroup, it cannot be greater than "*n*". This proportion "*p*" is sometimes expressed as a percentage and is calculated as follows:

$$\% = \left(\frac{x}{n}\right) 100\%$$

Example 1.1

A study, published several years ago by the Urban Coalition of Minneapolis and the University of Minnesota Adolescent Health Program, surveyed 12,915 students in Grades 7 through 12 in Minneapolis and St. Paul public schools. The report said minority students, about one-third of the group, were much less likely to have had a recent routine physical checkup. Among Asian students, 25.4% said they had not seen a doctor or a dentist in the last two years, followed by 17.7% of American Indians, 16.1% of Blacks, and 10% of Hispanics. Among Whites, it was 6.5%.

Proportion is a number used to *describe* a group of individuals according to a dichotomous characteristic under investigation. The following are a few illustrations of its use in the health sciences.

1.1.1. Comparative Studies

Comparative studies are intended to show possible *differences* between two or more groups. For example, the same survey of Example 1.1 also provided the following figures concerning boys in the surveyed group who use tobacco at least weekly. Among Asians, it was 9.7%, followed by 11.6% of Blacks, 20.6% of Hispanics, 25.4% of Whites, and 38.3% of American Indians.

In addition to surveys which are cross-sectional, as seen in the above example, data for comparative studies may come from different sources; the two fundamental designs being *retrospective* and *prospective*. Retrospective studies gather past data from selected *cases* and *controls* to determine differences, if any, in the exposure to a suspected *risk factor*. They are commonly referred to as *case–control studies*. In a case–control study, cases of a specific disease are ascertained as they arise from population-based registers or lists of hospital admissions and controls are sampled either as disease-free individuals from the population at risk, or as hospitalized patients having a diagnosis other than the one under study. The advantages of a retrospective study are that it is *economical* and it provides answers to research questions relatively quickly because the cases are already available. Major limitations are due to the inaccuracy of the *exposure histories* and uncertainty about the appropriateness of the control sample; these problems sometimes hinder retrospective studies and make them less preferred than prospective studies. The following is an example of a retrospective study in the field of occupational health.

Example 1.2

A case–control study was undertaken to identify reasons for the exceptionally high rate of *lung cancer* among male residents of coastal Georgia. Cases were identified from these sources:

(a) Diagnoses since 1970 at the single large hospital in Brunswick.
(b) Diagnoses during 1975–1976 at three major hospitals in Savannah.
(c) Death certificates for the period 1970–1974 in the area.

Controls were selected from admissions to the four hospitals and from death certificates in the same period for diagnoses other than lung cancer, bladder cancer, or chronic lung cancer. Data are tabulated separately for smokers and nonsmokers as follows:

Smoking	Shipbuilding	Cases	Controls
No	Yes	11	35
	No	50	203
Yes	Yes	84	45
	No	313	270

The exposure under investigation, "Shipbuilding," refers to employment in shipyards during World War II. By a separate tabulation, with the first half of the table for nonsmokers and the second half for smokers, we treat *smoking* as a potential *confounder*. A confounder is a factor may be an exposure by itself, not under investigation but related to the disease (in this case, lung cancer) and the exposure (shipbuilding); previous studies have linked smoking to lung cancer and construction workers are more likely to be smokers. The term *exposure* is used here to emphasize that employment in shipyards is a *risk factor*; however, the term would be also even used in studies where the factor under investigation has beneficial effects.

In an examination of the smokers in the above data set, the numbers of people employed in shipyards, 84 and 45, tell us little because the sizes of the two groups, cases and controls, are different. Adjusting these absolute numbers for the group sizes, we have

(1a) For the controls,

$$\text{Proportion of exposure} = \frac{45}{315}$$

$$= .143 \text{ or } 14.3\%$$

(2a) For the cases,

$$\text{Proportion of exposure} = \frac{84}{397}$$
$$= .212 \text{ or } 21.2\%$$

The results reveal different exposure histories: the proportion of exposure among cases was higher than that among controls. It is not in any way yet a conclusive proof, but it is a good clue indicating a possible relationship between the disease (lung cancer) and the exposure (employment in shipbuilding industry—a possible occupational hazard).

Similar examination of the data for nonsmokers shows that, by taking into consideration the numbers of cases and of controls, we have the following figures for employment:

(1b) For the controls,

$$\text{Proportion of exposure} = \frac{35}{238}$$
$$= .147 \text{ or } 14.7\%$$

(2b) For the cases,

$$\text{Proportion of exposure} = \frac{11}{61}$$
$$= .180 \text{ or } 18.0\%$$

Again, the results also reveal different exposure histories: the proportion of exposure among cases was higher than that among controls.

The above analyses also show that the difference (cases versus controls) between proportions of exposure among smokers, that is,

$$21.2\% - 14.3\% = 6.9\%$$

is different from the difference (cases versus controls) between proportions of exposure among nonsmokers, which is

$$18.0\% - 14.7\% = 3.3\%$$

The differences, 6.9 and 3.3% are measures of the *strength of the relationship* between the disease and the exposure, one for each of the two strata—the two groups of smokers and nonsmokers, respectively. The above calculation shows that the possible effects of employment in shipyards (as a suspected risk factor) are different for smokers and nonsmokers. This difference of differences (6.9% versus 3.3%), if confirmed, is called an "interaction" or an *effect modification*, where smoking alters the effect of employment in shipyards as a risk for lung cancer. In that case smoking is not only a confounder, it is an *effect modifier*, which modifies the effects of shipbuilding (on the possibility of having lung cancer).

Another example is provided in the following example concerning glaucomatous blindness.

Example 1.3

Persons registered blind from glaucoma

	Number of Cases	Cases	Cases per 100,000
White	32,930,233	2832	8.6
Nonwhite	3,933,333	3227	82.0

For these disease *registry* data, direct calculation of a proportion would result in a very tiny fraction that is the number of cases of the disease per person at risk. For convenience, this is multiplied by 100,000 and hence the result expresses the number of cases per 100,000 individuals. This data set also provides an example of the use of proportions as *disease prevalence*, which is defined as

$$\text{Prevalence} = \frac{\text{Number of diseased individuals at the time of investigation}}{\text{Total number of individuals tested}}$$

More details on disease prevalence and related concepts are in Section 1.2.2.

For blindness from glaucoma, calculations in this example reveal a striking difference between the races: the blindness prevalence among Nonwhites was over 8 times that among Whites. The number "100,000" was selected arbitrarily; any power of 10 would be suitable so as to obtain a result between 1 and 100, sometimes between 1 and 1000; it is easier to state the result "82 cases per 100,000" than saying that the prevalence was .00082.

1.1.2. Screening Tests

Other uses of proportions can be found in the evaluation of *screening tests* or *diagnostic procedures*. Following these procedures, clinical observation or laboratory techniques, individuals are classified as healthy or as falling into one of a number of disease categories. Such tests are important in medicine and epidemiologic studies, and may form the basis of early interventions. Almost all such tests are imperfect, in the sense that healthy individuals would occasionally be classified wrongly as being ill, while some individuals who are really ill may fail to be detected. That is, misclassification—in either way—is unavoidable. Suppose that each individual in a large population can be classified as truly positive or negative for a particular disease; this true diagnosis may be based on more refined methods than are used in the test; or it may be based on evidence which emerges after passage of time, for instance at autopsy. For each class of individuals, diseased and healthy, the test is applied and results are depicted as follows:

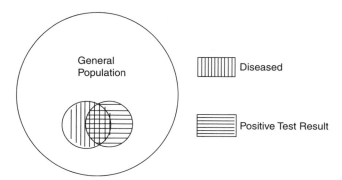

The two proportions fundamental to evaluating diagnostic procedures are *sensitivity* and *specificity*. The sensitivity is the proportion of diseased individuals detected as positive:

$$\text{Sensitivity} = \frac{\text{Number of diseased individuals who screen positive}}{\text{Total number of diseased individuals}}$$

(the corresponding errors are *false negatives*), where as the specificity is the proportion of healthy individuals detected as negative:

$$\text{Specificity} = \frac{\text{Number of healthy individuals who screen negative}}{\text{Total number of healthy individuals}}$$

(the corresponding errors are *false positives*). Clearly, it is desirable that a test or screening procedure be highly sensitive and highly specific. However, the two types of errors go in opposite directions; for example, an effort to increase sensitivity may lead to more false positives.

Example 1.4

A cytological test was undertaken to screen women for cervical cancer. Consider a group of 24,103 women consisting of 379 women whose cervices are abnormal (to an extent sufficient to justify concern with respect to possible cancer) and 23,724 women whose cervices are acceptably healthy. A test was applied and results are tabulated in the table below (This study was performed for a rather old test; it is used here only for illustration.):

	Test		
Truth	Negative	Positive	Total
Negative	23,362	362	23,724
Positive	225	154	379

The following calculations

$$\text{Sensitivity} = \frac{154}{379}$$
$$= .406 \quad \text{or} \quad 40.6\%$$

$$\text{Specificity} = \frac{23,362}{23,724}$$
$$= .985 \quad \text{or} \quad 98.5\%$$

show that the above test is highly specific (98.5%) but not very sensitive (40.6%); there were more than half ($100\% - 40.6\% = 59.4\%$) false negatives. The implications of the use of this test are

1. if a woman without cervical cancer is tested, the result would almost surely be negative, but
2. if a woman with cervical cancer is tested the chance is that the disease would go undetected because 59.4% of these cases would lead to false negatives.

Finally, it is important to note that throughout this section, proportions have been defined so that both the numerator and the denominator are counts or frequencies, and the numerator corresponds to a subgroup of the larger group involved in the denominator resulting in a number between 0 and 1 (or between 0 and 100%). It is straightforward to generalize this concept for use with characteristics having more than two outcome categories; for each category we can define a proportion, and these category-specific proportions add up to 1 (or 100%).

Example 1.5

An examination of the 668 children reported living in crack/cocaine households shows 70% Blacks, followed by 18% Whites, 8% American Indians, and 4% other or unknown.

1.1.3. Displaying Proportions

Perhaps the most effective and most convenient way of organizing, summarizing, and then presenting data, especially discrete or categorical data (observations or outcomes belong to one of two or several categories), is through the use of *graphs*. Graphs convey the information, the general patterns in a set of data, at a single glance. Graphs are often easier to read than *tables*; the most informative graphs are simple and self-explanatory. Of course, in order to achieve that objective, graphs should be carefully constructed. Like tables, they should be clearly labeled and units of measurement and/or magnitude of quantities should be included. Remember that graphs must tell their own story; they should be complete in themselves with *title* and *label*, and they should require little or no additional explanation in the main text.

Bar Charts

Bar charts are a very popular type of graph used to *display several proportions*—one for each of several groups—for quick comparison. In a bar chart, the various groups are represented along the horizontal axis; they may be arranged alphabetically, or by the size of their proportions, or on some other rational basis. A vertical bar is drawn above each group such that the height of the bar is the proportion associated with that group. The bars should be of equal width and should be separated from one another so as not to imply continuity.

Example 1.6

We can present the data set on kids without a recent physical checkup (Example 1.1) by a bar chart as follows:

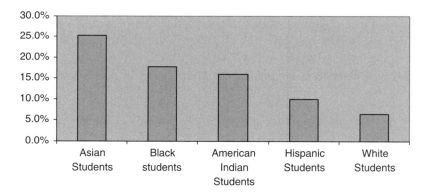

Adolescents without a recent physical checkup

Pie Charts

Pie charts are another popular type of graph. A pie chart consists of a circle; the circle is divided into wedges that correspond to the magnitude of the proportions for various categories. A pie chart shows the differences between the sizes of various categories or subgroups as a decomposition of the total. It is suitable, for example, for use in presenting a budget where we can easily see the difference between expenditures on health care and defense in the United States. In other words, a bar chart is a suitable graphic device when we have several groups, each associated with a different proportion; whereas a pie chart is more suitable when we have one group, which is divided into several categories. The proportions of various categories in a pie chart should add up to 100%. Like bar charts, the categories in a pie chart are usually arranged by the size of the proportions. They may also be arranged alphabetically, or on some other rational basis.

Example 1.7

We can present the data set on the crack kids of Example 1.5 by a pie chart as follows:

Who are the crack kids?

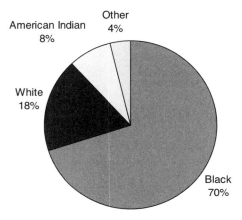

Example 1.8

The following table provides the number of deaths due to different causes among Minnesota residents for the year 1975.

Cause of Death	Number of Deaths
Heart disease	12,378
Cancers	6,448
Cerebrovascular disease	3,958
Accidents	1,814
Others	8,088
Total	32,686

After calculating the proportion of deaths due to each cause, for example

$$\text{Deaths due to cancers} = \frac{6,448}{32,686}$$

$$= .197 \text{ or } 19.7\%$$

We can present the results as in the following pie chart:

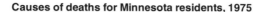

Causes of deaths for Minnesota residents, 1975

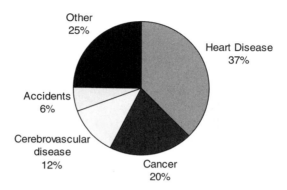

Line Graphs

A *line graph* is similar to a bar chart but the horizontal axis represents *time*. Different "groups" are consecutive years so that a line graph is suitable to illustrate how certain *proportions change over time*. In a line graph, the proportion associated with each year is represented by a point at the appropriate height; the points are then connected by straight lines.

Example 1.9

Between the years 1984 and 1987, the *crude death rates* for females in the United States are as follows:

Year	Crude Death Rate Per 100,000 Population
1984	792.7
1985	806.6
1986	809.3
1987	813.1

The change in crude death rate, per 100,000 population, for U.S. females can be represented by the following line graph:

American Female death Rates, 1984–1987

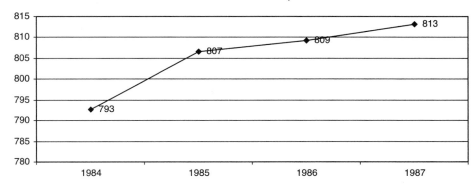

In addition to their use with proportions, line graphs can also be used to describe changes in the number of occurrences and with continuous measurements.

Example 1.10

The following line graph displays the trend in the reported rates of malaria that occurred in the United States between 1940 and 1989 (proportion times 100,000 as above).

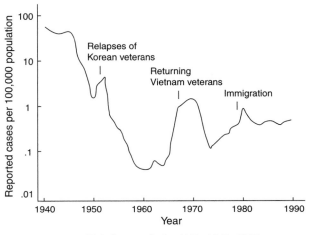

Malaria rates in the U.S., 1940–1989

1.2. RATES

The term *rate* is kind of confusing; sometimes it is used interchangingly with the term *proportion* as defined in the previous section, sometimes it refers to a quantity of very different nature. Section on the *change rate* covers this special use and the next two Sections 1.2.2 and 1.2.3 focus on rates used interchangingly with proportions as *measures of morbidity and mortality*. Even when they refer to the same things—measures of morbidity and mortality, there is still some degree of difference between these two terms; as contrast to the *static* nature of proportions, rates are aimed at measuring the *occurrences of events* during or after a certain time period.

1.2.1. Changes

Familiar examples of rates include their use to describe changes after a certain period of time. The change rate is defined by:

$$\text{Change rate} = \frac{\text{New value} - \text{old value}}{\text{Old value}} \times (100)\%$$

In general, change rates could exceed 100%. They are *not* proportions (a proportion is a number between 0 and 1, or 0 and 100%). *Change rates* are mostly used for description and not involved in common *statistical analyses*.

Example 1.11

The following is a typical paragraph of a *news report*:

A total of 35,238 new AIDS cases were reported in 1989 by the Centers for Disease Control (CDC), compared to 32,196 reported during 1988. The 9% increase is the smallest since the spread of AIDS began in the early 1980s. For example, new AIDS cases were up 34% in 1988 and 60% in 1987.

In 1989, 547 cases of AIDS transmissions from mothers to newborns were reported, up 17% from 1988; while females made up just 3971 of the 35,238 new cases reported in 1989 that was an increase of 11% over 1988.

In this example:

(1) The change rate for new AIDS cases was calculated as

$$\frac{35{,}238 - 32{,}196}{32{,}196} \times (10)\% = 9.4\%$$

(this was rounded *down* to the reported figure of 9% in the news report).

(2) For the new AIDS cases transmitted from mothers to newborns, we have

$$17\% = \frac{547 - (\text{Number of cases in 1988})}{\text{Number } of \text{ cases in 1988}} \times (100)\%$$

leading to

$$\text{Number of cases in 1988} = \frac{547}{1.17}$$

$$= 468$$

(a figure obtainable, as shown above, but usually not reported because of redundancy). Similarly, the number of new AIDS cases for the year 1987 is calculated as follows:

$$34\% = \frac{32,196-(\text{Number of cases in 1987})}{\text{Number of cases in 1987}} \times (100)\%$$

or

$$\text{Number of cases in 1987} = \frac{32,196}{1.34}$$

$$= 24,027$$

(3) Among the 1989 new AIDS cases, the proportion of females is

$$\frac{3,971}{35,238} = .113 \quad \text{or} \quad 11.3\%$$

and the proportion of males is

$$\frac{35,238-3,971}{35,238} = .887 \quad \text{or} \quad 88.7\%$$

The proportions of females and males add up to 1.0% or 100%.

1.2.2. Measures of Morbidity and Mortality

The field of *vital statistics* makes use some special applications of rates, three kinds of which are commonly mentioned: crude, specific, and adjusted (or standardized). Unlike change rates, these measures are proportions. *Crude rates* are computed for an entire large group or population; they disregard factors such as age, sex, and race. *Specific rates* consider these differences among subgroups or categories of diseases. *Adjusted* or *standardized rates* are used to make valid summary comparisons between two or more groups possessing different age distributions.

The annual *crude death rate* is defined as the number of deaths in a calendar year, divided by the population on July 1 of that year (which is usually an estimate); the quotient is often multiplied by 1000, or another suitable power of 10, resulting in a number between 1 and 100, or 1 and 1000. For example, the 1980 population of California was 23,000,000 (as estimated by July 1) and there were 190,247 deaths during 1980, leading to

$$\text{Crude death rate} = \frac{190,247}{23,000,000} \times (1000)$$

$$= 8.3 \text{ deaths per 1000 persons per year}$$

The age-specific and cause-specific death rates are similarly defined.

As for *morbidity*, the *disease prevalence*, as defined in the previous section, is a proportion used to describe the population at a certain point in time, whereas incidence is a rate used in connection with new cases:

$$\text{Incidence rate} = \frac{\text{Number of individuals who developed the disease over a defined period of time (a year, say)}}{\text{Number of individuals initially without the disease who were followed for the defined period of time}}$$

In other words, prevalence presents a snapshot of the population's morbidity experience at certain time point whereas the *incidence* is aimed to investigate possible time trends. For example, the 35,238 new AIDS cases in Example 1.7 and the national population without AIDS at the start of 1989 could be combined according to the above formula to yield an incidence of AIDS for the year.

Another interesting use of rates is in connection with *cohort studies*. Cohort studies are *epidemiological designs* in which one enrolls a group of persons and follows them over certain periods of time; examples include occupational mortality studies among others. The cohort study design focuses on a particular exposure rather than a particular disease as in case–control studies. Advantages of a longitudinal approach include the opportunity for more accurate measurement of exposure history and a careful examination of the time relationships between exposure and any disease under investigation. Each member of the cohort belongs to one of three types of termination:

(1) Subjects still alive on the analysis date.
(2) Subjects who died on a known date within the study period.
(3) Subjects who are lost to follow-up after a certain date (these cases are a potential source of bias effort should be expended on reducing the number of subjects in this category).

The contribution of each member is the length of *follow-up time* from enrollment to his or her termination. The quotient defined as the observed number of deaths for the cohort, divided by the total follow-up times (in *person-years*, say) is the *rate* to characterize the mortality experience of the cohort:

$$\text{Follow-up death rate} = \frac{\text{Number } of \text{ deaths}}{\text{Total person-years}}$$

Rates may be calculated for total deaths and for separate causes of interest and they are usually multiplied by an appropriate power of 10, say 1000, to result in a single-digit or double-digit figure; for example, deaths per 1000 months of follow-up. Follow-up death rates maybe used to measure effectiveness of medical treatment programs.

Example 1.12

In an effort to provide a complete analysis of the survival of patients with end-stage renal disease (ESRD), data were collected for a sample that included 929 patients who initiated hemodialysis for the first time at the Regional Disease Program in Minneapolis, Minnesota between 1 January 1976 and 30 June 1982; all patients were followed until 31 December 1982. Of these 929 patients, 257 are diabetics; among the 672 nondiabetics, 386 are classified as low-risk (without comorbidities such as arteriosclerotic heart disease, peripheral vascular disease, chronic obstructive pulmonary, and cancer). Results from these two subgroups were as follows (only some summarized figures are given here for illustration; details such as numbers of deaths and total treatment months for subgroups are not included—some detailed data can be found in Exercise 1.30):

Group	Age Group	Deaths/1000 Treatment Months
Low risk	1–45	2.75
	46–60	6.93
	61 +	13.08
Diabetics	1–45	10.29
	46–60	12.52
	61 +	22.16

For example, for the low-risk patients over 60 years of age, there were 38 deaths during 2906 treatment months leading to:

$$\frac{38}{2906} \times (1000) = 13.08 \text{ deaths per 1000 treatment months}$$

1.2.3. Standardization of Rates

Crude rates, as measures of morbidity or mortality, can be used for population description and may be suitable for investigations of their variations over time; however, the comparisons of crude rates are often invalid because the populations may be different with respect to an important characteristic such as age, sex or race (these are *potential confounders*). To overcome this difficulty, adjusted (or standardized) rates are used in the comparison; the adjustment removes the difference in composition with respect to a confounder, which is often *age*.

Example 1.13

The following table provides mortality data for Alaska and Florida for the year 1977.

	Alaska			Florida		
Age Group	No. of Deaths	Persons	Deaths/100,000	No. of Deaths	Persons	Deaths/100,000
0–4	162	40,000	405.0	2,049	546,000	375.3
5–19	107	128,000	83.6	1,195	1,982,000	60.3

(*continued*)

(*Continued*)

Age Group	Alaska			Florida		
	No. of Deaths	Persons	Deaths/100,000	No. of Deaths	Persons	Deaths/100,000
20–44	449	172,000	261.0	5,097	2,676,000	190.5
45–64	451	58,000	777.6	19,904	1,807,000	1101.5
65 +	444	9,000	4933.3	63,505	1,444,000	4397.9
Total	1613	407,000	396.3	91,750	8,455,000	1085.2

This example shows that the 1977 crude death rate per 100,000 population for Alaska was 396.8 and for Florida was 1085.7—almost a threefold difference. However, a closer examination shows:

(1) Alaska had higher *age-specific death rates* for 4 of the 5 age groups, the only exception being 45–64 years.

(2) Alaska had a higher percentage of its population in the younger age groups.

The findings make it essential to adjust the death rates of the two states in order to make a valid comparison. A simple way to achieve this, called the direct method, is to apply to a common *standard population*, age-specific rates observed from the two populations under investigation. For this purpose, the population of the United States as of the last decennial census is frequently used. The procedure consists of the following steps:

(1) The standard population is listed by the same age groups.

(2) *Expected number of deaths* in the standard population is computed for each age group of each of the two populations being compared. For example, for age group 0–4, the U.S. population for 1970 was 84,416 (per 1 million); therefore, we have:

(i) Alaska rate $= 405.0$ per 100,000

The expected number of deaths is

$$\frac{(84,416)(405.0)}{100,000} = 341.9$$

$$\cong 342$$

(ii) Florida rate $= 375.3$ per 100,000

The expected number of deaths is

$$\frac{(84,416)(375.3)}{100,000} = 316.8$$

$$\cong 317$$

(iii) The expected number of deaths for Florida is lower than the expected number of deaths for Alaska obtained for the same age group.

(iv) Obtain total number of expected deaths.

(v) Age-adjusted death rate is

$$\text{Adjusted death rate} = \frac{\text{Total number of expected deaths}}{\text{Standard population size}} \times (100{,}000)$$

Detailed calculations are, using the U.S. population in 1970 as the common standard:

Age Group	Standard	Alaska		Florida	
		Age-Specific Rate	Expected Deaths	Age-specific Rate	Expected Deaths
0–4	84,416	405.0	342	375.3	317
5–19	294,353	83.6	246	60.3	177
20–44	316,744	261.0	827	190.5	603
45–64	205,745	777.6	1600	1101.5	2266
65+	98,742	4933.3	4871	4397.9	4343
Total	1,000,000		7886		7706

The age-adjusted death rate per 100,000 population for Alaska is 788.6 and for Florida is 770.6. These age-adjusted rates are much closer than as shown by the crude rates, and the adjusted rate for Florida is *lower*. It is important to keep in mind that any population could be chosen as "standard" and, because of this, an adjusted rate is *artificial*; it does not reflect data from an actual population. The values of the adjusted rates depend in large part on the *choice of the standard population*. They have real meaning only for comparisons.

The advantage of using the U.S. population as the standard is that we can adjust death rates of many states and compare them with each other. Any population could be selected and used as "standard." In the above example, it does not mean that there were only 1 million people in the United States in the year 1970; it only presents the *age distribution* of 1 million U.S. residents for that year. If all we want to do is to compare Florida versus Alaska, we could choose either one of the states as standard and adjust the death rate of the other; this practice would save half of the labor. For example, if we choose Alaska as the standard population then the adjusted death rate for the state of Florida is calculated as follows:

Age Group	(Alaska as) Standard	Florida	
		Specific Rate/100,000	Expected Deaths
0–4	40,000	375.3	150
5–9	128,000	60.3	77
20–44	172,000	190.5	328
45–64	58,000	1101.5	639
65+	9,000	4397.9	396
Total	407,000		1590

The new adjusted rate

$$\frac{(1,590)(100,000)}{407,000} = 390.7 \text{ per } 100,000$$

is not the same as that obtained using the 1970 U.S. population as standard (it was 770.6), but it also shows that after age-adjustment the death rate in Florida (390.7 per 100,000) is somewhat lower than that of Alaska (396.8 per 100,000; there is no need for adjustment here because we use Alaska's population as the standard population).

1.3. RATIOS

In many cases, such as disease prevalence and disease incidence, proportions and rates are defined very similarly and the two terms, proportion and rate may even be used interchangeably. *Ratio* is a completely different term; it is a computation of the form

$$\text{Ratio} = \frac{a}{b}$$

where "a" and "b" are *similar quantities* measured from *different groups* or under *different circumstances*. An example is the male-to-female ratio of smoking rates; such a ratio is positive but may well exceed 1.0.

1.3.1. Relative Risk

One of the most often used ratios in epidemiological studies is the *Relative Risk* (RR), a concept for the comparison of two groups or populations with respect to a certain unwanted event (disease or death). The traditional method of expressing it in prospective studies is simply the ratio of the incidence rates:

$$\text{Relative } risk = \frac{\text{Disease incidence in group 1}}{\text{Disease incidence in group 2}}$$

However, ratio of disease prevalences as well as follow-up death rates can also be formed. Usually, group 2 is under standard conditions—such as nonexposure to a certain risk factor—against which group 1 (exposed) is measured. A relative risk, which is greater than 1.0 indicates harmful effects whereas a relative risk, which is less than 1.0 indicates beneficial effects. For example, if group 1 consists of smokers and group 2 nonsmokers, then we have a *relative risk due to smoking*. Using the data on ESRD of Example 1.12, we can obtain the following relative risks due to diabetes:

Age Group	Relative Risk
1–45	3.74
46–60	1.81
61 +	1.69

All three numbers are greater than 1 (indicating higher mortality for diabetics) and form a decreasing trend with increasing age.

1.3.2. Odds and Odds Ratio

The *relative risk*, also called *risk ratio*, is an important index in epidemiological studies because in such studies it is often useful to measure the *increased* risk (if any) of incurring a particular disease if a certain factor is present. In cohort studies such an index is readily obtained by observing the experience of groups of subjects with and without the factor as shown above. In a case–control study, the data do not present an immediate answer to this type of question, and we now consider how to obtain an useful short-cut solution.

Suppose that each subject in a large study, at a particular time, is classified as positive or negative according to some risk factor, and as having or not having a certain disease under investigation. For any such categorization the population may be enumerated in a 2×2 table, as follows:

	Disease		
Factor	Yes $(+)$	No $(-)$	Total
Exposed $(+)$	A	B	A + B
Unexposed $(-)$	C	D	C + D
Total	A + C	B + D	$N = A + B + C + D$

The entries A, B, C and D in the table are sizes of the four combinations of disease presence-and-absence and factor presence-and-absence and the number N at the lower right corner of the table is the total population size. The relative risk is

$$RR = \frac{A}{A+B} \div \frac{C}{C+D}$$
$$= \frac{A(C+D)}{C(A+B)}$$

In many situations, the number of subjects classified as disease positive is very small as compared to the number classified as disease negative, that is,

$$C + D \cong D$$
$$A + B \cong B$$

($\cong$ means "almost equal to") and, therefore, the relative risk can be approximated as follows:

$$RR \cong \frac{AD}{BC}$$
$$= \frac{A/B}{C/D} = \frac{A/C}{B/D}$$

where the slash denotes division. The resulting ratio, AD/BC, is an approximate relative risk, but it is often referred to as *odds ratio* because

(i) A/B and C/D are the *odds* in favor of having disease from groups with or without the factor;
(ii) A/C and B/D are the odds in favor of having exposed to the factors from groups with or without the disease.

The two odds in (ii) can be easily estimated using case–control data, by using sample frequencies. For example, the odds A/C can be estimated by a/c where "a" is the number of exposed cases and "c" the number of exposed controls in the sample of cases in a case–control design.

For the many diseases that are rare—the terms "relative risk" and "odds ratio" are used interchangeably because of the above-mentioned approximation. The relative risk is an important epidemiological index used to measure seriousness, or the magnitude of the harmful effect of suspected risk factors. For example, if we have

$$RR = 3.0$$

then we can say that the exposed individuals have a risk of contracting the disease, which is approximately three times the risk of unexposed individuals. A perfect 1.0 indicates no effect and beneficial factors result in relative risk values which are smaller than 1.0. From data obtained by a case–control or retrospective study, it is impossible to calculate the relative risk that we want, but if it is reasonable to assume that the disease is rare (prevalence is less than .05, say), then we can calculate the *odds ratio* as a "stepping stone" and use it as an approximate *relative risk* (we use the notation "$\cong$", meaning *almost equal to*, for this purpose). In these cases, we interpret the calculated odds ratio just as we would do with the relative risk.

Example 1.14

The role of smoking in the etiology of pancreatitis has been recognized for many years. In order to provide estimates of the quantitative significance of these factors, a hospital-based study was carried out in eastern Massachusetts and Rhode Island between 1975 and 1979. Ninety-eight patients who had a hospital discharge diagnosis of pancreatitis were included in this unmatched case–control study. The control group consisted of 451 patients admitted for diseases other than those of the pancreas and biliary tract. Risk factor information was obtained from a standardized interview with each subject, conducted by a trained interviewer. The following are some data for the males:

Use of Cigarettes	Cases	Controls
Never	2	56
Ex-smokers	13	80
Current smokers	38	81
Total	53	217

For the above data for this example, the approximate relative risks or odds ratios are calculated as follows:

(i) For ex-smokers,

$$RR_e = \frac{13/2}{80/56}$$

$$= \frac{(13)(56)}{(80)(2)}$$

$$= 4.55$$

(The subscript "e" in the notation RR_e indicates that we are calculating the RR for ex-smokers.)

(ii) For current smokers,

$$RR_c = \frac{38/2}{81/56}$$

$$= \frac{(38)(56)}{(81)(2)}$$

$$= 13.14$$

(The subscript "c" in the notation RR_c indicates that we are calculating the RR for current smokers). In these calculations, the nonsmokers (who never smoke) are used as references. These values indicate that the risk of having pancreatitis for current smokers is approximately 13.14 times the same risk for people who never smoke. The effect for ex-smokers is smaller (4.55 times) but it is still very high (as compared to 1.0—the no-effect baseline for relative risks and odds ratios). In other words, if the smokers quit smoking they would reduce their own risk (from 13.14 times to 4.55 times), but *not* to the normal level for people who never smoke.

1.3.3. The Mantel–Haenszel Method

In most in investigation, we are concerned with one primary outcome, such as a disease, and focusing on one primary (risk) factor, such as an exposure with a possible harmful effect. There are situations, however, where an investigator may want to adjust for a *confounder* that could influence the outcome of a statistical analysis. A confounder, or a confounding variable, is a variable that may be associated with either the disease or exposure or both. For example, in Example 1.2, a case–control study was undertaken to investigate the relationship between lung cancer and employment in shipyards during World War II among male residents of coastal Georgia. In this case, smoking is a possible confounder; it has been found to be associated with lung cancer and it may be associated with employment because construction workers are likely to be smokers. Specifically, we want to know the following:

(i) Among smokers, whether or not shipbuilding and lung cancer are related.
(ii) Among nonsmokers, whether or not shipbuilding and lung cancer are related.

In fact, the original data were tabulated separately for three smoking levels (none, moderate, and heavy); in Example 1.2, the last two tables were combined and presented together for simplicity. Assuming that the confounder, smoking, is not an effect modifier (i.e., smoking does not alter the relationship between lung cancer and shipbuilding); however, we do not want to reach separate conclusions, one at each level of smoking. In those cases, we want to pool data for a combined decision. When both the disease and the exposure are binary, a popular method is achieve this task is the *Mantel–Haenszel method*. This method provides one single estimate for the common odds ratio and can be summarized as follows:

(1) We form 2×2 tables, one at each level of the confounder.

(2) At a particular level of the confounder, we have

Exposure	Disease Classification		Total
	Yes (+)	No (−)	
Yes (+)	a	b	$a + b$
No (−)	c	d	$c + d$
Total	$a + c$	$b + d$	n

Because we assume that the confounder is not an effect modifier, the odds ratio is constant across its levels. The odds ratio at each level is estimated by *ad/bc*; the Mantel–Haenszel procedure pools data across levels of the confounder to obtain a combined estimate (some kind of weighted average of level-specific odds ratios):

$$\text{OR}_{\text{MH}} = \frac{\sum ad/n}{\sum bc/n}$$

The summations, in both numerator and denominator, are across all levels of the confounder.

Example 1.15

A case–control study was conducted to identify reasons for the exceptionally high rate of lung cancer among male residents of coastal Georgia as first presented in Example 1.2. The primary risk factor under investigation was employment in shipyards during World War II, and data are tabulated separately for three levels of smoking as follows:

Smoking	Shipbuilding	Cases	Controls
No	Yes	11	35
	No	50	203
Moderate	Yes	70	42
	No	217	220
Heavy	Yes	14	3
	No	96	50

There are three 2×2 tables, one for each level of smoking.

(1) We begin with the 2×2 table for *nonsmokers*:

Smoking	Shipbuilding	Cases	Controls	Total
No	Yes	11 (*a*)	35 (*b*)	46
	No	50 (*c*)	203 (*d*)	253
	Total	51	238	299 (*n*)

we have, for the nonsmokers,

$$\frac{ad}{n} = \frac{(11)(203)}{299}$$
$$= 7.47$$

$$\frac{bc}{n} = \frac{(35)(50)}{299}$$
$$= 5.85$$

The process is repeated for each of the other two smoking levels.

(2) For moderate smokers

Smoking	Shipbuilding	Cases	Controls	Total
Moderate	Yes	70 (*a*)	42 (*b*)	112
	No	217 (*c*)	220 (*d*)	437
	Total	287	262	549 (*n*)

$$\frac{ad}{n} = \frac{(70)(220)}{549}$$
$$= 28.05$$

$$\frac{bc}{n} = \frac{(42)(217)}{549}$$
$$= 16.60$$

(3) And for heavy smokers

Smoking	Shipbuilding	Cases	Controls	Total
Heavy	Yes	14 (*a*)	3 (*b*)	17
	No	96 (*c*)	50 (*d*)	146
	Total	110	53	163 (*n*)

$$\frac{ad}{n} = \frac{(14)(50)}{163}$$
$$= 4.29$$

$$\frac{bc}{n} = \frac{(3)(96)}{163}$$
$$= 1.77$$

The above results from the three levels of the confounder (smoking) are combined to estimate the common odds ratio:

$$OR_{MH} = \frac{7.47 + 28.05 + 4.28}{5.85 + 16.60 + 1.77}$$
$$= 1.64$$

This combined estimate of the odds ratio, 1.64, represents an approximate increase of 64% in lung cancer risk for those employed in the shipbuilding industry.

The following is another similar example aiming at the possible effects of oral contraceptive (OC) use on myocardial infarction (MI).

Example 1.16

A case–control study was conducted to investigate the relationship between MI and OC use. The data, stratified by cigarette smoking, were

Smoking	OC Use	Cases	Controls
No	Yes	4	52
	No	34	754
Yes	Yes	25	83
	No	171	853

There are two 2 × 2 tables, one for each level of smoking.

(1) We begin with the 2×2 table for *nonsmokers*:

Smoking	OC Use	Cases	Controls	Total
No	Yes	4 (*a*)	52 (*b*)	56
	No	34 (*c*)	754 (*d*)	788
	Total	38	806	844

$$\frac{ad}{n} = \frac{(4)(754)}{844}$$
$$= 3.57$$

$$\frac{bc}{n} = \frac{(52)(34)}{845}$$
$$= 2.09$$

(2) And for smokers,

Smoking	OC Use	Cases	Controls	Total
Yes	Yes	25 (*a*)	83 (*b*)	108
	No	171 (*c*)	853 (*d*)	1024
	Total	196	936	1132

$$\frac{ad}{n} = \frac{(25)(853)}{1132}$$
$$= 18.84$$

$$\frac{bc}{n} = \frac{(83)(171)}{1132}$$
$$= 12.54$$

The above results from the two levels of the confounder (smoking) are combined to estimate the common odds ratio:

$$OR_{MH} = \frac{3.57 + 18.84}{2.09 + 12.54}$$
$$= 1.53$$

This combined estimation of the odds ratio, 1.53, represents an approximate increase of 53% in myocardial infarction risk for OC users.

1.4. COMPUTATIONAL AND VISUAL AIDS

Much of this book is concerned with arithmetic and algebraic procedures for data analysis. In many biomedical investigations, particularly those involving large quantities of data, most analyses—for example, regression analysis of Chapter 8—give rise quickly to difficulties in computational implementation. In these investigations it will be necessary to use statistical software specially designed to do these jobs. All calculations described in this book, or any other introductory books can be readily carried out using statistical packages, and any student or practitioner of data analysis will find the use of such packages essential.

There are many specialized packages for statistical analyses; some are very well-known, such as SAS, SPSS, and BMDP. However, students and investigators contemplating to use of one of these commercial programs should read the specifications of each program—may be with help from course instructor—before choosing options needed or suitable for any particular arithmetic or algebraic procedure. But our book is very different; all calculations described in this book can be readily carried out using *Microsoft Excel*, very user-friendly and very popular software available in every personal computer. Notes on the use of Excel are included in separate sections at the end of each chapter.

A *worksheet* or *spreadsheet* is a (blank) sheet where you do your work. An Excel *file* holds a stack of worksheets in a *workbook*. You can *name* a sheet, put data on it and *save*; later, *open* and use it. You can *move* or size your windows by dragging the borders. You can also scroll up and down, or left and right through an Excel worksheet using the *scroll bars* on the right side and at the bottom.

An Excel worksheet consists of *grid lines* forming *columns* and *rows*; columns are *lettered* (A, B, C, AA, BB, . . .) and rows are *numbered* (1, 2, . . .). The intersection of each column and row is a box called a *cell* (a square). Every cell has an *address*, also called *cell reference*; to refer to a cell, enter the column letter followed by the row number. For example, the intersection of column C and row 3 is *cell C3*. Cells hold numbers, text, or formulas. To refer to a range of cells, enter the cell in the *upper left corner* of the range followed by a colon (:) and then the *lower right corner of the range. For example A1:B20* refers to the first 20 rows in both column A and B.

You can click a cell to make it *active* (for use, for example, to type a number in it); an active cell is where you enter or edit your data, and it is identified by a heavy border. You can also *define* or *select* a range by left clicking on the upper left most cell and dragging the mouse to the lower right most cell. To move around inside a selected range, press Tab or Enter to move forward one cell at a time.

Excel is software to handle numbers; so, get a project and start typing. Conventionally, files for data analysis use rows for subjects and columns for factors. For example, you conduct a survey using a 10-item questionnaire and receive returns from 75 people; your data require a file with 75 rows and 10 columns—not counting labels or other identifications (a column for subjects' ID and a row for factors' names). If you made an error, it can fixed; for example, to hit the *Del key* that wipes out the cell contents. You can change your mind again, deleting the delete by clicking the *Undo button* (or *backspace*, reversed curved arrow). Remember, you can widen your columns by double-clicking their right borders or dragging a right border further to the right.

1.4.1. Computer Screen

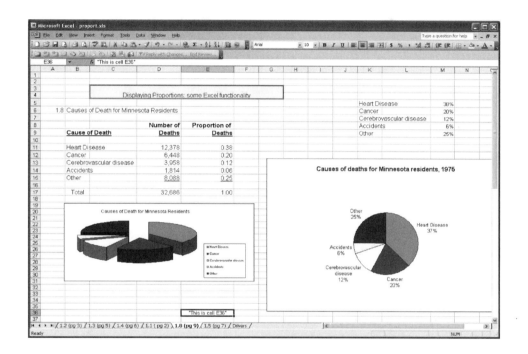

1.4.2. Formula Bar

The formula bar (near the top, next to an "=" sign) is a common way to provide the content of an active cell. Excel executes a formula from left to right and performs multiplication ("*") and division ("/") before addition (" + ") and subtraction ("−"). Parentheses can and should be used to change the order of calculations. To use formulas (e.g., for data transformation), do it in one of two ways: (i) click the cell you want to fill, then type an "=" sign followed by the formula in the formula bar (e.g., click C5, then type "=" A5 + B5); or (ii) click the cell you want to fill, then click the paste function icon, marked as "f*", which will give you—in a box—a list Excel functions available for your use.

1.4.3. Cut and Paste

The *cut and paste* procedure greatly simplifies the typing necessary to form a chart or table or write numerous formulas. The procedure involves highlighting the cells that contain the information you want to copy, clicking on the cut button (scissors icon) or copy button (two page icon), selecting the cell or cells to which the information is to be placed, and clicking on the paste button (clipboard and page icon).

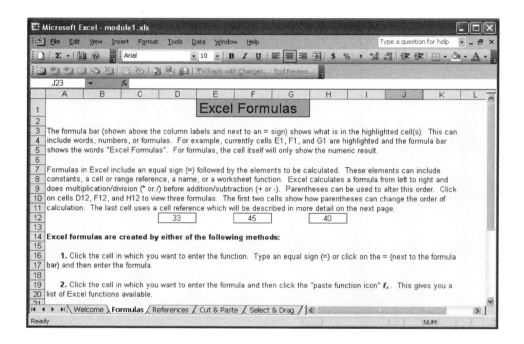

1.4.4. Select and Drag

The *select and drag* is very efficient for *data transformation.* Suppose you have the weight and height of 15 men, the weights are in C6:C20 and the heights are in D6:D20; and you need their body mass index. You can use the formula bar, for example, clicking E6 and typing = C6/(D6^2). The content of E6 now has the body mass index for the first man in your sample, but you do not have to repeat this process 15 times. Notice when you click on E6, there is a little box in the lower right corner of the cell boundary. If you move the mouse over this box, the cursor changes to a smaller plus sign. If you click on this box, you can then drag the mouse over the remaining cells and once you release the button, the cells will be filled.

1.4.5. Bar and Pie Charts

Forming a *bar chart* or pie to display proportions is a very simple task. Just click any blank cell to start (you have to do this so the computer knows where to put your resulting figure—even tough you can move it elsewhere later), you will be able to move your chart to any location when done. With data ready, click the *ChartWizard icon* (the one with multiple colored bars on the *standard toolbar* near the top). A box appears with choices including bar chart, pie chard, and line chart; the list is on the left side. Choose your chart type and follow instructions. There are many choices, including three-dimensional (3D) ones. You can put data and charts side by side for impressive presentation.

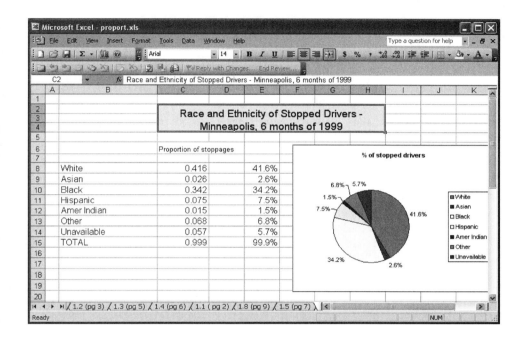

1.4.6. Rate Standardization

This is a good problem to practice with Excel: use it as a calculator. Recall this example:

(i) Florida's rate = 1085.3

(ii) Alaska's rate = 396.8

If Florida has Alaska's population:

		Florida	
Age Group	Alaska's	Age-Specific Rate	Expected Deaths
0–4	40,000	375.3	150
5–9	128,000	60.3	77
20–44	172,000	190.5	328
45–64	58,000	1101.5	639

(continued)

(Continued)

			Florida
65 +	9,000	4397.9	396
Total	407,000		1590
Age adjusted rate for Florida =			390.6

You proceed with these steps:

(1) Use *formula* to calculate the first expected number.

(2) Use *drag and fill* to obtain other expected numbers.

(3) Select last column, then click *Autosum icon* (Σ) to add the numbers of expected deaths.

1.4.7. Forming 2×2 Tables

Recall that in a *data file* you have one row for each subject and one column for each variable. Suppose two of those variables are *categorical*, say binary (with two categories coded as 1 for "yes" and 0 for "no"), and you want to form a 2×2 table (a table for 2 rows for Factor A, and 2 columns for Factor B) so you can study their relationship—for example, to calculate an odds ratio to measure the strength of the association between factors A and B. To achieve that, you can simply follow the following steps; as noted later, step 0 is only optional:

(0) Create a (dummy factor), call it—say- *fake* or any other name, and fill up that column with "1" (you can enter "1" for the first subject, then select and drag).

(1) Step 1: Activate a cell (by clicking it), then click *Data* (on the bar above the standard toolbar, near the end); when a box appears, choose *PivotTable Report*. Click "next" (to indicate that data are here, in Excel, then *highlight* the area containing your data (including variable names on first row—use the mouse; or you could identify the *range of cells*—say, C5:E28, as a response to question on "range." Then click "next" to bring in the *PivotTable Wizard*, which shows two groups of things:

(a) A *frame* for a 2×2 table with places identified as *row*, *column*, and *data*.

(b) Names of the factors you chose, say, *exposure*, *disease*, and *fake*.

(2) Drag "exposure" to merge with row (or column), drag "disease" to merge with column (or row), and drag "fake" to merge with data. Then click Finish, a 2×2 table appears in the active cell you identified, complete with *cell frequencies*, row and column totals, and grand total.

Note: If you have another factor, besides exposure and disease, available in the data set; even a column for names or ID; then there is no need to create the dummy factor "fake." Complete step 1; then, in step 2, drag that third factor, say ID, to merge with "data" in the frame shown by the PivotTable Wizard; it appears as *sum* ID. Click on that item and then choose "count" (to replace "sum").

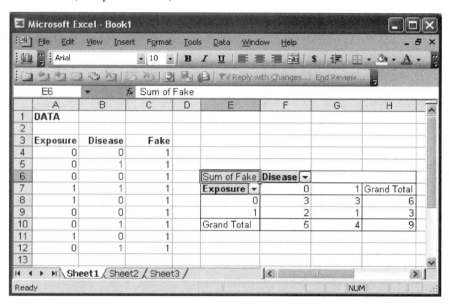

EXERCISES

1.1. Self-reported injuries among left-handed and right-handed people were compared in a survey of 1896 college students in British Columbia, Canada. Ninety-three of the 180 left-handed students reported at least one injury and 619 of the 1716 right-handed students reported at least one injury in the same period. Arrange the data into a 2 × 2 table and calculate the proportion of people with at least one injury during the period of observation for each group.

1.2. A study was conducted in order to evaluate the hypothesis that tea consumption and premenstrual syndrome are associated. One hundred eighty-eight nursing students and 64 tea factory workers were given questionnaires. The prevalence of premenstrual syndrome was 39% among the nursing students and 77% among the tea factory workers. How many people in each group have premenstrual syndrome? Arrange the data into a 2 × 2 table.

1.3. The relationship between prior condom use and tubal pregnancy was assessed in a population-based case–control study at Group Health Cooperative of Puget Sound during 1981–1986. The results are:

Condom Use	Cases	Controls
Never	176	488
Ever	51	186

Compute the proportion of subjects in each group who never used condoms.

1.4. Epidemic keratoconjunctivitis (EKC) or "shipyard eye" is an acute infectious disease of the eye. A case of EKC is defined as an illness

(a) consisting of redness, tearing, and pain in one or both eyes for more than 3 days duration,

(b) having diagnosed as EKC by an ophthalmologist.

In late October 1977, one of the two ophthalmologists (Physician A) providing the majority of specialized eye care to the residents of a central Georgia county (population 45,000) saw a 27-year-old nurse who had returned from a vacation in Korea with severe EKC. She received symptomatic therapy and was warned that her eye infection could spread to others; nevertheless, numerous cases of an illness similar to hers soon occurred in the patients and staff of the nursing home (Nursing Home A) where she worked (these individuals came to Physician A for diagnosis and treatment). The following table provides exposure history of 22 persons with EKC between October 27, 1977 and January 13, 1978 (when the outbreak stopped after proper control techniques were initiated). Nursing Home B, included in this table, is the only other area chronic-care facility.

Exposed Cohort	Number Exposed	Number Positive
Nursing Home A	64	16
Nursing Home B	238	6

Compute and compare the proportions of cases from the two nursing homes; what would be your conclusion?

1.5. In August 1976, tuberculosis was diagnosed in a high school student (index case) in Corinth, Mississippi. Subsequently, laboratory studies revealed that the student's disease was caused by drug-resistant tubercule bacilli. An epidemiologic investigation was conducted at the high school.

The following table gives the rate of positive tuberculin reactions, determined for various groups of students according to degree of exposure to the index case.

Exposure Level	Number Tested	Number Positive
High	129	63
Low	325	36

(a) Compute and compare the proportions of positive cases for the two exposure levels; what would be your conclusion?

(b) Calculate the odds ratio associated with high exposure; does this result support your conclusion in (a)

1.6. Consider the data taken from a study that attempts to determine whether the use of electronic fetal monitoring (EFM) during labor affects the frequency of caesarean section deliveries. Of the 5824 infants included in the study, 2850 were electronically monitored and 2974 were not. The outcomes are as follows:

Caesarean Delivery	EFM Exposure		Total
	Yes	No	
Yes	358	229	587
No	2492	2745	5237
Total	2850	2974	5824

(a) Compute and compare the proportions of caesarean delivery for the two exposure groups; what would be your conclusion?

(b) Calculate the odds ratio associated with EFM exposure; does this result support your conclusion in (a)

1.7. A study was conducted to investigate the effectiveness of bicycle safety helmets in preventing head injury. The data consist of a random sample of 793 individuals who were involved in bicycle accidents during a 1-year period.

Head Injury	Wearing Helmet		Total
	Yes	No	
Yes	17	218	237
No	130	428	558
Total	147	646	793

(a) Compute and compare the proportions of head injury for the group with helmets versus the group without helmets; what would be your conclusion?

(b) Calculate the odds ratio associated with not using helmet; does this result support your conclusion in (a)

1.8. A case–control study was conducted in Auckland, New Zealand to investigate the effects of alcohol consumption on both nonfatal myocardial infarction and coronary death in the 24 h after drinking, among regular drinkers. Data were tabulated separately for men and women.

(1) Data for Men

Drink in the Last 24 h	Myocardial Infarction		Coronary Death	
	Controls	Cases	Controls	Cases
No	197	142.	135	103
Yes	201	136	159	69

(2) Data for Women

	Myocardial Infarction		Coronary Death	
Drink in the Last 24 h	Controls	Cases	Controls	Cases
No	144	41	89	12
Yes	122	19	76	4

(a) Refer to myocardial infarction (tables on the left); calculate the odds ratio associated with drinking, separately for men and women.

(b) Compare the two odds ratios in (a); when the difference is properly confirmed, we have an effect modification.

(c) Refer to coronary deaths (tables on the right); calculate the odds ratio associated with drinking, separately for men and women.

(d) Compare the two odds ratios in (c); when the difference is properly confirmed, we have an effect modification.

1.9. Data taken from a study to investigate the effects of smoking on cervical cancer are stratified by the number of sexual partners. Results are as follows:

		Cancer	
Number of Partners	Smoking	Yes	No
Zero or one	Yes	12	21
	No	25	118
Two or more	Yes	96	142
	No	92	150

(a) Calculate the odds ratio associated with smoking, separately for the two groups, those with zero or one partners and those with two or more partners.

(b) Compare the two odds ratios in (a); when the difference is properly confirmed, we have an effect modification.

(c) Assuming that the odds ratios for the two groups, those with zero or one partners and those with two or more partners, are equal (in other words, the number of partners is not an effect modifier), calculate the Mantel–Haenszel estimate of this common odds ratio.

1.10. The following table provides the proportions of currently married women having an unplanned pregnancy; data are tabulated for several different methods of contraception.

Method of Contraception	Proportion with Unplanned Pregnancy
None	.431
Diaphragm	.149
Condom	.106
IUD	.071
Pill	.037

Display these proportions in a bar chart.

1.11. The following table summarizes the coronary heart disease (CHD) and lung cancer mortality rates per 1000 person-years by number of cigarettes smoked per day at baseline for men participating in Multiple Risk Factor Intervention Trial (MRFIT, a very large controlled clinical trial focusing on the relationship between smoking and cardiovascular diseases).

Smoking Status	CHD Deaths/1000 years	Lung Cancer Deaths/1000 years
Never-smoker	2.22	0
Ex-smoker	2.44	.43
Smoker 1–19 cigarettes/day	2.56	.22
Smoker 20–29 cigarettes/day	4.45	1.29
Smoker 40+ cigarettes/day	3.08	1.45

For each cause of death, display the rates in a bar chart.

1.12. The following table provides data taken from a study on the association between race and use of medical care by adults experiencing chest pain in the past year.

Response	Blacks	Whites
MD seen in past year	35	67
MD not seen in past year	45	38
MD never seen	78	39
Total	158	144

Display the proportions of the three response categories for each group, Blacks and Whites, in separate pie charts.

1.13. The following frequency distribution provides the number of cases of pediatric AIDS between 1983 and 1989.

Year	Number of Cases
1983	122
1984	250
1985	455
1986	848
1987	1412
1988	2811
1989	3098

Display the trend of numbers of cases using a line graph.

1.14. A study was conducted to investigate the changes between 1973 and 1985 in women's use of three preventive health services. The data were obtained from the National Health Survey; women were divided into subgroups according to age and race. The percentages (%) of women receiving a breast exam within the past two years are given below.

Age	Race	Percent with Breast Exam	
		1973	1985
Total	Black	61.7	74.8
	White	65.9	69.0
20–39 years	Black	77.0	83.9
	White	77.6	77.0
40–59 years	Black	54.8	67.9
	White	62.9	67.5
60–79 years	Black	39.1	64.5
	White	44.7	55.4

Separately for each group, Blacks and Whites, display the proportions of women receiving a breast exam within the past two years in a bar chart so as to show the relationship between the examination rate and age. Display the same data using a line graph.

1.15. Consider the following data:

X-Ray	Tuberculosis		Total
	No	Yes	
Negative	1739	8	1747
Positive	51	22	73
Total	1790	30	1820

Calculate the sensitivity and specificity of X-ray as a screening test for tuberculosis.

1.16. Sera from a T-lymphotropic virus type (HTLV-I) risk group (prostitute women) were tested with two commercial "research" enzyme-linked immuno-absorbent assays (EIA) for HTLV-I antibodies. These results were compared with a gold standard, and outcomes are shown below.

Truth	Dupont's EIA		Cellular Product's EIA	
	Positive	Negative	Positive	Negative
Positive	15	1	16	0
Negative	2	164	7	179

Calculate and compare the sensitivity and specificity of these two EIAs.

1.17. The following table provides the number of deaths for several leading causes among Minnesota residents for the year 1991; only the death rate for heart disease is given (number of deaths per 100,000 population).

Cause of Death	Number of Deaths	Deaths/100,000
Heart disease	10,382	294.5
Cancer	8,299	?
Cerebrovascular disease	2,830	?
Accidents	1,381	?
Other causes	11,476	?
Total	34,368	?

(a) Calculate the percent of total deaths for deaths from each cause and display the results in a pie chart.

(b) From death rate (per 100,000 population) for heart disease, calculate the population for Minnesota for the year 1991.

(c) From the result of (b), fill in the missing death rates (per 100,000 population) at the question marks in the above table.

1.18. The survey described in Example 1.1, continued in Section 1.1.1, provided percentages of boys from various ethnic groups who use tobacco at least weekly. Display these proportions in a bar chart similar to the one in Example 1.6.

1.19. A case–control study was conducted relating to the epidemiology of breast cancer and the possible involvement of dietary fats, along with other vitamins and nutrients. It included 2024 breast cancer cases that were admitted to Roswell Park Memorial Institute, Erie County, New York, from 1958 to 1965. A control group of 1463 was chosen from the patients having no neoplasms and no pathology of gastrointestinal or reproductive systems. The primary factors being investigated were vitamins A and E (measured in international units per month). The following are data for 1500 women over 54 years of age.

Vitamin A (IU/month)	Cases	Controls
<150,500	893	392
>150,500	132	83
Total	1025	475

Calculate the odds ratio associated with a decrease in ingestion of foods containing vitamin A.

1.20. Refer to the data set in Example 1.2,

Smoking	Shipbuilding	Cases	Controls
No	Yes	11	35
	No	50	203
Yes	Yes	84	45
	No	313	270

(a) calculate the odds ratio associated with employment in shipyards for nonsmokers,

(b) calculate the same odds ratio for smokers. Compare the results with those of (a); when the difference is properly confirmed, we have an "effect modification," where smoking alters the effect of employment in shipyards as a risk for lung cancer, and

(c) assuming that the odds ratios for the two groups, nonsmokers and smokers, are equal, calculate the Mantel–Haenszel estimate of this common odds ratio.

1.21. Although cervical cancer is not a major cause of death among American women, it has been suggested that virtually all such deaths are preventable. In an effort to find out who is being screened for the disease, data from the 1973 National Health Interview (a sample of the U.S. population) were used to examine the relationship between Pap testing and some socioeconomic factors. The following table provides the percentages (%) of women who reported *never having had* a Pap test (these are from metropolitan areas):

Age	Income	Whites	Blacks
25–44	Poor	13	14.2
	Nonpoor	5.9	6.3
45–64	Poor	30.2	33.3
	Nonpoor	13.2	23.3
65 and over	Poor	47.4	51.5
	Nonpoor	36.9	47.4

(a) Calculate the odds ratios associated with race (Black versus White) among

(i) 25–44 nonpoor,

(ii) 45–64 nonpoor, and

(iii) 65 + nonpoor.

Briefly discuss a possible effect modification if any.

(b) Calculate the odds ratios associated with income (poor versus nonpoor) among

(iv) 25–44 Black,

(v) 45–64 Black, and

(vi) 65 + Black.

Briefly discuss a possible effect modification if any.

(c) Calculate the odds ratios associated with race (Black versus White) among

(vii) 65 + Poor and

(viii) 65 + Nonpoor

and briefly discuss a possible effect modification.

1.22. Since incidence rates of most cancers rise with age, this must always be considered a confounder. The following are stratified data for an unmatched case–control study; the disease was esophageal cancer among men and the risk factor was alcohol consumption.

| Age | Sample | Daily Alcohol Consumption | |
		80 + g	0–79 g
25–44	Cases	5	5
	Controls	35	270
45–64	Cases	67	55
	Controls	56	277
65 and over	Cases	24	44
	Controls	18	129

(a) Calculate the odds ratio associated with high alcohol consumption, separately for the three age groups.

(b) Compare the three odds ratios in (a); when the difference is properly confirmed, we have an effect modification.

Assuming that the odds ratios for the three age groups are equal (in other words, age is not an effect modifier), calculate the Mantel–Haenszel estimate of this common odds ratio.

1.23. Postmenopausal women who develop endometrial cancer are, on the average, heavier than women who do not develop the disease. One possible explanation is that heavy women are more exposed to endogenous estrogens, which are produced in post-menopausal women by conversion of steroid precursors to active estrogens in peripheral fat. In the face of varying levels of endogenous estrogen production one might ask whether the carcinogenic potential of exogenous estrogens would be the same in all women. A case–control study has been conducted to examine the relation between weight, replacement estrogen therapy, and endometrial cancer; results are as follows.

Weight (kg)	Sample	Estrogen Replacement	
		Yes	No
<57	Cases	20	12
	Controls	61	183
[0,1-4]			
57–75	Cases	37	45
	Controls	113	378
[0,1-4]			
>75	Cases	9	42
	Controls	23	140

(a) Calculate the odds ratio associated with estrogen replacement, separately for the three weight groups.

(b) Compare the three odds ratios in (a); when the difference is properly confirmed, we have an effect modification.

(c) Assuming that the odds ratios for the three weight groups are equal (in other words, weight is not an effect modifier), calculate the Mantel–Haenszel estimate of this common odds ratio.

1.24. The role of menstrual and reproductive factors in the epidemiology of breast cancer has been reassessed using pooled data from three large case–control studies of breast cancer from several Italian regions. The following are summarized data for age at menopause and age at first live birth.

	Cases	Controls
Age at first Live Birth		
<22	621	898
22–24	795	909
25–27	791	769
>27	1043	775
Age at Menopause		
<45	459	543
45–49	749	803
>49	1378	1167

For each of the two factors (age at first live birth and age at menopause), choose the lowest level as the baseline and calculate the odds ratio associated with each other level.

1.25. Risk factors of gallstone disease were investigated in male self-defense officials who received, between October 1986 and December 1990, a retirement health examination at the Self-Defense Forces Fukuoka Hospital, Fukuoka, Japan. The following are parts of the data:

Factor	Level	No. of Men Surveyed	
		Total	No. with Gallstone
Smoking	Never	621	11
	Past	776	17
	Current	1342	33
Alcohol	Never	447	11
	Past	113	3
	Current	2179	47
BMI (kg/m^2)	<22.5	719	13
	22.5–24.9	1301	30
	>24.9	719	18

(a) For each of the three factors (smoking, alcohol, and body mass index), rearrange the data into a 3 × 2 table; the other column is for those without gallstone.
(b) For each of the three 3 × 2 tables in (a), choose the lowest level as the baseline and calculate the odds ratio associated with each other level.

1.26. Data were collected from 2197 white ovarian cancer patients and 8893 white controls in 12 different U.S. case–control studies conducted by various investigators in the period 1956–1986. These were used to evaluate the relationship of invasive epithelial ovarian cancer to reproductive and menstrual characteristics, exogenous estrogen use, and prior pelvic surgeries. The following are parts of the data related to unprotected intercourse and to history of infertility.

	Cases	Controls
Duration of Unprotected Intercourse (years)		
<2	237	477
2–9	166	354
10–14	47	91
15 and over	133	174
History of Infertility		
No	526	966
Yes, no drug use	76	124
Yes, drug use	20	11

For each of the two factors (duration of unprotected intercourse and history of infertility; treating the latter as ordinal: no history, history but no drug use, and history with drug use), choose the lowest level as the baseline and calculate the odds ratio associated with each other level.

1.27. Post-neonatal mortality due to respiratory illnesses is known to be inversely related to maternal age, but the role of young motherhood as a risk factor for respiratory morbidity in infants has not been thoroughly explored. A study was conducted in Tucson, Arizona aimed at the incidence of lower respiratory tract illnesses during the first year of life. In this study, over 1200 infants were enrolled at birth between 1980 and 1984 and the following data are concerned with wheezing lower respiratory tract illnesses (wheezing LRI: No/Yes).

Maternal Age (years)	Boys		Girls	
	No	Yes	No	Yes
<21	19	8	20	7
21–25	98	40	128	36
26–30	160	45	148	42
Over 30	110	20	116	25

For each of the two groups, boys and girls, choose the lowest age group as the baseline and calculate the odds ratio associated with each other age group.

1.28. An important characteristic of glaucoma, an eye disease, is the presence of classical visual field loss. Tonometry is a common form of glaucoma screening whereas, for example, an eye is classified as positive if it has an intraocular pressure of 21 mmHg or higher at a single reading. Given the following data,

Field Loss	Test Result		Total
	Positive	Negative	
Yes	13	7	20
No	413	4567	4980

calculate the sensitivity and specificity of this screening test.

1.29. Recall the news report of Example 1.11: "A total of 35,238 new AIDS cases were reported in 1989 by the Centers for Disease Control (CDC), compared to 32,196 reported during 1988. The 9% increase is the smallest since the spread of AIDS began in the early 1980s. For example, new AIDS cases were up 34% in 1988 and 60% in 1987."
"In 1989, 547 cases of AIDS transmissions from mothers to newborns were reported up 17% from 1988; while females made up just 3971 of the 35,238 new cases reported in 1989 that was an increase of 11% over 1988."

From the above information, calculate:

(a) The number of new AIDS cases for the years 1987 and 1986.

(b) The number of cases of AIDS transmission from mothers to newborns for 1988.

1.30. In an effort to provide a complete analysis of the survival of patients with ESRD, data were collected for a sample that included 929 patients who initiated hemodialysis for the first time at the Regional Disease Program in Minneapolis, Minnesota between 1 January 1976 and 30 June 1982; all patients were followed until 31 December 1982. Of these 929 patients, 257 are diabetics; among the 672 nondiabetics, 386 are classified as low-risk (without comorbidities such as arteriosclerotic heart disease, peripheral vascular disease, chronic obstructive pulmonary, and cancer). For the low-risk ESRD patients, we had the following follow-up data (in addition to those in Example 1.12):

Age (years)	Deaths	Treatment Months
21–30	4	1012
31–40	7	1387
41–50	20	1706
51–60	24	2448
61–70	21	2060
Over 70	17	846

Compute the follow-up death rate for each age group, then choose "21–30" as the baseline and calculate the relative risk associated with each other age group.

1.31. Given the following mortality data for the State of Georgia for the year 1977:

Age Group	No. Deaths	Persons
0–4	2,483	424,600
5–19	1,818	1,818,000
20–44	3,656	1,126,500
45–64	12,424	870,800
65+	21,405	360,800

(a) From the above mortality table, calculate the crude death rate for the State of Georgia.

(b) From the above mortality table and the mortality data for Alaska and Florida for the year 1977 (same data as given in Example 1.13 but shown again below),

Age Group	Alaska			Florida		
	No. Deaths	Persons	Deaths/100,000	No. Deaths	Persons	Deaths/100,000
0–4	162	40,000	405.0	2,049	546,000	375.3
5–19	107	128,000	83.6	1,195	1,982,000	60.3
20–44	449	172,000	261.0	5,097	2,676,000	190.5
45–64	451	58,000	777.6	19,904	1,807,000	1101.5
65 +	444	9,000	4933.3	63,505	1,444,000	4397.9
Total	1613	407,000	396.3	91,750	8,455,000	1085.2

calculate the age-adjusted death rate for Georgia and compare them to those for Alaska and Florida, the U.S. population given in Example 1.13, reproduced below, being used as standard.

Age Group	Persons
U.S. Standard Population	
0–4	84,416
5–19	294,353
20–44	316,744
45–64	205,745
65 +	98,742
Total	1,000,000

(c) Calculate, again, the age-adjusted death rate for Georgia with the Alaska population serving as the standard population. How does this adjusted death rate compare to the crude death rate of Alaska?

1.32. Refer to the same set of mortality data as in the above Exercise 1.30. Calculate and compare the age-adjusted death rates for the states of Alaska and Florida with the Georgia population serving as the standard population. How do mortality in these two states compare to the state of Georgia?

1.33. A long-term follow-up study of diabetes has been conducted among Pima Indian residents of the Gila River Indian Community of Arizona since 1965. Subjects of this study, at least 5 years old and of at least half Pima ancestry, were examined approximately every two years; examinations included measurements of height and weight, and a number of other factors. The following table relates diabetes incidence rate (new cases/1000 person-years) to body mass index (BMI, a measure of obesity defined as weight/(height)^2).

Body Mass Index	Incidence Rate
<20	.8
20–25	10.9
25–30	17.3
30–35	32.6
35–40	48.5
Over 40	72.2

Display these rates by means of a bar chart.

1.34. In the course of selecting controls for a study to evaluate effect of caffeine-containing coffee on the risk of myocardial infarction among women 30–49 years of age, a study noted appreciable differences in coffee consumption among hospital patients admitted for illnesses not known to be related to coffee use. Among potential controls, the coffee consumption of patients who had been admitted to hospital by conditions having an acute onset (such as fractures) was compared to that of patients admitted for chronic disorders.

	Cups of Coffee Per Day			
Admission by	0	1–4	5 or more	Total
Acute condition	340	457	183	980
Chronic condition	2440	2527	868	5835

(a) Each of the above 6815 subject is considered as belonging to one of the three groups defined by the number of cups of coffee consumed per day (the three columns). Calculate, for each of the three groups, the proportion of subjects admitted because of an acute onset. Display these proportions by means of a bar chart.

(b) For those admitted because of their chronic conditions, express their coffee consumption by means of a pie chart.

1.35. In a seroepidemiologic survey of health workers representing a spectrum of exposure to blood and patients with hepatitis B virus (HBV), it was found that infection increased as a function of contact. The following table provides data for hospital workers with uniform socioeconomic status at an urban teaching hospital in Boston, Massachusetts.

Personnel	Exposure	No. Tested	HBV Positive
Physicians	Frequent	81	17
	Infrequent	89	7
Nurses	Frequent	104	22
	Infrequent	126	11

(a) Calculate the proportion of HBV positive workers in each subgroup.

(b) Calculate the odds ratios associated with frequent contacts (as compared to infrequent contacts); do this separately for physicians and nurses.

(c) Compare the two ratios obtained in (b); a large difference would indicate a "three-term interaction" or "effect modification," where frequent effects are different for physicians and nurses.

(d) Assuming that the odds ratios for the two groups, physicians and nurses, are equal (in other words, type of personnel is not an effect modifier), calculate the Mantel–Haenszel estimate of this common odds ratio.

1.36. The results of the Third National Cancer Survey have shown substantial variation in lung cancer incidence rates for White males within Allegheny County, Pennsylvania, which may be due to different smoking rates. The following table gives the percentages (%) of current smokers by age for two study areas.

	Lawrenceville		South Hills	
Age (years)	No. Surveyed	Smoking Rate	No. Surveyed	Smoking Rate
35–44	71	54.9	135	37.0
45–54	79	53.2	193	28.5
55–64	119	43.7	138	21.7
Over 65	109	30.3	141	18.4

(a) Display the age distribution for Lawrenceville by means of a pie chart.

(b) Display the age distribution for South Hills by means of a pie chart.

(c) Display the smoking rates for Lawrenceville and South Hills, side by side, by means of a bar chart.

1.37. Prematurity, which ranks as the major cause of neonatal morbidity and mortality, has traditionally been defined on the basis of a birth weight under 2500 g. But this definition encompasses two distinct types of infants: infants who are small because they are born early, and infants who are born at or near term but are small because their growth was retarded. "Prematurity" has now been replaced by

(i) "low birth weight" to describe the second type

(ii) "preterm" to characterize the first type (babies born before 37 weeks of gestation)

A case–control study of the epidemiology of preterm delivery was undertaken at Yale-New Haven Hospital in Connecticut during 1977. The study population consisted of 175 mothers of singleton preterm infants and 303 mothers of singleton full-term infants. The following tables give the distributions of age (first table) and socioeconomic status (second table).

Age	Cases	Controls
14–17	15	16
18–19	22	25
20–24	47	62
25–29	56	122
30 or over	35	78

Socioeconomic Level	Cases	Controls
Upper	11	40
Upper-middle	14	45
Middle	33	64
Lower-middle	59	91
Lower	53	58
Unknown	5	5

(a) Refer to the age data (first table) and choose the "30 or over" group as baseline; calculate the odds ratio associated with each other age group. Is this true, in general, that the younger the mother the higher the risk?

(b) Refer to the socioeconomic data (second table) and choose the "lower" group as the baseline, calculate the odds ratio associated with each other group. Is this true, in general, that the poorer the mother the higher the risk?

1.38. Adult male residents of 13 counties of western Washington State, in whom testicular cancer had been diagnosed during 1977–1983 were interviewed over the telephone regarding their history of genital tract conditions, including vasectomy. For comparison, the same interview was given to a sample of men selected from the population of these counties by dialing telephone numbers at random. The following data are tabulated by religious background.

Religion	Vasectomy	Cases	Controls
Protestant	Yes	24	56
	No	205	239
Catholic	Yes	10	6
	No	32	90
Others	Yes	18	39
	No	56	96

Calculate the odds ratio associated with vasectomy for each religious group. Is there any evidence of an effect modification? If not, calculate the Mantel–Haenszel estimate of the common odds ratio.

1.39. The role of menstrual and reproductive factors in the epidemiology of breast cancer has been reassessed using pooled data from three large case–control studies of breast cancer from several Italian regions. The following are summarized data for age at menopause and age at first live birth.

	Cases	Controls
Age at First Live Birth		
<22	621	898
22–24	795	909
25–27	791	769

(continued)

(Continued)

	Cases	Controls
>27	1043	775
Age at Menopause		
<45	459	543
45–49	749	803
>49	1378	1167

Find a way (or ways) to further summarize the data so as to express the observation that the risk of breast cancer is lower for women with younger ages at first live birth and younger ages at menopause.

1.40. It has been hypothesized that dietary fiber decreases the risk of colon cancer, while meats and fats are thought to increase this risk. A large study was undertaken to confirm these hypotheses. Fiber and fat consumptions are classified as "low" or "high" and data are tabulated separately for males and females as follows ("low" means below median):

	Males		Females	
Diet	Cases	Controls	Cases	Controls
Low fat, high fiber	27	38	23	39
Low fat, low fiber	64	78	82	81
High fat, high fiber	78	61	83	76
High fat, low fiber	36	28	35	27

For each group (males and females), using "low fat, high fiber" as the baseline, calculate the odds ratio associated with each other dietary combination. Any evidence of an effect modification (interaction between consumption of fat and consumption of fiber)?

1.41. In 1979, the U.S. Veterans Administration conducted a health survey of 11,230 veterans. The advantages of this survey are that it includes a large random sample with a high interview response rate and it was done before the recent public controversy surrounding the issue of the health effects of possible exposure to Agent Orange. The following are data relating Vietnam service to eight post-traumatic stress disorder symptoms among the 1787 veterans who entered the military service between 1965 and 1975.

		Service in Vietnam	
Symptom	Level	Yes	No
Nightmares	Yes	197	85
	No	577	925
Sleep problems	Yes	173	160

(continued)

(Continued)

Symptom	Level	Service in Vietnam	
		Yes	No
	No	599	851
Troubled memories	Yes	220	105
	No	549	906
Depression	Yes	306	315
	No	465	699
Temper control problem	Yes	176	144
	No	595	868
Life goal association	Yes	231	225
	No	539	786
Omit feelings	Yes	188	191
	No	583	821
Confusion	Yes	163	148
	No	607	864

Calculate the odds ratio for each symptom.

1.42. The following table compiles data from different studies designed to investigate the accuracy of death certificates. The results of 5373 autopsies were compared to the causes of death listed on the certificates. The results are:

Date of Study	Accurate Certificate		Total
	Yes	No	
1955–1965	2040	694	2734
1970–1971	437	203	640
1975–1978	1128	599	1727
1980	121	151	272

Find a graphical way to display the downward trend of accuracy over time.

1.43. A study was conducted to ascertain factors that influence a physician's decision to transfuse a patient. A sample of 49 attending physicians was selected. Each physician was asked a question concerning the frequency with which an unnecessary transfusion was give because another physician suggested it. The same question was asked of a sample of 71 residents. The data were as follows:

Type of Physician	Frequency of Unnecessary Transfusion				
	Very Frequent (1/week)	Frequent (1/2 weeks)	Occasionally (1/month)	Rarely (1/2 months)	Never
Attending	1	1	3	31	13
Resident	2	13	28	23	5

Choose "never" as the baseline and calculate the odds ratio associated with each other frequency and "residency."

1.44. When a patient is diagnosed as having cancer of the prostate, an important question in deciding on treatment strategy for the patient is whether or not the cancer has spread to the neighboring lymph nodes. The question is so critical in prognosis and treatment that it is customary to operate on the patient (i.e., perform a laparotomy) for the sole purpose of examining the nodes and removing tissue samples to examine under the microscope for evidence of cancer. However, certain variables that can be measured without surgery are predictive of the nodal involvement; and the purpose of the study presented here was to examine the data for 53 prostate cancer patients receiving surgery, to determine which of five preoperative variables are predictive of nodal involvement. The following table presents the complete data set. For each of the 53 patients, there are two continuous independent variables, age at diagnosis and level of serum acid phosphatase (multiplied by 100; called "acid"), and three binary variables, X-ray reading, pathology reading (grade) of a biopsy of the tumor obtained by needle before surgery, and a rough measure of the size and location of the tumor (Stage) obtained by palpation with the fingers via the rectum. For these three binary independent variables a value of one signifies a positive or more serious state and a zero denotes a negative or less serious finding. In addition, the sixth column presents the finding at surgery—the primary outcome of interest, which is binary, a value of 1 denoting nodal involvement, and a value of 0 denoting no nodal involvement found at surgery. In this exercise we investigate the effects of the three binary preoperative variables (X-ray, Grade, and Stage); the effects of the two continuous factors (age and acid phosphatase) will be studied in an exercise in the next chapter.

(a) Arrange the data on Notes and X-ray into a 2×2 table, calculate the odds ratio associated with X-ray and give your interpretation.

(b) Arrange the data on Notes and Grade into a 2×2 table, calculate the odds ratio associated with Grade and give your interpretation.

(c) Arrange the data on Notes and Stage into a 2×2 table, calculate the odds ratio associated with Stage and give your interpretation.

(This is a very long data file; its electronic version is available from the author upon request. Two-by-two tables can be easily formed using the method for Excel as explained in Section 1.4)Data

Case	X-Ray	Grade	Stage	Age	Acid	Nodes
1	0	1	1	64	40	0
2	0	0	1	63	40	0
3	1	0	0	65	46	0
4	0	1	0	67	47	0
5	0	0	0	66	48	0
6	0	1	1	65	48	0
7	0	0	0	60	49	0
8	0	0	0	51	49	0
8	0	0	0	66	50	0

(continued)

(Continued)

Case	X-Ray	Grade	Stage	Age	Acid	Nodes
10	0	0	0	58	50	0
11	0	1	0	56	50	0
12	0	0	1	61	50	0
13	0	1	1	64	50	0
14	0	0	0	56	52	0
15	0	0	0	67	52	0
16	1	0	0	49	55	0
17	0	1	1	52	55	0
18	0	0	0	68	56	0
19	0	1	1	66	59	0
20	1	0	0	60	62	0
21	0	0	0	61	62	0
22	1	1	1	59	63	0
23	0	0	0	51	65	0
24	0	1	1	53	66	0
25	0	0	0	58	71	0
26	0	0	0	63	75	0
27	0	0	1	53	76	0
28	0	0	0	60	78	0
29	0	0	0	52	83	0
30	0	0	1	67	95	0
31	0	0	0	56	98	0
32	0	0	1	61	102	0
33	0	0	0	64	187	0
34	1	0	1	58	48	1
35	0	0	1	65	49	1
36	1	1	1	57	51	1
37	0	1	0	50	56	1
38	1	1	0	67	67	1
39	0	0	1	67	67	1
40	0	1	1	57	67	1
41	0	1	1	45	70	1
42	0	0	1	46	70	1
43	1	0	1	51	72	1
44	1	1	1	60	76	1
45	1	1	1	56	78	1
46	1	1	1	50	81	1
47	0	0	0	56	82	1
48	0	0	1	63	82	1
49	1	1	1	65	84	1
50	1	0	1	64	89	1
51	0	1	0	59	99	1
52	1	1	1	68	126	1
53	1	0	0	61	136	1

2

Organization, Summarization, and Presentation of Data

A class of measurements or a characteristic on which individual observations or measurements are made is called a *variable*; examples include weight, height, and blood pressure, among others. Suppose we have a set of numerical values for a variable:

(i) If each element of this set may lie only at a few isolated points, we have a *discrete data* set. Examples are race, sex, counts of events, or some sort of artificial grading.

(ii) If each element of this set may theoretically lie anywhere on the numerical scale, we have a *continuous data* set. Examples are blood pressure, cholesterol level, or time to a certain event such as death.

The previous chapter deals with the organization, summarization, and presentation of discrete data; in this chapter the focus is on the same tasks for continuous measurements, research outcomes that can be put on a numerical scale.

2.1. TABULAR AND GRAPHICAL METHODS

There are different ways of organizing and presenting data; simple *tables* and *graphs*, however, are still very effective methods. They are designed to help the reader obtain an intuitive feeling for the data *at a glance*.

2.1.1. One-Way Scatter Plots

This method is the simplest type of graph that can be used to summarize a set of continuous observations. A *one-way scatter plot* uses a single horizontal axis to display the relative position of each data point. As an example, Figure 2.1 depicts the crude death

Health and Numbers: A Problems-Based Introduction to Biostatistics, Third Edition, by Chap T. Le
Copyright © 2009 John Wiley & Sons, Inc.

393.9   Rate per 100,000 population   1,242.1

Figure 2.1. Crude death rates for the United States, 1988.

rates for all 50 states and the District of Columbia, from a low of 393.9 per 100,000 population to a high of 1242.1 per 100,000 population.

An advantage of a one-way scatter plot is that, since each observation is represented individually, no information is lost; a disadvantage is that it may be difficult to read (and to construct!) if values are close to each other.

2.1.2. Frequency Distribution

There is no difficulty if the data set is small, for we can arrange those few numbers and write them, say, in increasing order; the result would be sufficiently clear; the above one-way scatter plot is an example. For fairly large data sets, a useful way to summarize a set of continuous data is to form a *frequency table* or *frequency distribution*. This is a table showing the number of observations called *frequency* within certain ranges of values of the variable under investigation. For example, taking the variable to be the age at death, we have the following example; the second column of the table provides the frequencies.

Example 2.1

The following table gives the number of deaths by age for the state of Minnesota in 1987.

Age (years)	No. of Deaths
<1	564
1–4	86
5–14	127
15–24	490
25–34	667
35–44	806
45–54	1,425
55–64	3,511
65–74	6,932
75–84	10,101
85 +	9,825
Total	35,534

If a data set is to be grouped to form a frequency distribution, difficulties should be recognized and an efficient strategy is needed for better communication. First, there is no clear-cut rule on the *number of intervals* or *classes*. With too many intervals, the data are not summarized enough for a clear visualization of how they are distributed. On the contrary, too few intervals are undesirable because the data are over-summarized and some of the details of the distribution may be lost. In general, between 5 and 15 intervals are acceptable; of course, this also depends on the number of observations.

The widths of the intervals must also be decided. Example 2.1 shows the special case of mortality data, where it is traditional to show infant deaths (deaths of persons who are born live but die before living 1 year). Without such specific reasons, intervals generally should be of the same width. This common width "*w*" may be determined by dividing the range "*R*" by "*k*", the number of intervals:

$$w = \frac{R}{k}$$

where the *range R* is the difference between the smallest and the largest numbers in the data set. In addition, a width should be chosen so that it is convenient to use or easy to recognize, such as a multiple of 5 (or 1, for example, if the data set has a narrower range). Similar considerations apply to the choice of the beginning of the first interval; it is a convenient number, which is low enough for the first interval to include the smallest observation. Finally, care should be taken in deciding in which interval to place an observation falling on one of the interval boundaries. For example, a consistent rule could be made so as to place such an observation in the interval of which the observation in question is the lower limit.

Example 2.2

The following are weights in pounds of 57 children at a daycare center:

Weights of Children in Daycare									
68	63	42	27	30	36	28	32	79	27
22	23	24	25	44	65	43	25	74	51
36	42	28	31	28	25	45	12	57	51
12	32	49	38	42	27	31	50	38	21
16	24	69	47	23	22	43	27	49	28
23	19	46	30	43	49	12			

From the above data set we have

(1) The smallest number is 12 and the largest is 79 so that

$$R = 79 - 12$$
$$= 67$$

If 5 intervals are used, we would have

$$w = \frac{67}{5}$$
$$= 13.4$$

And if 15 intervals are used we would have

$$w = \frac{67}{15}$$
$$= 4.5$$

Between these two values, 4.5 and 13.4, there are two convenient (or conventional) numbers: 5 and 10. Since the sample size of 57 is not large, a width of 10 should be an apparent choice because it results in fewer intervals (the usual concept of "large" could be like "100 or more").

(2) Since the smallest number is 12, we may begin our first interval at 10. These considerations, (1) and (2), lead to the following seven intervals:

$$10-19$$
$$20-29$$
$$30-39$$
$$40-49$$
$$50-59$$
$$60-69$$
$$70-79$$

(3) Determining the frequencies or the number of values or measurements for each interval is merely a matter of examining the values one by one and of placing a tally mark beside the appropriate interval. When we do this we have Table 2.1 (for which the temporary column of tallies was already deleted).

Table 2.1. Frequency Distribution of Weights of 57 Children

Weight Intervals (lb)	Frequency	Relative Frequency (%)
10–19	5	8.8
20–29	19	33.3
30–39	10	17.5
40–49	13	22.8
50–59	4	7.0
60–60	4	7.0
70–79	2	3.5
Total	57	100.0

(4) An optional, but recommended, step in the formulation of a frequency distribution is to present the proportion or *relative frequency* in addition to frequency, for each interval. These proportions, defined by

$$\text{Relative frequency} = \frac{\text{Frequency}}{\text{Total number of observations}}$$

were shown in the third column of the above table (as %) and would be very useful if we need to compare two data sets of different sizes.

Example 2.3

A study was conducted to investigate the possible effects of exercise on the menstrual cycle. From the data collected from that study, we obtained the menarchal age (in years) of 56 female swimmers who began their swimming training after they had reached menarche; these served as controls in order to compare with those who began their training *prior to* menarche.

Age at Menarche							
14.0	16.1	13.4	14.6	13.7	13.2	13.7	14.3
12.9	14.1	15.1	14.8	12.8	14.2	14.1	13.6
14.2	15.8	12.7	15.6	14.1	13.0	12.9	15.1
15.0	13.6	14.2	13.8	12.7	15.3	14.1	13.5
15.3	12.6	13.8	14.4	12.9	14.6	15.0	13.8
13.0	14.1	13.8	14.2	13.6	14.1	14.5	13.1
12.8	14.3	14.2	13.5	14.1	13.6	12.4	15.1

From this data set we have

The smallest number is 12.4 and the largest is 16.1 so that

$$R = 16.1 - 12.4$$
$$= 3.7$$

If 5 intervals are used, we would have

$$w = \frac{3.7}{5}$$
$$= .74$$

And if 15 intervals are used we would have

$$w = \frac{3.7}{15}$$
$$= .25$$

Between these two values, .25 and. 74, .5 seems to be a convenient (or conventional) number to use for the width;.25 is another choice but it would create many more intervals (15) for such a small data set. (Another alternative is to express ages in months and not to deal with decimal numbers.)

(1) Because the smallest number is 12.4, we may begin our first interval at 12.0 leading to the following nine intervals:

$$12.0–12.4$$
$$12.5–12.9$$
$$13.0–13.4$$
$$13.5–13.9$$
$$14.0–14.4$$
$$14.5–14.9$$
$$15.0–15.4$$
$$15.5–15.9$$
$$16.0–16.4$$

(2) Count the number of swimmers whose ages belong to each of the above nine intervals, the frequencies, and obtain Table 2.2—completed with the last column for relative frequencies expressed as percentages (%).

2.1.3. Histogram and the Frequency Polygon

A convenient way of displaying a frequency table is by means of a *histogram* and/or a *frequency polygon*. A histogram is a diagram in which

(1) The horizontal scale represents the value of the variable marked at interval boundaries.

Table 2.2. Frequency Distribution of Menarchal Age of 56 Swimmers

Chosen Interval	Frequency	Relative Frequency (%)
12.0–12.4	1	1.8
12.5–12.9	8	14.3
13.0–13.4	5	8.9
13.5–13.9	12	21.4
14.0–14.4	16	28.6
14.5–14.9	4	7.2
15.0–15.4	7	12.5
15.5–15.9	2	3.6
16.0–16.4	1	1.8
Total	56	100

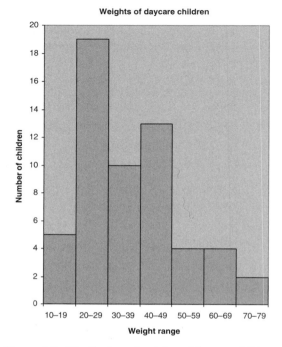

Figure 2.2. Distribution of weights of daycare children.

(2) The vertical scale represents the frequency or relative frequency in each interval (see exceptions below). For example, we have the following histogram for data in Example 2.1 and Figure 2.2 for data in Example 2.2 (weights of 57 children).

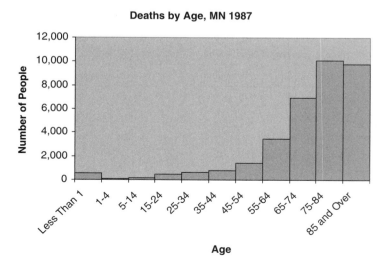

The histogram presents us with a graphic picture of the distribution of measurements. This picture consists of rectangular bars joining each other, one for each interval as shown in Figure 2.2 for the data set of Example 2.2. If disjoint intervals are used such as in Table 2.1, the horizontal axis is marked with true boundaries. A true boundary is the average of the upper limit of one interval and the lower limit of the next higher interval. For example, 19.5 serves as the true upper boundary of the first interval and true lower boundary for the second interval. In cases where we need to compare the shapes of the histograms representing different data sets, or if intervals are of unequal widths, the height of each rectangular bar should represent the density of the interval, where the interval density is defined by

$$\text{Density} = \frac{\text{Relative frequency}(\%)}{\text{Interval width}}$$

The unit for density is "percent per unit (of measurement)," for example, percent per year. If we do this, the relative frequency is represented by the area of the rectangular bar and the total area under the histogram is 100%. It may be a good practice to always graph densities on the vertical axis with or without having equal class width; when class widths are equal, the shape of the histogram looks similar to the graph with relative frequencies on the vertical axis.

To draw a *frequency polygon*, we first place a dot at the midpoint of the upper base of each rectangular bar. The points are connected with straight lines. At the ends, the points could be connected to the midpoints of the previous and succeeding intervals (these are make-up intervals with zero frequency, where widths are the widths of the first and last intervals, respectively). A frequency polygon as thus constructed is another way to portray graphically the distribution of a data set:

 (i) The frequency polygon can be shown without the histogram (see Figure 2.3).

(ii) The frequency polygon can also be imposed on top of a histogram.

The frequency table and its graphical relatives, the histogram, and the frequency polygon, have a number of applications, as seen below; the first leads to a research question and the second leads to a new analysis strategy.

(1) When data are homogeneous, the table and graphs usually show a *uni-modal pattern*, a histogram or frequency polygon with one peak in the middle part. A *bi-modal pattern* might indicate possible influence or effect of certain hidden factor or factors.

Example 2.4

The following table provides data on age and percentage saturation of bile for 31 male patients. Using equal-width (10%) intervals, the data set can be represented by a histogram or a frequency polygon as shown in Figure 2.4. This picture shows an apparent bi-modal distribution; however, a closer examination shows that among the nine patients with over 100% saturation, eight (or 89%) are over 50 years of age. On the contrary, only 4 of 22 (or 18%)

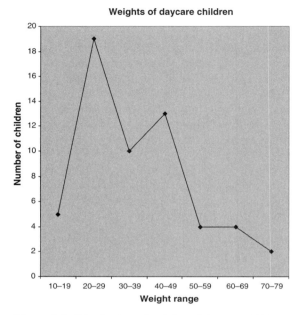

Figure 2.3. Distribution of weights of daycare children.

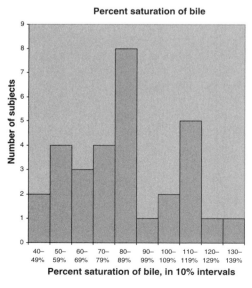

Figure 2.4. Frequency polygon for percentage saturation of bile in men.

patients with less than 100% saturation are over 50 years of age. The two peaks in the diagram might correspond to the two age groups.

Percent Saturation of Bile (Age)				
40 (23)	90 (48)	88 (20)	106 (53)	58 (36)
86 (31)	112 (29)	65 (23)	110 (59)	88 (29)
111 (58)	52 (26)	79 (43)	78 (48)	73 (27)
86 (25)	88 (64)	87 (27)	80 (27)	118 (65)
106 (63)	137 (55)	56 (63)	47 (32)	67 (42)
66 (43)	88 (31)	110 (66)	74 (62)	57 (60)
123 (67)				

Chosen Interval (%)	Frequency
40–49	2
50–59	4
60–69	3
70–79	4
80–89	8
90–99	1
100–109	2
110–119	5
120–129	1
130–139	1
Total	31

(2) Another application concerns the *symmetry* of the distribution as depicted by the table or its graphs. A symmetric distribution is one in which the distribution has the same shape on both sides of the peak location. If there are more extremely large values, the distribution is then skewed to the right, or *positively skewed.* Examples include family income, antibody level after vaccination, and drug dose to produce a predetermined level of response, among others. It is common that for positively skewed distributions, subsequent statistical analyses should be performed on the log scale; for example, to compute and/or to compare averages of log(dose).

Example 2.5

The distribution of family income for the United States in 1983 by race is shown below. It is obvious that the distribution is not symmetric; it is very skewed to the right.

Income ($)	Percent of Families	
	White	Nonwhite
0–14,999	13	34
15,000–19,999	24	31
20,000–24,999	26	19
25,000–34,999	28	13
35,000–59,999	9	3
60,000 +	1	0
Total	100	100

The distribution for Nonwhite families is represented in the histogram in Figure 2.5, where the vertical axis represents the density (percent per thousand dollars). In this histogram, we graph the densities on the vertical axis. For example, for the second income interval (15,000–19,999), the relative frequency is 31% and the width of the interval is $5000 (31% per $5000), or 6.2% per $1000 (we arbitrarily multiply by 1000—or any power of 10—just to obtain a larger number for easy reading and graphing).

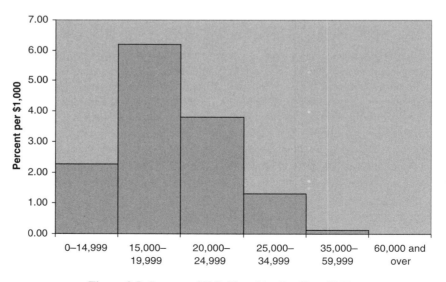

Figure 2.5. Income of U.S. Nonwhite Families, 1983.

2.1.4. The Cumulative Frequency Graph and Percentiles

Cumulative relative frequency, or cumulative percentage, gives the percentage of individuals having a measurement less than or equal to the upper boundary of the class interval. Data from Table 2.1 are here with a column for cumulative relative frequency (Table 2.3) as follows:

Table 2.3. Distribution of Weights of 57 Children

Weight Intervals (lb)	Frequency	Relative Frequency (%)	Cumulative Relative Frequency (%)
10–19	5	8.8	8.8
20–29	19	33.3	42.1
30–39	10	17.5	59.6
40–49	13	22.8	82.4
50–59	4	7.0	89.4
60–60	4	7.0	96.4
70–79	2	3.5	100
Total	57	100.0	

This last column is easy to form; you do it by successively cumulating the relative frequencies of each of the various intervals. In the above example, the cumulative percentage for the first three intervals is

$$8.8 + 33.3 + 17.5 = 59.6$$

and we can say that 59.6% of the children in the data set have a weight of 39.5 lb or less. Or, as another example, 96.4% of children weigh 69.5 lb or less, and so on.

The cumulative relative frequency can be presented graphically as in Figure 2.6. This type of curve is called a *cumulative frequency graph*, or cumulative frequency polygon. To construct a cumulative frequency graph, we place a point with horizontal axis marked at the *upper class boundary* and vertical axis marked at the corresponding cumulative frequency. Each point represents the cumulative relative frequency for that interval and the points are connected with straight lines. At the left end, it is connected to the lower boundary of the first interval. If disjoint intervals, such as

10-19
20-29

are used, points are placed at the *true boundaries* (Table 2.4). We have, for data of Example 2.2:

Table 2.4. True Upper Boundaries

Weight Interval	True Upper Boundary	Relative Cumulative Frequency (%)
10–19	19.5	8.8
20–29	29.5	42.1
30–39	39.5	59.6
40–49	49.5	82.4
50–59	59.5	89.4
60–69	69.5	96.4
70–79	79.5	100.0

Cumulative frequency polygons or graphs, constructed as the one shown in Figure 2.6, give us an approximate idea what such a graph should look like, with just a few points marked at the upper boundaries on intervals of a histogram. If you want to use all raw data in a data set to form a graph with more accuracy, follow these steps:

(1) Enter the raw data in a single column, one value in each row.
(2) Sort the data; to do this, begin by highlighting the column of data from step 1 then exercise menu commands by clicking *Data* (on a bar above the standard toolbar) and selecting *Sort*.
(3) Create a column that numbers the children or subjects from 1 to 57.
(4) Calculate the cumulative percentages from numbers in step 3 to form a new column.
(5) Create a *line graph* using output from step 2 as the *x*-axis and output from step 4 as the *y*-axis (see more details on line graph formation using Excel in Section 2.4).

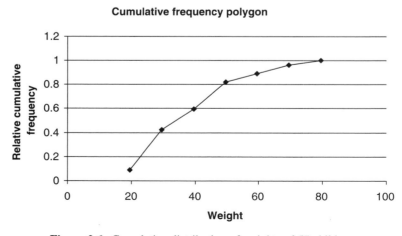

Figure 2.6. Cumulative distribution of weights of 57 children.

The result will be a smoother curve as shown below—especially for larger samples.

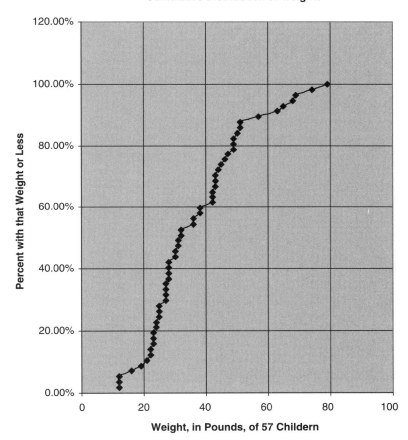

Cumulative Distribution of Weights

The cumulative percentages and their graphical representation, the cumulative frequency graph, have a number of applications.

(1) When two cumulative frequency graphs, representing two different data sets, are placed on the same graph, they provide a rapid visual comparison without any need to compare individual intervals. Figure 2.7 gives such a comparison of family incomes using data of Example 2.4.

(2) The cumulative frequency graph provides a class of important *statistics* known as *percentiles* or *percentile scores*. The 90th percentile, for example, is the numerical value that exceeds 90% of the values in the data set and is exceeded by only 10% of them. Or, as another example, the 80th percentile is that numerical value that exceeds 80% of the values contained in the data set and is exceeded by 20% of them, and so on.

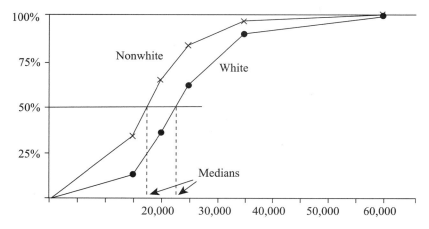

Figure 2.7. Distribution of family income for The United States in 1983.

The 50th percentile is especially important, popular, and is commonly called the *median*; the median is the numerical value that exceeds exactly 50% of the values in the data set and is exceeded by the other 50%. In our example of Figure 2.7, the median family income in 1983 for Nonwhites was about $17,500 as compared to a median of about $22,000 for White families. In order to get the median, we start at the 50% point on the vertical axis, and go horizontally until meeting the cumulative frequency graph; the projection of this intersection on the horizontal axis is the median. For a smaller data set, one can simply sort the raw data and the median is the value in the middle or average of the two values in the middle. Other percentiles are obtained similarly.

The cumulative frequency graph also provides an important application in the formation of *health norms* for the monitoring of physical progress of infants and children. Here, the same percentiles, say 90th, of weight or height of groups of children at different ages are joined by a curve. There are three set of curves, one for heights, one for weights, and one for head circumferences; two are shown here in Figure 2.8a and b. These health norms form standard references used in pediatrics well visits to monitor the consistency of growths of infants and children—especially in the first 3 years of life. Example 2.6 and Figure 2.9 illustrate a simple application in health research.

Example 2.6

Figure 2.9 provides results from a study of Hmong refugees in the Minneapolis—St. Paul area where each dot represents the average weight of five refugee girls of the same age. The graph shows that even though the refugee girls are small, mostly in the lowest 25%, they grow at the same rate as measured by the American standard. However, the pattern changes by the age of 15 years, when their average weight drops to a level below the 5th percentile. As a comparison, most Caucasians are growing until the age of 17 or 18. In this example, we plot the average height of five girls instead of individual weights; because the Hmongs are small, individual weights are likely to be out of the chart. This concept of *average* or *mean* will be further explained in the next Section 2.2.

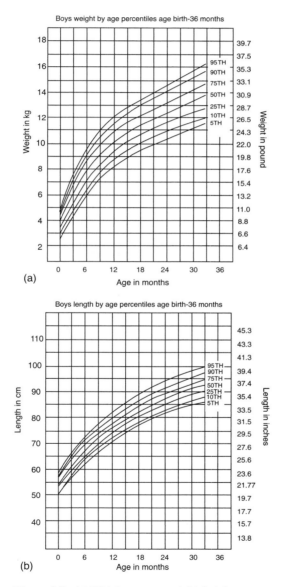

Figure 2.8. (a) Weight curves and (b) height curves.

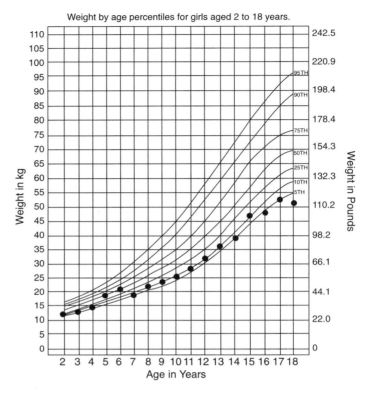

Figure 2.9. Average weight by age for refugee girls.

2.2. NUMERICAL METHODS

Although tables and graphs serve useful purposes, there are many situations that require other types of *data summarization*. What we need in many applications is the ability to summarize data by means of just a few numerical measures, particularly before inferences or generalizations are drawn from the data. Measures for describing the *location* (or typical value) of a set of measurements and their *variation* or *dispersion* are used for these purposes.

First, let us suppose we have *n* measurements in a data set; for example, {8, 2, 3, 5} with $n = 4$, *n* being the sample size (the number of observations or data points). We usually denote these numbers as x_i's; thus we have for the above example: $x_1 = 8$, $x_2 = 2$, $x_3 = 3$, and $x_4 = 5$. If we add all the x_i's in the above data set, we obtain 18 as the sum. This addition process is recorded as

$$\sum x = 18$$

where the Greek letter "sigma" ($\sum$) is the *summation sign*.

With the summation notation, we are now able to define a number of important summarized measures starting with the *arithmetic average* or *mean*.

2.2.1. Mean

Given a data set of size n,

$$\{x_1, x_2, \ldots, x_n\}$$

the *mean* of the x's will be denoted by $\bar{x}$ ("x-bar") and is computed by summing all the x's and dividing the sum by n, the *sample size* or number of observations. Symbolically,

$$x = \frac{\sum x}{n}$$

It is important to know that $\sum$ ("sigma") stands for an operation (that of obtaining the sum of the quantities that follow), rather than a quantity itself. For example, considering the data set

$$\{8, 5, 4, 12, 15, 5, 7\}$$

we have

$$\sum_{n=7} x = 56$$

$$\bar{x} = \frac{56}{7}$$

$$= 8$$

As earlier indicated, a characteristic of some interest is the symmetry or lack of symmetry of a distribution and it was recommended that for very positively skewed distributions, analyses are commonly done on the log scale. After obtaining a mean on the log scale, we should take the *antilog* to return to the original scale of measurement; the result is called the *geometric mean* of the x's. The effect of this process is to minimize the influences of *extreme observations* (very large numbers in the data set).

For example, considering the data set

$$\{8, 5, 4, 12, 15, 7, 28\}$$

with one unusually large measurement, we have Table 2.5 with natural logs presented in the second column:

Table 2.5. Calculation of a Geometric Mean

	x	$\ln x$
	8	2.08
	5	1.61
	4	1.39
	12	2.48
	15	2.71
	7	1.95
	28	3.33
Total	79	15.55

The (arithmetic) mean is:

$$x = \frac{79}{7}$$

$$= 11.3$$

while on the log scale, we have

$$\sum_n \ln x = \frac{15.55}{7}$$

$$= 2.22$$

leading to a geometric mean of 9.22, which is less affected by the large measurements. Geometric mean is used extensively in microbiological and serological research in which distributions are often positively skewed.

Example 2.7

In some studies, the important number is the time to an event, such as death; it is called the survival time. The term *survival time* is conventional even though the primary event could be nonfatal such as a relapse or the appearance of the first disease symptom. Similar to the cases of income and antibody level, the distributions of survival times are often positively skewed. Therefore, data are often summarized using median or geometric mean. The following is a typical example:

The remission times of 42 patients with acute leukemia were reported from a clinical trial undertaken to assess the ability of a drug called 6-mercaptopurine (6-MP) to maintain remission. Each patient was randomized to receive either 6-MP or placebo. The study was terminated after 1 year; patients have different follow-up time because they were enrolled sequentially at different times. Times to relapse in weeks for the 21 patients in the Placebo group were:

$$\{1, 1, 2, 2, 3, 4, 4, 5, 5, 8, 8, 8, 8, 11, 11, 12, 12, 15, 17, 22, 23\}$$

The mean is

$$\bar{x} = 8.67 \text{ weeks}$$

while on the log scale, we have

$$\frac{\sum \ln x}{n} = 1.826$$

leading to a geometric mean of 6.21 weeks, which is less affected by a few large survival times.

2.2.2. Other Measures of Location

Another useful measure of location is the median. If the observations in the data set are arranged in increasing or decreasing order, the median is the middle observation, which divides the set into equal halves:

(1) If the number of observations n is odd there will be a unique median.

(2) If n is even there is strictly no middle observation, but the median is conventionally defined as the average of the two middle observations.

In the previous Section 2.1, we showed a quicker way to get an approximate value for the median using the cumulative frequency graph (see Figure 2.6).

The two data sets {8, 5, 4, 12, 15, 7, 28} and {8, 5, 4, 12, 15, 7, 49}, for example, have different means but the same median, 8. Therefore, the advantage of the median as a measure of location is that it is less affected by extreme observations. However, the median has some disadvantages in comparison with the mean:

(1) In large data sets, the median requires more work to calculate than the mean.
(2) It takes no account of the precise magnitude of most of the observations, and is therefore less efficient than the mean because it wastes information.
(3) If two groups of observations are pooled, the median of the combined group cannot be expressed in terms of the medians of the two component groups. However, the mean can be so expressed. If component groups are of sizes n_1 and n_2 and have means $\bar{x}_1$ and $\bar{x}_2$, respectively, the mean of the combined group is

$$\bar{x} = \frac{n_1\bar{x}_1 + n_2\bar{x}_2}{n_1 + n_2}$$

A third measure of location, the *mode*, was briefly introduced in the histogram and frequency polygon section. It is a value at which the frequency polygon reaches a peak. The mode is not widely used in analytical statistics, other than as a descriptive measure, mainly because of the ambiguity in its definition as the fluctuations of small frequencies are apt to produce spurious modes. Because of these reasons, the rest of this book is focused on only one measure of location, the *mean*.

2.2.3. Measures of Dispersion

When the mean of a set of measurements has been obtained it is usually a matter of considerable interest to measure the *degree of variation* or *dispersion* around this mean. Are the x's all rather close to the mean or are some of them dispersed widely in each direction? This question is important for purely descriptive reasons, but it is also important because the measurement of dispersion or variation plays a central part in the methods of statistical inference, which will be described in subsequent chapters of this book.

An obvious candidate for the measurement of dispersion is the *range R*, defined as the difference between the largest value and the smallest value, which was introduced in the histogram section, Section 2.1.3. However, there are a few difficulties about the use of the range. The first is that the value of the range is determined by only two of the original observations. Secondly, the interpretation of the range depends, in a complicated way, on the number of observations, which is an undesirable feature.

An alternative approach is to make use of the *deviations from the mean* $(x-\bar{x})$; it is obvious that the greater the variation in the data set, the larger will be the magnitude of these deviations tend to be. From these deviations, the variance s^2—a popular measure of variation, is computed by squaring each deviation, adding them, and dividing their sum by 1 less than n:

$$s^2 = \frac{\sum (x - \bar{x})^2}{n - 1}$$

The use of the divisor $(n - 1)$ instead of n is clearly not very important when n is large. It is more important for small values of n and its justification will be briefly explained later in this section.

It should be noted that

(1) It would be no use to take the mean of deviations because

$$\sum (x - \bar{x}) = 0$$

(2) Taking the mean of the *absolute values*, for example

$$\frac{\sum |x - \bar{x}|}{n}$$

is a possibility. However, this measure has the drawback of being difficult to handle mathematically, and we will not consider it further in this book.

The variance s^2 is measured in the square of the units in which the x's are measured. For example, if x is the time in seconds, the variance is measured in seconds squared $(s)^2$. It is convenient, therefore, to have a measure of variation expressed in the same units as the x's, and this can be easily done by taking the square root of the variance. This quantity is known as the *standard deviation*, and its formula is

$$s = \sqrt{\frac{\sum (x - \bar{x})^2}{n - 1}}$$

For example, consider again the data set:

$$\{8, 5, 4, 12, 15, 5, 7\}$$

calculations of the variance, s^2, and standard deviation "s" are illustrated as in Table 2.6.

Table 2.6. Calculation of Variance and Standard Deviation

x	$x - \bar{x}$	$(x - \bar{x})^2$
8	0	0
5	−3	9
4	−4	16
12	4	16
15	7	49
5	−3	9
7	−1	1
$\sum x = 56$	$\sum (x - \bar{x})^2 = 100$	
$n = 7$	$s^2 = 100/6 = 16.67$	
$\bar{x} = 8$	$s = \sqrt{16.67} = 4.08$	

Table 2.7. Use of Short-cut Formula for Variance

x	x^2
8	64
5	25
4	16
12	144
15	225
5	25
7	49
56	**548**

In general, this "hand calculation" process is likely to cause some trouble. If the mean is not a "round" number, say $\bar{x} = 10/3$, it will need to be rounded off and errors arise in the subtraction of this figure from each x. This difficulty can be easily overcome with the use of the following "short-cut formula" for the variance:

$$s^2 = \frac{\sum x^2 - (\sum x)^2 / n}{n-1}$$

The previous example is re-worked in Table 2.7 yielding identical results.

$$s^2 = \frac{(548) - (56)^2 / 7}{6} = 16.67$$

It is often not clear to beginners why we use $(n-1)$ instead of n as the denominator for the variance. This number $(n-1)$ in the denominator is called the *degree of freedom* representing the "amount of information" in a sample contained in the sample for the calculation of the variance.

The variance is calculated from the *n deviations from the mean* but these deviations add up to zero. Another explanation for this degree of freedom n could be seen as follows. What we are trying to do with "s" is to provide a "measure of the degree of variability," a measure of the average *gap* or average *distance* between numbers in the sample—and there are $(n-1)$ such gaps between n numbers. When $(n=2)$ there is only one gap or distance between the two numbers, and when $(n=1)$ there is no variability to measure.

Finally, it is occasionally useful to describe the variation by expressing the standard deviation as a proportion or percentage of the mean. The resulting measure

$$CV = \frac{s}{\bar{x}} \times 100\%$$

is called the *coefficient of variation*. It is an index, a dimensionless quantity because the standard deviation is expressed in the same units as the mean and, therefore, could be used to compare the difference in variation between two types of measurements. However, its use is rather limited and we will not present it in subsequent parts of this book.

2.3. COEFFICIENT OF CORRELATION

Methods discussed in the previous two sections of this chapter have been directed to the analyses of data where a *single* continuous measurement was made on each element of a sample. However, in many important investigations we may have *two measurements* made, that is, where the sample consists of pairs of values and the research objective is concerned with the *association* between these variables. For example, what is the relationship between a mother's weight and her baby's weight? Section 1.3 was focused on the association between two dichotomous variables. For example, if we want to investigate the relationship between a disease and a certain risk factor, we could calculate an odds ratio to represent the strength of the relationship. This section deals with continuous measurements and the method is referred to as the *correlation analysis*. Correlation is a concept, with common colloquial usage of association, such as "height and weight are correlated." The statistical procedure will give a technical meaning to it; we can actually calculate a number that tells the "strength of the association."

When dealing with the relationship between two continuous variables, we first have to distinguish between a deterministic relationship and a statistical *relationship*. For a deterministic relationship, values of the two variables are related through an exact mathematical formula. For example, consider the relationship between hospital cost and number of days in hospital. If the costs are 100 dollars for admission and 150 dollars per day, then we can easily calculate the total cost given the number of days in hospital and if any set of data is plotted, say cost versus number of days, all data points fall perfectly on a straight line. A statistical relationship, unlike a deterministic one, is not a perfect one. In general, the points do not fall perfectly on any line or curve. Table 2.8 gives the values for the birth weight (x) and the increase in weight between 70th and 100th days of life, expressed as a percentage of the birth weight (y) for ($n = 12$) infants:

Table 2.8. Birth Weight Data

Birth Weight, x (oz)	Percent Increase, y (%)
112	63
111	66
107	72
119	52
92	75
80	118
81	120
84	114
118	42
106	72
103	90
94	91

If we let each pair of numbers (x, y) be represented by a dot in a diagram with the x's on the horizontal axis, we have the figure shown below (Figure 2.10). The dots do not

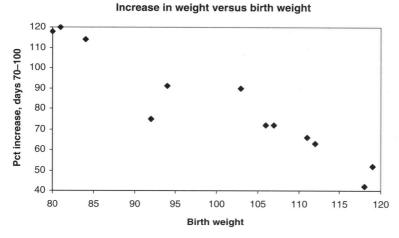

Figure 2.10. Scatter diagram for birth weight data.

fall perfectly on a straight line, but rather scatter around one, very typical for statistical relationships. Because of this scattering of dots, the diagram is called a *scatter diagram*. The positions of the dots provide some information about the direction as well as the strength of the association under the investigation. If they tend to go from lower left to upper right, we have a *positive association*; in a positive association a large value of *x* tends to go with a large value of *y* (upper right quadrant of the graph) and a small value of *x* tends to go with a small value of *y* (lower left quadrant of the graph). If the dots tend to go from upper left to lower right, we have a *negative association*; in a negative association a small value of *x* tends to go with a large value of *y* (upper left quadrant of the graph) and a large value of *x* tends to go with a small value of *y* (lower right quadrant of the graph). In addition, the relationship is strong when most of the dots lie close to the line. The relationship becomes weaker and weaker as the distribution of the dots clusters less closely around the line, and becomes virtually no correlation when the distribution approximates a circle or oval (keep in mind that the method is ineffective for measuring a relationship that is not linear where the dots form a curve instead of a straight line).

The graph in Figure 2.10 shows a negative association between birth weight and a child's growth.

Consider again a scatter diagram, as shown in Figure 2.10. In Figure 2.11, we added a vertical and a horizontal line through the point $(\overline{x}\,\overline{y})$ and label the four quarters as I, II, III and IV.

It can be seen from Figure 2.11 that:

(1) In quarters I and III,

$$(x - \bar{x})(y - \bar{y}) > 0$$

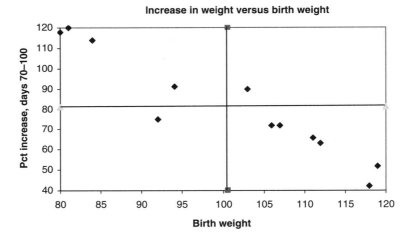

Figure 2.11. Scatter diagram divided into quadrants.

So that for positive association, we have:

$$\sum (x - \bar{x})(y - \bar{y}) > 0$$

Furthermore, this sum is large for stronger relationships because most of the dots, being closely clustered around the line, are in these two quarters I and III.

(2) Similarly, in quarters II and IV,

$$(x - \bar{x})(y - \bar{y}) > 0$$

leading to

$$\sum (x - \bar{x})(y - \bar{y}) > 0$$

for a negative association.

With a proper standardization, we obtain

$$r = \frac{\sum (x - \bar{x})(y - \bar{y})}{\sqrt{\left[\sum (x - \bar{x})^2\right]\left[\sum (y - \bar{y})^2\right]}}$$

This statistic "r" is called the *correlation coefficient* or *Pearson's correlation coefficient*, and is a popular measure for the *strength* of a statistical relationship; the following is a short-cut formula:

$$r = \frac{\sum xy - \{[(\sum x)(\sum y)]/n\}}{\sqrt{\{\sum x^2 - [(\sum x)^2/n]\}\{\sum y^2 - [(\sum y)^2/n]\}}}$$

Meaningful interpretation of the correlation coefficient r is rather complicated at this level; we will re-visit the topic in Chapter 8 in the context of *regression analysis*, a statistical method, which is closely connected to correlation. Generally,

(1) Values near 1 indicate a strong positive association.
(2) Values near (-1) indicate a strong negative association.
(3) Values around 0 indicate a weak association.

Interpretation of r should be made cautiously, however. It is true that a scatter plot of data, which results in a correlation number of $(+1)$ or (-1) has to lie in a perfectly straight line. But correlation of 0 does not mean that there is no association. It means there is no linear association. You can have a correlation near 0, and yet have a very strong association, such as the case when the data fall neatly on a sharply bending curve.

Example 2.8

Consider again the previous birth weight problem. We have

x (oz)	y (%)	x^2	y^2	xy
112	63	12544	3969	7056
111	66	12321	4356	7326
107	72	11449	5184	7704
119	52	14161	2704	6188
92	75	8464	5625	6900
80	118	6400	13924	9440
81	120	6561	14400	9720
84	114	7056	12996	9576
118	42	13924	1764	4956
106	72	11236	5184	7632
103	90	10609	8100	9270
94	91	8836	8281	8554
1207	**975**	**123561**	**86487**	**94322**

Using these five totals, we obtain

$$r = \frac{94{,}322 - \{[(1207)(975)]/12\}}{\sqrt{[123{,}561 - \{(1207)^2/12\}][86{,}487 - \{(975)^2/12\}]}} = .946$$

indicating a very strong negative association.

The following example presents a problem with similar data structure where the target of investigation is a possible relationship between a woman's age and her systolic blood pressure.

Example 2.9

The following data represent systolic blood pressure readings on 15 women:

Age (x)	SBP (y)
42	130
46	115
42	148
71	100
80	156
74	162
70	151
80	156
85	162
72	158
64	155
81	160
41	125
61	150
75	165

The corresponding scatter diagram is shown below indicating that we would have a positive association, positive but may not very strong:

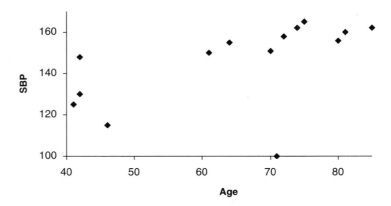

We set up a work table, shown below, as in the previous example and add up numbers in each column to obtain the totals as shown in the last row; using these totals, we obtain $r = .566$ confirming a *moderately* positive association:

$$r = \frac{146{,}269 - \{[(984)(2193)]/15\}}{\sqrt{\{67{,}954 - [(984)^2/15]\}\{325{,}929 - [(2193)^2/15]\}}} = .566$$

Age (x)	SBP (y)	x^2	y^2	xy
42	130	1764	16900	5460
46	115	2116	13225	5290
42	148	1764	21904	6216
71	100	5041	10000	7100
80	156	6400	24336	12480
74	162	5476	26244	11988
70	151	4900	22801	10570
80	156	6400	24336	12480
85	162	7225	26244	13770
72	158	5184	24964	11376
64	155	4096	24025	9920
81	160	6561	25600	12960
41	125	1681	15625	5125
61	150	3721	22500	9150
75	165	5625	27225	12375
984	**2193**	**67954**	**325929**	**146260**

2.4. VISUAL AND COMPUTATIONAL AIDS

Section 1.4 covered basic techniques for Microsoft's Excel and graphical methods for discrete data—such as how to open and or how to form a spreadsheet, save, and retrieve it. Topics included data entry steps—such as select and drag, use of formula bar, and bar and pie charts. This section focuses on continuous data covering topics, such as the construction of histograms, basic descriptive statistics, and correlation analysis. Many of the products have been used and shown in the last three sections of this chapter.

2.4.1. Histograms

With a frequency table ready, click the *ChartWizard icon* (the one with multiple colored bars on the standard toolbar near the top). A box appears with choices (exactly as when you learned to form a bar chart or pie chart—for more details, review Section 1.4); select the column chart type. Then click on "next."

(1) For the data range, highlight the frequency column; this can be done by clicking on the first observation and dragging the mouse to the last observation (you could highlight the data before clicking the ChartWizard icon). Then click on "next."

(2) To remove the gridlines, click on the gridline tab and uncheck the box. To remove the legend, you can do the same using the legend tab. Now click "finish."

(3) The problem is that you do not have a histogram yet; what you get is just a *bar chart*, there are still *gaps* between the vertical rectangles. To remove these, double click on a

bar of the graph and a new set of options should appear. Click on the options tab and change the gap width from 150 to 0.

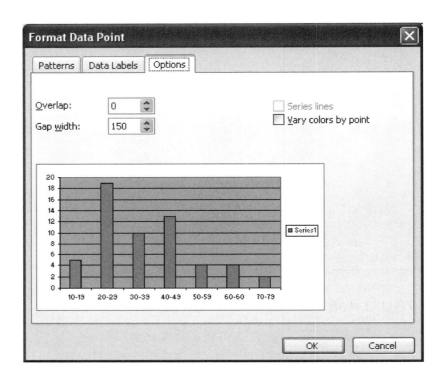

2.4.2. Descriptive Statistics

(1) First, click the cell you want to fill, then click the *paste function icon*, f*, which will give you—in a box—a list Excel functions available for your use.

(2) The item you need in this list is *Statistical*; upon hitting this, a new list appears with *function names*, each for a statistical procedure.

(3) The following procedures or *names* we learn in this chapter (alphabetically): AVERAGE, GEOMEAN, MEDIAN, STDEV, and VAR:

  (i) AVERAGE: provides the *sample mean*,

  (ii) GEOMEAN: provides the *geometric mean*,

  (iii) MEDIAN: provides the sample *median*,

  (iv) STDEV: provides the standard deviation, and

  (v) VAR: provides the variance.

In each case, you can only obtain one statistic at a time. First, you have to enter the *data range* (location on the spreadsheet) containing your sample, for example D6:D20 (you can see what you are entering on the *formula bar*); the computer will return with numerical value for the requested statistic in a preselected cell.

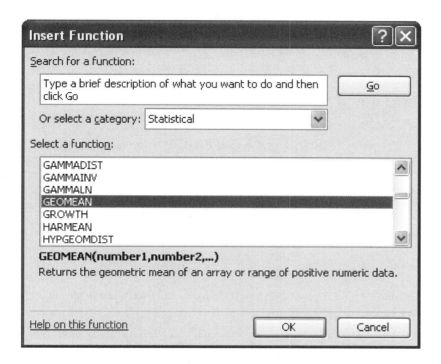

2.4.3. Pearson's Coefficient of Correlation

The formula for the (Pearson's) *correlation coefficient* r (even the "short-cut formula") is quite complicated, hard to remember and use for hand calculation. However, you could easily obtain the numerical result with the help of Excel as follows:

(1) First, click the cell you want to fill, then click the *paste function icon*, f*, which will give you—in a box—a list Excel functions available for your use.
(2) The item you need in this list is *Statistical* as in previous step for descriptive statistics (mean, variance, so on); upon hitting this, a new list appears with *function names*, each for a statistical procedure. Click "CORREL," for correlation.
(3) In the newly appeared box, move the cursor to fill in the X and Y ranges in the two rows marked as "Array 1" and "Array 2." The computer will return with numerical value for the requested statistic, the Pearson's correlation coefficient r, in a preselected cell. In the formula for the (Pearson's) correlation coefficient r, the roles of X and Y are interchangeable, you could name either one factor as "Array 1" (and the other one as "Array 2").

Function Arguments ⊠

CORREL

Array1		= array
Array2		= array

=

Returns the correlation coefficient between two data sets.

Array1 is a cell range of values. The values should be numbers, names, arrays, or references that contain numbers.

Formula result =

Help on this function — OK — Cancel

EXERCISES

2.1. The following table gives the values of serum cholesterol levels for 1067 U.S. men, aged 25–34 years.

Cholesterol Level (mg/100 ml)	Number of Men
80–119	13
120–159	150
160–199	442
200–239	299
240–279	115
280–319	34
320–399	14
Total	1067

(a) Plot the histogram, the frequency polygon, and the cumulative frequency graph.

(b) Find, approximately, the median using your cumulative frequency graph.

2.2. The following table provides the relative frequencies of blood lead concentrations for two groups of workers in Canada, one examined in 1979 and the other in 1987.

Blood Lead (μg/dl)	Relative Frequency (%)	
	1979	1987
0–19	11.5	37.8
20–39	12.1	14.7
30–39	13.9	13.1

(*Continued*)

(*Continued*)

Blood Lead (µg/dl)	Relative Frequency (%)	
	1979	1987
40–49	15.4	15.3
50–59	16.5	10.5
60–69	12.8	6.8
70–79	8.4	1.4
80+	9.4	.4

(a) Plot the histogram and frequency polygon for each year on separate graphs.

(b) Plot the two cumulative frequency graphs in one figure.

(c) Find and compare the medians.

2.3. A study on the effects of exercise on the menstrual cycle provides the following ages (years) of menarche (the beginning of menstruation) for 96 female swimmers who began training prior to menarche:

15.0	17.1	14.6	15.2	14.9	14.4	14.7	15.3
13.6	15.1	16.2	15.9	13.8	15.0	15.4	14.9
14.2	16.5	13.2	16.8	15.3	14.7	13.9	16.1
15.4	14.6	15.2	14.8	13.7	16.3	15.1	14.5
16.4	13.6	14.8	15.5	13.9	15.9	16.0	14.6
14.0	15.1	14.8	15.0	14.8	15.3	15.7	14.3
13.9	15.6	15.4	14.6	15.2	14.8	13.7	16.3
15.1	14.5	13.6	15.1	16.2	15.9	13.8	15.0
15.4	14.9	16.2	15.9	13.8	15.0	15.4	14.9
14.2	16.5	13.4	16.5	14.8	15.1	14.9	13.7
16.2	15.8	15.4	14.7	14.3	15.2	14.6	13.7
14.9	15.8	15.1	14.6	13.8	16.0	15.0	14.6

(a) Form a frequency distribution including relative frequencies and cumulative relative frequencies.

(b) Plot the frequency polygon and the cumulative frequency graph.

(c) Find the median and 95th percentile.

2.4. The following are the menarchal ages (in years) of 56 female swimmers who began training after they had reached menarche.

Age at Menarche							
14.0	16.1	13.4	14.6	13.7	13.2	13.7	14.3
12.9	14.1	15.1	14.8	12.8	14.2	14.1	13.6
14.2	15.8	12.7	15.6	14.1	13.0	12.9	15.1
15.0	13.6	14.2	13.8	12.7	15.3	14.1	13.5
15.3	12.6	13.8	14.4	12.9	14.6	15.0	13.8
13.0	14.1	13.8	14.2	13.6	14.1	14.5	13.1
12.8	14.3	14.2	13.5	14.1	13.6	12.4	15.1

(a) Form a frequency distribution using the same age intervals as in Exercise 2.3.

(b) Display in the same graph two cumulative frequency graphs, one for the group trained before and one for the group trained after menarche. Compare these two graphs and draw your conclusion.

(c) Find the median and compare it to the result of the previous exercise.

2.5. The following table shows the daily fat intake (grams) of a group of 150 adult males.

22	62	77	84	91	102	117	129	137	141
42	56	78	73	96	105	117	125	135	143
37	69	82	93	93	100	114	124	135	142
30	77	81	94	97	102	119	125	138	142
46	89	88	99	95	100	116	121	131	152
63	85	81	94	93	106	114	127	133	155
51	80	88	98	97	106	119	122	134	151
52	70	76	95	107	105	117	128	144	150
68	79	82	96	109	108	117	120	147	153
67	75	76	92	105	104	117	129	148	164
62	85	77	96	103	105	116	132	146	168
53	72	72	91	102	101	128	136	143	164
65	73	83	92	103	118	127	132	140	167
68	75	89	95	107	111	128	139	148	168
68	79	82	96	109	108	117	130	147	153

(a) Form a frequency distribution including relative frequencies and cumulative relative frequencies.

(b) Plot the frequency polygon and investigate the symmetry of the distribution.

(c) Plot the cumulative frequency graph and find the 25th and 75th percentiles. Also calculate the mid-range, which is the distance from the 25th percentile to the 75th percentile (this is another good descriptive measure of variation; it is similar to the range but is less affected by extreme observations).

2.6. Refer to the data on daily fat intake of Exercise 2.5, calculate the mean fat intake.

2.7. Using the income data of Example 2.5,

(a) Plot the histogram for the White families. Does it have the same shape as that for Nonwhite families as seen in Figure 2.5?

(b) Plot and compare the two cumulative frequency graphs, Whites versus Nonwhites.

2.8. Refer to the percentage saturation of bile for the 31 *male* patients in Example 2.4.

(a) Compute the mean, the variance, and the standard deviation.

(b) The frequency polygon of Figure 2.3 is based on the following grouping (arbitrary choices). Plot the cumulative frequency graph and obtain, approximately, the median from this graph. How does the answer compare to the exact median (the 16th largest saturation percentage)?

Interval (%)	Frequency
40–49	2
50–59	4
60–69	3
70–79	4
80–89	8
90–99	1
100–109	2
110–119	5
120–129	1
130–139	1
140–149	0

2.9. The same study referenced in Example 2.4 also provided data (percentage saturation of bile) for 29 *women*. These percentages were

65	58	52	91	84	107
86	98	35	128	116	84
76	146	55	75	73	120
89	80	127	82	87	123
142	66	77	69	76	

(a) Form a frequency distribution using the same intervals as in Example 2.4 and Exercise 2.8.

(b) Plot in the same graph and compare the two frequency polygons and cumulative frequency graphs: men and women.

(c) Compute the mean, the variance and the standard deviation using these new data for women and compare the results to those for men in Exercise 2.8.

(d) Compute and compare the two coefficients of variation, men versus women.

2.10. The following frequency distribution was obtained for the preoperational percentage hemoglobin values of a group of subjects from a village where there has been a malaria eradication program (MEP):

Frequency	Hemoglobin Interval (%)
2	30–30
7	40–49
14	50–59
10	60–69
8	70–79
2	80–89
2	90–99

The results for another group was obtained after MEP and are given below:

43	63	63	75	95	75	80	48	62	71	76	90
51	61	74	103	93	82	74	65	63	53	64	67
80	77	60	69	73	76	91	55	65	69	84	78
50	68	72	89	75	57	66	79	85	70	59	71
87	67	72	52	35	67	99	81	97	74	61	62

(a) Form a frequency distribution using the same intervals as in the first table.

(b) Plot in the same graph and compare the two cumulative frequency graphs: before and after the MEP.

2.11. In a study of water pollution, a sample of mussels was taken and lead concentration (milligrams per gram dry weight) was measured from each one. The following data were obtained:

$$\{113.0, 140.5, 163.3, 185.7, 202.5, 207.2\}$$

Calculate the mean, variance, and standard deviation.

2.12. Consider this data taken from a study that examines the response to ozone and sulfur dioxide among adolescents suffering from asthma. The following are measurements of forced expiratory volume (liters) for 10 subjects:

$$\{3.50, 2.60, 2.75, 2.82, 4.05, 2.25, 2.68, 3.00, 4.02, 2.85\}$$

Calculate the mean, variance, and standard deviation.

2.13. The percentage of ideal body weight was determined for 18 randomly selected insulin-dependent diabetics. The outcomes (%) are:

$$\{107, 119, 99, 114, 120, 104, 124, 88, 114, 116, 101, 121, 152, 125, 100, 114, 95, 117\}$$

Calculate the mean, variance, and standard deviation.

2.14. A study on birth weight provided the following data (in ounces) on 12 newborns:

$$\{112, 111, 107, 119, 92, 80, 81, 84, 118, 106, 103, 94\}$$

Calculate the mean, variance, and standard deviation.

2.15. The following are the activity values (micromoles per minute per gram of tissue) of a certain enzyme measured in normal gastric tissue of 35 patients with gastric carcinoma:

$$\{.360, 1.189, .614, .788, .273, 2.464, .571, 1.827, .537, .374, .449, .262, .448,$$
$$.971, .372, .898, .411, .348, 1.925, .550, .622, .610, .319, .406, .413, .767, .385,$$
$$.674, .521, .603, .533, , .662, \ 1.177, .307, 1.499\}$$

Calculate the mean, variance, and standard deviation.

2.16. The following data represent systolic blood pressure readings on 15 women:

Age (x)	SBP (y)
42	130
46	115
42	148
71	100
80	156
74	162
70	151
80	156
85	162
72	158
64	155
81	160
41	125
61	150
75	165

Calculate the mean, variance, and standard deviation for systolic blood pressure and age.

2.17. The ages (in days) at time of death for samples of 11 girls and 16 boys who died of sudden infant death syndrome are shown below:

Girls	{53, 56, 60, 60, 78, 87, 102, 117, 134, 160, 277}
Boys	{46, 52, 58, 59, 77, 78, 80, 81, 84, 103, 114, 115, 133, 134, 175, 175}

Calculate the mean, variance, and standard deviation for each group.

2.18. A study was conducted to investigate whether oat bran cereal helps to lower serum cholesterol in men with high cholesterol levels. Fourteen men were randomly placed on a diet which included either oat bran or corn flakes; after 2 weeks, their low-density lipoprotein cholesterol levels (LDL) were recorded. Each man was then switched to the alternative diet. After a second 2-week period, the LDL cholesterol level of each individual was again recorded. The data were:

Subject	LDL (mmol/l)	
	Corn Lakes	Oak Bran
1.00	4.61	3.84
2.00	6.42	5.57
3.00	5.40	5.85
4.00	4.54	4.84
5.00	3.98	3.68
6.00	3.82	2.96
7.00	5.01	4.41

(*Continued*)

(Continued)

	LDL (mmol/l)	
Subject	Corn Lakes	Oak Bran
8.00	4.34	3.72
9.00	3.80	3.49
10.00	4.56	3.84
11.00	5.35	5.26
12.00	3.89	3.73
13.00	2.25	1.84
14.00	4.24	4.14

Calculate the LDL difference (Corn flake–Oat bran) for each of the 14 men, then the mean, variance, and standard deviation for this sample of differences.

2.19. An experiment was conducted at the University of California at Berkeley to study the psychological environment effect on the anatomy of the brain. A group of 19 rats was randomly divided into two groups. Twelve animals in the treatment group lived together in a large cage, furnished with playthings, which were changed daily, while animals in the control group lived in isolation with no toys. After a month, the experimental animals were killed and dissected. The following table gives the cortex weights (the thinking part of the brain) in milligrams:

Treatment	{707, 740, 745, 652, 649, 676, 699, 696, 712, 708, 749, 690}
Control	{669, 650, 651, 627, 656, 642, 698}

Calculate the mean, variance, and standard deviation of the cortex weight separately for each group.

2.20. Ozone levels around Los Angeles have been measured as high as 220 parts per billion (ppb). Concentrations this high can cause the eyes to burn and are a hazard to both plant and animal life. But what about the other cities? The following are data (in ppb) on the ozone level obtained in a forested area near Seattle, Washington:

160	165	170	172	161
176	163	196	162	160
162	185	167	180	168
163	161	167	173	162
169	164	179	163	178

(a) Calculate the mean, variance, and standard deviation; compare the mean to that of Los Angeles.

(b) Calculate the coefficient of variation.

2.21. The systolic blood pressures (in mmHg) of 12 women between the ages of 20 and 35 were measured before and after administration of a newly developed oral contraceptive. Focus on the column of differences in the following table; calculate the mean, variance, and standard deviation:

Subject	Before	After	After–Before Difference, d
1	122	127	5
2	126	128	2
3	132	140	8
4	120	119	−1
5	142	145	3
6	130	130	0
7	142	148	6
8	137	135	−2
9	128	129	1
10	132	137	5
11	128	128	0
12	129	133	4

2.22. A group of 12 hemophiliacs, all under 41 years of age at the time of HIV seroconversion, were followed from primary AIDS diagnosis until death (ideally we should take, as a starting point, the time at which an individual contracts AIDS rather than the time at which the patient is diagnosed, but this information is unavailable). Survival times (in months) from diagnosis until death of these hemophiliacs were:

$$\{2, 3, 6, 6, 7, 10, 15, 15, 16, 27, 30, 32\}$$

Calculate the mean, geometric mean, and median.

2.23. Suppose that we are interested in studying patients with systemic cancer who subsequently develop a brain metastasis; our ultimate goal is to prolong their lives by controlling the disease. A sample of 23 such patients, all of whom were treated with radiotherapy, was followed from the first day of their treatment until recurrence of the original tumor. Recurrence is defined as the reappearance of a metastasis in exactly the same site, or, in the case of patients whose tumor never completely disappeared, enlargement of the original lesion. Times to recurrence (in weeks) for the 23 patients were:

$$\{2, 2, 2, 3, 4, 5, 5, 6, 7, 8, 9, 10, 14, 14, 18, 19, 20, 22, 22, 31, 33, 39, 195\}$$

Calculate the mean, geometric mean, and median.

2.24. A laboratory investigator interested in the relationship between diet and the development of tumors divided 90 rats into three groups and fed them with low-fat, saturated-, and unsaturated-fat diets, respectively. The rats were the same age and species, and were in similar physical condition. An identical amount of tumor cells were injected into a foot pad of each rat. The tumor-free time is the time from injection of tumor cells to the time that a tumor develops. All 30 rats in the unsaturated-fat diet group developed tumors; tumor-free times (in days) were:

{112, 68, 84, 109, 153, 143, 60, 70, 98, 164, 63, 63, 77, 91, 91, 66, 70, 77, 63, 66, 66, 94, 101, 105, 108, 112, 115, 126, 161, 178}

Calculate the mean, geometric mean, and median.

2.25. The following data are taken from a study that compares adolescents who have bulimia to healthy adolescents with similar body compositions and levels of physical activity. The following table provides measures of daily caloric intake for random samples of 23 bulimic adolescents and 15 healthy ones:

Daily Calorie Intake (kcal/kg)				
Mulimic Adolescents			Healthy Adolescents	
15.90	17.00	18.90	30.60	40.80
16.00	17.60	19.60	25.70	37.40
16.50	28.70	21.50	25.30	37.10
18.90	28.00	24.10	24.50	30.60
18.40	25.60	23.60	20.70	33.20
18.10	25.20	22.90	22.40	33.70
30.90	25.10	21.60	23.10	36.60
29.20	24.50		23.80	

(a) Calculate and compare the means.

(b) Calculate and compare the variances.

2.26. Two drugs, Amantadine and Rimantadine are being studied for use in combating the influenza virus. A single 100-mg dose is administered orally to healthy adults. The response variable is the time (in minutes) required to reach maximum concentration. Results are:

Amantadine	{105, 126, 120, 119, 133, 145, 200, 123, 108, 112, 132, 136, 156, 124, 134, 130, 130, 142, 170}
Rimantadine	{221, 261, 250, 230, 253, 256, 227, 264, 236, 246, 273, 271, 280, 238, 240, 283, 616}

(a) Calculate and compare the means.

(b) Calculate and compare the variances and the standard deviations.

(c) Calculate and compare the medians.

2.27. Data are shown below for two groups of patients who died of acute myelogenous leukemia. Patients were classified into the two groups according to the presence or absence of a morphologic characteristic of white cells. Patients termed "AG Positive" were identified by the presence of Auer rods and/or significant granulature of the leukemic cells in the bone marrow at diagnosis. For the AG Negative patients these factors were absent. Leukemia is a cancer characterized by an over-proliferation of white blood cells; the higher the white blood count (WBC), the more severe the disease.

AG Positive, $n = 17$		AG Negative, $n = 16$	
White Blood Count (WBC)	Survival Time (weeks)	White Blood Count (WBC)	Survival Time (weeks)
2,300	65	4,400	56
750	156	3,000	65
4,300	100	4,000	17
2,600	134	1,500	7
6,000	16	9,000	16
10,500	108	5,300	22
10,000	121	10,000	3
17,000	4	19,000	4
5,400	39	27,000	2
7,000	143	28,000	3
9,400	56	31,000	8
32,000	26	26,000	4
35,000	22	21,000	3
100,000	1	79,000	30
100,000	1	100,000	4
52,000	5	100,000	43
100,000	65		

(a) Calculate the mean, variance, and standard deviation for *survival time*, separately for each group (AG Positive and AG Negative).

(b) Calculate the mean, geometric mean, and median for white blood count, separately for each group (AG Positive and AG Negative).

2.28. Refer to the survival data for acute myelogenous leukemia patients of previous Exercise 2.27, calculate the (Pearson's) coefficient of correlation measuring the strength of the correlation between white blood count and survival time, separately for each group (AG Positive and AG Negative).

2.29. Refer to the data on systolic blood pressure (in mmHg) of 12 women in Exercise 2.21. Calculate the Pearson's correlation coefficient representing the strength of the relationship between systolic blood pressures measured before and after administration of the oral contraceptive.

2.30. The following are the heights (measured to the nearest 2 cm) and the weights (measured to the nearest kg) of 10 men and 10 women.

Men

Height	162	168	174	176	180	180	182	184	186	186
Weight	65	65	84	63	75	76	82	65	80	81

Women

Height	152	156	158	160	162	162	164	164	166	166
Weight	52	50	47	48	52	55	55	56	60	60

(a) Draw a scatter diagram, for men and women separately, to show the association, if any, between the height and the weight.

(b) Calculate the Pearson's correlation coefficient between height and weight for men and women separately.

2.31. The following data give the net food supply (x that is the number of calories per person per day) and the infant mortality rate (y, number of infant deaths per 1000 live births) for certain selected countries before World War II:

Country	X	Y
Argentina	2730	98.8
Australia	3300	39.1
Austria	2990	87.4
Belgium	3000	83.6
Burma	1080	202.1
Canada	3070	67.4
Chile	2240	240.8
Cuba	2610	116.8
Egypt	2450	162.9
France	2880	66.1
Germany	2960	63.3
Iceland	3160	42.4
India	1970	161.6
Ireland	3390	69.6
Italy	2510	102.7
Japan	2180	60.6
New Zealand	3260	32.2
Netherlands	3010	37.4
Sweden	3210	43.3
England	3100	53.3
USA	3150	53.2
Uraguay	2380	94.1

(a) Draw a scatter diagram to show the association, if any, between the average daily number of calories per person and the infant mortality rate.

(b) Calculate the Pearson's correlation coefficient.

2.32. In an assay of heparin, a standard preparation is compared with a test preparation by observing the log clotting times (y, in seconds) of blood containing different doses of heparin (x is log dose, replicate readings are made at each dose level):

Log Clotting Times				
Standard		Test		Log Dose
1.81	1.76	1.80	1.76	.72
1.85	1.79	1.83	1.83	.87
1.95	1.93	1.90	1.88	1.02
2.12	2.00	1.97	1.98	1.17
2.26	2.16	2.14	2.10	1.32

(a) Draw a scatter diagram to show the association, if any, between the *log clotting times* and *log dose* separately for the standard preparation and the test preparation. Do they appear to be linear?

(b) Calculate the (Pearson's) correlation coefficient for log clotting times and log dose separately for the standard preparation and the test preparation. Do they appear to be different?

2.33. When a patient is diagnosed as having cancer of the prostate, an important question in deciding on treatment strategy for the patient is whether or not the cancer has spread to the neighboring lymph nodes. The question is so critical in prognosis and treatment that it is customary to operate on the patient (i.e., perform a laparoscopy) for the sole purpose of examining the nodes and removing tissue samples to examine under the microscope for evidence of cancer. However, certain variables that can be measured without surgery are predictive of the nodal involvement; and the purpose of the study presented here was to examine the data for 53 prostate cancer patients receiving surgery, to determine which of five preoperative variables are predictive of nodal involvement. The following table presents the complete data set. (This is a very long data file; its electronic version is available from the author upon request.) For each of the 53 patients, there are two continuous independent variables, age at diagnosis and level of serum acid phosphatase (multiplied by 100; called "acid"), and three binary variables, X-ray reading, pathology reading (grade) of a biopsy of the tumor obtained by needle before surgery, and a rough measure of the size and location of the tumor (stage) obtained by palpation with the fingers via the rectum. For these three binary independent variables, a value of 1 signifies a positive or more serious state and a 0 denotes a negative or less serious finding. In addition, the sixth column presents the finding at surgery—the primary outcome of interest, which is binary, a value of 1 denoting nodal involvement, and a value of 0 denoting no nodal involvement found at surgery. In the last exercise of Chapter 1 (Exercise 1.43), we investigated the effects of the three binary preoperative variables (X-ray, grade, and stage); in this exercise, we focus on the effects of the two continuous factors (age and acid phosphatase). The 53 patients are divided into two groups by the finding at surgery, a group with nodal involvement and a group without (denoted by 1 or 0 in the sixth column). For each group and for each of the two factors, age at diagnosis and level of serum acid phosphatase, calculate the mean, the variance, and the standard deviation.

Data

Case	X-Ray	Grade	Stage	Age	Acid	Nodes
1	0	1	1	64	40	0
2	0	0	1	63	40	0
3	1	0	0	65	46	0
4	0	1	0	67	47	0
5	0	0	0	66	48	0
6	0	1	1	65	48	0
7	0	0	0	60	49	0
8	0	0	0	51	49	0
8	0	0	0	66	50	0
10	0	0	0	58	50	0
11	0	1	0	56	50	0
12	0	0	1	61	50	0
13	0	1	1	64	50	0
14	0	0	0	56	52	0
15	0	0	0	67	52	0
16	1	0	0	49	55	0
17	0	1	1	52	55	0
18	0	0	0	68	56	0
19	0	1	1	66	59	0
20	1	0	0	60	62	0
21	0	0	0	61	62	0
22	1	1	1	59	63	0
23	0	0	0	51	65	0
24	0	1	1	53	66	0
25	0	0	0	58	71	0
26	0	0	0	63	75	0
27	0	0	1	53	76	0
28	0	0	0	60	78	0
29	0	0	0	52	83	0
30	0	0	1	67	95	0
31	0	0	0	56	98	0
32	0	0	1	61	102	0
33	0	0	0	64	187	0
34	1	0	1	58	48	1
35	0	0	1	65	49	1
36	1	1	1	57	51	1
37	0	1	0	50	56	1
38	1	1	0	67	67	1
39	0	0	1	67	67	1
40	0	1	1	57	67	1

(continued)

(*Continued*)

Case	X-Ray	Grade	Stage	Age	Acid	Nodes
41	0	1	1	45	70	1
42	0	0	1	46	70	1
43	1	0	1	51	72	1
44	1	1	1	60	76	1
45	1	1	1	56	78	1
46	1	1	1	50	81	1
47	0	0	0	56	82	1
48	0	0	1	63	82	1
49	1	1	1	65	84	1
50	1	0	1	64	89	1
51	0	1	0	59	99	1
52	1	1	1	68	126	1
53	1	0	0	61	136	1

2.34. Refer to the data on cancer of the prostate in Exercise 2.33, investigate the relationship between age at diagnosis and level of serum acid phosphatase by calculating the Pearson's correlation coefficient and draw your conclusion. Repeat this analysis but analyzing data separately for the two groups, the group with nodal involvement and the group without nodal involvement. Does the nodal involvement seem to have any effect on the strength of this relationship?

2.35. The purpose of this study was to examine the data for 44 physicians working for an emergency at a major hospital so as to determine which of a number of factors are related to the number of complaints (X) received during the previous year. In addition to the number of complaints, data available consist of the number of visits—which serves as the "size" for the observation unit, the physician—and four other factors under investigation. The following table presents the complete data set. For each of the 44 physicians there are two continuous explanatory factors, the revenue (dollars per hour) and work load at the emergency service (hours) and two binary variables, sex (female/male) and residency training in emergency services ("Rcy," No/Yes).

Number of Visits	X	Rcy	Sex	Revenue	Hours
2014	2	Y	F	263.03	1287.25
3091	3	N	M	334.94	1588.00
879	1	Y	M	206.42	705.25
1780	1	N	M	226.32	1005.50
3646	11	N	M	288.91	1667.25
2690	1	N	M	275.94	1517.75
1864	2	Y	M	295.71	967.00
2782	6	N	M	224.91	1609.25
3071	9	N	F	249.32	1747.75
1502	3	Y	M	269	906.25
2438	2	N	F	225.61	1787.75

(*continued*)

(*Continued*)

Number of Visits	X	Rcy	Sex	Revenue	Hours
2278	2	N	M	212.43	1480.50
2458	5	N	M	211.05	1733.50
2269	2	N	F	213.23	1847.25
2431	7	N	M	257.3	1433.00
3010	2	Y	M	326.49	1520.00
2234	5	Y	M	290.53	1404.75
2906	4	N	M	268.73	1608.50
2043	2	Y	M	231.61	1220.00
3022	7	N	M	241.04	1917.25
2123	5	N	F	238.65	1506.25
1029	1	Y	F	287.76	589.00
3003	3	Y	F	280.52	1552.75
2178	2	N	M	237.31	1518.00
2504	1	Y	F	218.7	1793.75
2211	1	N	F	250.01	1548.00
2338	6	Y	M	251.54	1446.00
3060	2	Y	M	270.52	1858.25
2302	1	N	M	247.31	1486.25
1486	1	Y	F	277.78	933.75
1863	1	Y	M	259.68	1168.25
1661	0	N	M	260.92	877.25
2008	2	N	M	240.22	1387.25
2138	2	N	M	217.49	1312.00
2556	5	N	M	250.31	1551.50
1451	3	Y	F	229.43	973.75
3328	3	Y	M	313.48	1638.25
2927	8	N	M	293.47	1668.25
2701	8	N	M	275.4	1652.75
2046	1	Y	M	289.56	1029.75
2548	2	Y	M	305.67	1127.00
2592	1	N	M	252.35	1547.25
2741	1	Y	F	276.86	1499.25
3763	10	Y	M	308.84	1747.50

Divide the number of complaints by the number of visits and use this ratio (number of complaints per visit) as the new primary outcome or *endpoint* called *ratio*.

(a) For each of the two binary factor, sex (female/male) and residency training in emergency services (No/Yes), which divide the 44 physicians into two subgroups—say men and women, calculate the mean and standard deviation for the new endpoint "Ratio."

(b) Investigate the relationship between the outcome, ratio or number of complaints per visit, and each of the two continuous explanatory factors, the revenue (dollars per hour) and work load at the emergency service (hours), by calculating the Pearson's correlation coefficient and draw your conclusion.

(c) Draw a scatter diagram to show the association, if any, between the number of complaints per visit and work load at the emergency service. Does it appear to be linear?

2.36. There have been times that the city of London experienced periods of dense fog. The following table shows such data for a 15-day very severe period which include the number of deaths in each day (Y), the mean atmospheric smoke (X_1, in mg/m^3), and the mean atmospheric sulfur dioxide content (X_2, in ppm):

Y	X_1	X_2
112	.30	.09
140	.49	.16
143	.61	.22
120	.49	.14
196	2.64	.75
294	3.45	.86
513	4.46	1.34
518	4.46	1.34
430	1.22	.47
274	1.22	.47
255	.32	.22
236	.29	.23
256	.50	.26
222	.32	.16
213	.32	.16

(a) Calculate Pearson's correlation coefficient for Y and X_1 alone.

(b) Calculate Pearson's correlation coefficient for Y and X_2 alone.

3

Probability and Probability Models

3.1. PROBABILITY

Most of Chapter 1 dealt with proportions. A proportion is defined to represent the relative size of the portion of a population with certain (binary) characteristic that is, for a particular member of the population, present or absent. For example, *disease prevalence* is the proportion of a population with a disease. Similarly, we can talk about the proportion of positive reactors to certain screening test, the proportion of males in colleges, and so on. A *proportion* is used as a *descriptive measure* for a target population with respect to a binary or dichotomous characteristic, the *relative size* of the subpopulation for which the characteristic is present. It is a number between 0 and 1 (or 100%), and the larger the number, the larger the subpopulation with the characteristic; for example, for a population with 70% male, there are more males than a population with 50% male.

Consider now a population with certain binary characteristic. A *random selection* is defined as one in which each individual has an equal *chance* of being selected. What is the chance that an individual with the characteristic being selected? For example, the chance to have, say, a diseased person. The answer depends on the size of the subpopulation that he or she belongs, that is, the proportion. The larger the proportion, the higher the chance (for such an individual being selected). This *chance is measured by the proportion*, a number between 0 and 1, but called the *probability*. Proportion measures *size* (of a subpopulation), a descriptive statistic; probability measures *chance*. When we are concerned about the outcome (still *uncertain* at this stage) with a random selection, a *proportion* (static, no action) becomes a *probability* (action about to be taken). Think of this simple example about a box containing 100 marbles, 90 of them are red and the other 10 are blue. If the question is: "Are there red marbles in the box?" and someone who saw the box's contents would answer "90%." But if the question is: "If I take one marble at

Health and Numbers: A Problems-Based Introduction to Biostatistics, Third Edition, by Chap T. Le
Copyright © 2009 John Wiley & Sons, Inc.

random, do you think I would have a red one?" the answer would be "90% chance." The first number, "90%," represents a proportion; the second number, still the same "90%," indicates the probability. In addition, if we keep taking random selections (called repeated sampling), the *accumulated long-term relative frequency* with which the event occurs (i.e., characteristic be observed) is equal to the proportion of the subpopulation with that characteristic. Because of this observation, sometimes the term *proportion* and the term *probability* are used interchangingly. Later, in Chapter 4, we will introduce another term, *degree of confidence*, which would have the same numerical value as proportion and probability but used in a different context with a different interpretation. This chapter deals with the concept of probability and some simple applications in making health decisions.

3.1.1. The Certainty of Uncertainty

Even science is uncertain. Scientists are sometimes wrong. They arrive at different conclusions in many different areas: the effects of certain food ingredients or of low-level radioactivity, the role of fats in diets, and so on. Many studies are inconclusive. For example, for decades surgeons believed that a radical mastectomy was the only treatment for breast cancer. Only later were carefully designed clinical trials conducted to show that less drastic treatments seem equally effective.

Why is science not always certain? The processes are certain (why things happen the way they do) but the end results may be not. Nature is complex and full of unexplained biological variability. In addition, almost all methods of observation and experiment are imperfect. Observers are subject to human bias and error. Science is a continuing story: subjects vary; measurements fluctuate. Biomedical science, in particular, contains controversy and disagreement; with the best of intentions, biomedical data—medical histories, physical examinations, interpretations of clinical tests, descriptions of symptoms and diseases—are somewhat inexact. But, most important of all, we always have to deal with *incomplete information*: it is impossible, too costly, or too time-consuming to study the entire population; we often have to rely on information gained from a *sample*—that is, a subgroup of the population under investigation. So some uncertainty in the results almost always prevails.

Science and scientists cope with uncertainty by using the concept of *probability*. By calculating probabilities, they are able to describe what has happened and predict what should happen in the future under similar conditions.

3.1.2. Probability

The *target population* of a specific research effort is the entire set of subjects at which the research is aimed. For example, in a screening for cancer in a community, the target population will consist of all persons in that community who are at risk for the disease. For one cancer site, the target population might be all women over the age of 35, and for another site, all men over the age of 50.

The probability of an event, such as a screening test being positive, in a target population is defined as the relative frequency (i.e., proportion) with which the event occurs in that target population. For example, the probability of having a disease (for a member selected at random from some particular target population) is the disease prevalence. For another example, suppose that out of $N = 100{,}000$ persons of a certain target population, a total of 5500 are positive reactors to a certain screening test, and then the probability of being positive, denoted by "Pr(positive)," is

$$\Pr(positive) = \frac{5500}{100{,}000}$$
$$= .005 \text{ or } 5.5\%$$

A *probability* is thus a descriptive measure for a target population with respect to a certain *event* of interest. It is a number between 0 and 1 (or 0 and 100%), and the larger the number, the larger the subpopulation with the event. For the case of a continuous measurement, we have the probability of being within a certain interval. For example, the probability of a serum cholesterol level between 180 and 210 (mg/100 ml) is the proportion of people in a certain target population having their cholesterol levels falling between 180 and 210 (mg/100 ml). This is measured, in the context of a histogram of Chapter 2, by the area of a rectangular bar for the class (180–210). Again, a proportion and a probability may have the same numerical value but different interpretation. Proportion measures size of a subpopulation, a number used to describe; probability measures the chance for event about to occur; when we are concerned about the outcome (still *uncertain* at this stage) with a random selection, a proportion (static, no action) becomes a probability (action about to be taken). Another way to help with the interpretation of probability is the concept of *random sampling*, which also links or associates the concept of *probability* with *uncertainty* and *chance*.

Let the size of the target population be N (usually a very large number), a *sample* is any subset, say, consisting of n members of the target population, and n is the sample size whereas N is the population size. Simple random sampling from the target population is the kind of selection of subjects so that every possible sample of size n has an equal chance of being selected. For simple random sampling

(1) Each individual selection is uncertain with respect to any event or characteristic under investigation (e.g. having a disease), but
(2) In repeated sampling from the same population, the accumulated long-run relative frequency with which the event occurs is the population relative frequency of the event.

We can now link the concepts of probability and random sampling as follows. In the above example of cancer screening in a community of $N = 100{,}000$ persons, the calculated probability of .055 is interpreted as "the probability of a randomly selected person from the target population having a positive test result .055 or 5.5%." The rationale is as follows. On an initial selection, the chosen subject may or may not be a positive reactor. However, *if* this process—of randomly selecting one subject at a time from the population and testing—is repeated over and over again a large number of times, the accumulated long-run relative frequency of positive receptors in the sample will be approximately .055.

3.1.3. Rules of Probabilities

The data from the cancer screening test of Example 1.4 are reproduced here as follows:

Disease Status, Y	Test Result, X Positive (+)	Test Result, X Negative (−)	Total
Positive (+)	154	225	379
Negative (−)	362	23,362	23,724
Total	516	23,587	24,103

In this design, each member of the population is characterized by two characteristics or variables: the test result "X" and the true disease status "Y." Following our above definition of simple random sampling, where the accumulated long-run relative frequency with which the event occurs is equal to the population relative frequency of the event, the probability of a positive test result, denoted by $\Pr(X=+)$, is

$$\Pr(X=-) = \frac{516}{24{,}103}$$
$$= .021 \text{ or } 2.1\%$$

And the probability of a negative test result, denoted by $\Pr(X=-)$, is

$$\Pr(X=-) = \frac{23{,}587}{24{,}103}$$
$$= .979 \text{ or } 97.9\%$$

Similarly the probabilities of having the disease and not having the disease are given by

$$\Pr(Y=+) = \frac{379}{24{,}103}$$
$$= .016 \text{ or } 1.6\%$$

$$\Pr(Y=-) = \frac{23{,}724}{24{,}103}$$
$$= .985 \text{ or } 98.5\%$$

Note that the sum of the probabilities for each variable is unity:

$$\Pr(X=+) + \Pr(X=-) = 1.0$$
$$\Pr(Y=+) + \Pr(Y=-) = 1.0$$

This is an example of the *addition rule* for probabilities of mutually exclusive events: The sum of probabilities is equal to 1.0, and one of the two events $(X=+)$ or $(X=-)$ is "certain to be true" for a randomly selected individual from the population.

Further, we can calculate the *joint probabilities*. These are the probabilities for two events—such as having the disease and also having a positive test result—occurring simultaneously. With two variables, X (for test result) and y (for disease status), there are four conditions of outcomes: $(X = +, Y = +)$, $(X = +, Y = -)$, $(X = -, Y = +)$, and $(X = -, Y = -)$; the notation $(X = +, Y = +)$ denotes the joint even that "X is positive and Y is positive." The associated joint probabilities for these four joint events are as follows:

$$\Pr(X = +, Y = +) = \frac{154}{24,103}$$

$$= .006 \text{ or } 0.6\%$$

$$\Pr(X = +, Y = -) = \frac{362}{24,103}$$

$$= .015 \text{ or } 1.5\%$$

$$\Pr(X = -, Y = +) = \frac{225}{24,103}$$

$$= .010 \text{ or } 1.0\%$$

$$\Pr(X = -, Y = -) = \frac{23,362}{24,103}$$

$$= .970 \text{ or } 97.0\%$$

The second of the four joint probabilities, .015, represents the probability of a randomly drawn person from the target population having a positive test result, but being healthy (i.e., a false positive). These four joint probabilities and the above marginal probabilities separately calculated for X and Y are summarized and can be displayed as follows:

	Test Result, X		
Disease Status, Y	Positive (+)	Negative (−)	Total
Positive (+)	0.006	0.010	0.016
Negative (−)	0.015	0.970	0.985
Total	0.021	0.980	1.000

Observe that the four cell probabilities add to unity; that is, one of the four events $(X = +, Y = -)$ or $(X = +, Y = -)$ or $(X = -, Y = +)$ or $(X = -, Y = -)$ is certain to be true for a randomly selected individual from the population. Also, note that the joint probabilities in each row (or column) add up to the above *marginal probability* or *univariate probability* (in calculating "univariate" probability, we consider or study "one variable at a time") at the margin of that row (or column). For example, we have for the first row

$$\Pr(X = +, Y = +) + \Pr(X = -, Y = +) = \Pr(Y = +)$$

$$= .016$$

We now consider a third type of probability. For example, the sensitivity is expressible as

$$Sensitivity = \frac{154}{379}$$

$$= .406 \text{ or } 40.6\%$$

This number, another probability, was also calculated for the event that $(X = +)$ but, different from the calculation of $\Pr(X = +)$, it is using the subpopulation having $(Y = +)$ instead of the whole population. It is "the probability that the test result is positive given that he/she has the disease." That is, of the total number of 379 individuals with cancer, the proportion with a positive test result is .406 or 40.6% (whereas only 2.1% of the population at large have positive test result, that is, $\Pr(X = +)$—the marginal probability). This number, denoted by $\Pr(X = +|Y = +)$, is called a *conditional probability* (where "$Y = +$" being the condition). A conditional probability is related to the other two types of probability as follows:

$$\Pr(X = +|Y = +) = \frac{\Pr(X = +, Y = +)}{\Pr(Y = +)}$$

or

$$\Pr(X = +, Y = +) = \Pr(X = +|Y = +)\Pr(Y = +)$$

This last equation is referred to as the *multiplication rule* for probabilities.

3.1.4. Statistical Relationship

When a conditional probability and the corresponding marginal (or "unconditional") probability are equal, say

$$\Pr(X = +|Y = +) = \Pr(X = +)$$

the condition (i.e. $(Y = +)$, in this example) is irrelevant and the two events $(X = +)$ and $(Y = +)$ are said to be *independent* (because the condition $(Y = +)$ does not change the probability of $(X = +)$), and we have the multiplication rule for probabilities of independent events

$$\Pr(X = +, Y = +) = \Pr(X = +)\Pr(Y = +)$$

If the two events are not independent, they have a statistical relationship or we say that they are *statistically associated*. For the above screening example,

$$\Pr(X = +|Y = +) = .406, \text{ but}$$

$$\Pr(X = +) = .021$$

It clearly indicates a strong statistical relationship (because $\Pr(X=+|Y=+)$ is very different from $\Pr(X=+)$). Of course, it makes sense to have a strong statistical relationship here, otherwise the screening is useless. However, it should be emphasized that a statistical association does not necessarily mean there is a cause and effect. Unless a relationship is so strong and so constantly repeated that the case is overwhelming, a statistical relationship, especially those observed from a sample (because the totality of population information is rarely available) is only a clue, meaning more study or confirmation is needed.

It should be noted that there are several different ways to check for the presence of a statistical relationship, and the most common way, as we learned from Chapter 1, is calculating the odds ratio. The *odds ratio* is defined as follows, and when X and Y are independent, or not statistically associated, the odds ratio equals 1.

$$\text{Odds ratio} = \frac{\dfrac{\Pr(X = + \,|\, Y = +)}{1 - \Pr(X = + \,|\, Y = +)}}{\dfrac{\Pr(X = + \,|\, Y = -)}{1 - \Pr(X = + \,|\, Y = -)}}$$

$$= \frac{\dfrac{\Pr(X = + \,|\, Y = +)}{\Pr(X = - \,|\, Y = +)}}{\dfrac{\Pr(X = + \,|\, Y = -)}{\Pr(X = - \,|\, Y = -)}}$$

The numerator represents the "odds" to have a positive test result among the subpopulation with the disease and the denominator represents the odds to have a positive test result among the subpopulation without the disease. This odds ratio, OR, can be expressed, equivalently, in terms of the joint probabilities as

$$\text{Odds ratio} = \frac{\Pr(X = +, Y = +)\Pr(X = -, Y = +)}{\Pr(X = +, Y = -)PR(X = -, Y = -)}$$

and the above example yields

$$\text{OR} = \frac{(.006)(.970)}{(.015)(.010)}$$

$$= 43.11$$

This result, OR > 1.0, clearly indicates a (strong and positive) statistical relationship.

The next two sections present some applications of the probability rules introduced: the problem of *when* to use screening tests and the problem of *how* to measure agreement.

3.1.5. Using Screening Tests

We have introduced the concept of conditional probability. However, it is important to distinguish the two conditional probabilities, $\Pr(X = + \,|\, Y = +)$ and $\Pr(Y = + \,|\, X = +)$. In Example 1.4, reintroduced in section 3.1.3, we have these very different numerical values:

$$\Pr(X = + \,|\, Y = +) = \frac{154}{379}$$

$$= .406$$

$$\Pr(Y = + \,|\, X = +) = \frac{154}{516}$$

$$= .298$$

Within the context of screening test evaluation, we interpret these conditional probabilities as follows:

(1) $\Pr(X=+|Y=+)$ and $\Pr(X=-|Y=-)$ are the *sensitivity* and *specificity*, respectively.
(2) $\Pr(Y=+|X=+)$ and $\Pr(Y=-|X=-)$ are called the *positive predictivity* and *negative predictivity*.

With positive predictivity (or also called *positive predictive value*), the question is, given that the test X suggests cancer, what is the probability that, in fact, cancer is present? And with negative predictivity (or also called *negative predictive value*), the question is, given that the test X suggests no cancer, what is the probability that, in fact, the person tested has no cancer?

Rationales for these predictive values are that a test passes through several stages. Initially, the original test idea occurs to some researcher. It then must go through a *developmental stage*. This may have many aspects (in biochemistry, microbiology, etc.), and one of which is in biostatistics, namely, trying the test out on a pilot population. From this developmental stage, efficiency of the test is characterized by the sensitivity and the specificity. An efficient test will then go through an *applicational stage* with an actual application of X to a target population, and here we are concerned with its predictive values. The following simple example shows that, unlike sensitivity and specificity, the positive and negative predictive values depend not only on the efficiency of the test but also on the disease prevalence of the target population.

| Population A | Test Result, X | | |
Disease Status, Y	Positive (+)	Negative (−)	Total
Positive (+)	45,000	5,000	50,000
Negative (−)	5,000	45,000	50,000
Total	50,000	50,000	100,000

| Population B | Test Result, X | | |
Disease Status, Y	Positive (+)	Negative (−)	Total
Positive (+)	9,000	1,000	10,000
Negative (−)	9,000	81,000	90,000
Total	18,000	82,000	100,000

In both cases, the test is 90% sensitive and 90% specific. However,

(1) Population A has a "disease prevalence," $\Pr(Y=+)$, of 50%, leading to a positive predictive value of 90%,

$$\Pr(Y=+|X=+) = \frac{45{,}000}{50{,}000}$$

$$= .90$$

(2) Population B has a prevalence of 10%, leading to a positive predictive value of only 50%,

$$\Pr(Y = + | X = +) = \frac{9000}{18,000}$$

$$= .50$$

The conclusion is clear: if a test—even a highly sensitive and highly specific one—is applied to a target population in which the disease prevalence is low (e.g., population screening for a rare disease), the positive predictive value is low. (How does this relate to an important public policy: Should we conduct *random testing* for AIDS?)

In the actual application of a screening test to a target population (the applicational stage), data on the disease status of individuals are not available (otherwise, screening would not be needed). However, disease prevalence is often available from national agencies and health surveys. Predictive values are then calculated from

$$Positive\ predictivity = \frac{(Prevalence)(Sensitivity)}{(Prevalence)(Sensitivity) + (1 - Prevalence)(1 - Specificity)}$$

$$Negative\ predictivity = \frac{(1 - Prevalence)(Specificity)}{(1 - Prevalence)(Specificity) + (Prevalence)(1 - Sensitivity)}$$

These formulas, referred to as "the Bayes' theorem," allow us to calculate the predictive values without having data from the application stage. All we need are the disease prevalence (obtainable from federal health agencies) and sensitivity and specificity; these were obtained after the developmental stage. It is not too hard to prove these formulas using the addition and multiplication rules of probability, but we skip the proof. You can see, instead of going through formal proofs, our illustration of their validity using the above population B data:

$$\Pr(Y = + | X = +) = \frac{(Prevalence)(Sensitivity)}{(Prevalence)(Sensitivity) + (1 - Prevalence)(1 - Specificity)}$$

$$= (.1)(.9) + \frac{(.1)(.9)}{(.1)(.9) + (1 - .1)(1 - .9)}$$

$$= .50$$

3.1.6. Measuring Agreement

Many research studies rely on an observer's judgment to determine whether a disease, a trait, or an attribute is present or absent. For example, results of ear examinations will surely have effects on a comparison of competing treatments for ear infection. Of course, the basic concern is the issue of *reliability*. Section 1.1.2 and the above section on screening tests dealt with an important aspect of reliability, the *validity* of the assessment. However, to judge a method's validity, an exact method for classification, or a *gold standard*, must be available for the calculation of sensitivity and specificity. When an exact method is not available, reliability can only be judged indirectly in terms of *reproducibility*; the most common way for doing this is by measuring the *agreement* between examiners.

For simplicity, assume that each of the two observers independently assigns each of n items or subjects to one of the two categories. The sample may then be enumerated in a 2×2 table of frequencies as follows:

| | Observer 2 | | |
Observer 1	Category 1	Category 2	Total
Category 1	n_{11}	n_{12}	n_{1+}
Category 2	n_{21}	n_{22}	n_{2+}
Total	n_{+1}	n_{+2}	$n = n_{2+}$

or, in terms of the cell probabilities;

| | Observer 2 | | |
Observer 1	Category 1	Category 2	Total
Category 1	p_{11}	p_{12}	p_{1+}
Category 2	p_{21}	p_{22}	p_{++}
Total	p_{+1}	p_{+2}	$1.0 = p_{++}$

Using these frequencies, we can define

(1) An overall proportion of *concordance*

$$C = \frac{n_{11} + n_{22}}{n}$$

(2) Two category-specific proportions of concordance

$$C_1 = \frac{2n_{11}}{2n_{11} + n_{12} + n_{21}}$$

$$C_2 = \frac{2n_{22}}{2n_{22} + n_{12} + n_{21}}$$

The distinction between *concordance* and *association* is that for two responses to be perfectly associated, we only require that we can predict the category on one response from the category of the other response, while for two responses to have a perfect concordance, they must fall into the identical category. However, the proportions of concordance, overall or category specific, do not measure agreement. Among other reasons, they are affected by the marginal totals. One possibility is to compare the *overall concordance*,

$$\theta_1 = \sum_i p_{ii}$$

where p's are the proportions in the above second 2×2 table, with the *chance concordance*,

$$\theta_2 = \sum_i p_{i+} p_{+i}$$

that occurs if the row variable is independent of the column variable, because if two events are independent, the probability of their joint occurrence is the product of their individual or marginal probabilities (the Multiplication Rule). This leads to a popular *measure of agreement*

$$\kappa = \frac{\theta_1 - \theta_2}{1 - \theta_2}$$

called the "Kappa statistic," $0 \leq \theta \leq 1$. With data in the following form

	Observer 2		
Observer 1	Category 1	Category 2	Total
Category 1	n_{11}	n_{12}	n_{1+}
Category 2	n_{21}	n_{22}	n_{2+}
Total	n_{+1}	n_{+2}	$n = n$

Kappa statistic can be expressed as

$$\kappa = \frac{2[n_{11}n_{22} - n_{12}n_{21}]}{n_{1+}n_{2+} + n_{+1}n_{+2}}$$

The following are guidelines for the evaluation of Kappa in clinical research:

$\kappa > .75$: excellent reproducibility
$.40 \leq \kappa \leq .75$: good reproducibility
$0 \leq \kappa < .40$: marginal/poor reproducibility

In general, reproducibility not good, indicating the need for multiple assessment.

Example 3.1

Two nurses perform ear examinations focusing on the color of the eardrum (tympanic membrane); each independently assigns each of the 100 ears to one of the two categories:

(i) normal or gray or (ii) normal or gray or (iii) not normal (white, pink, orange, or red). The data were

		Nurse 2	
Nurse 1	Normal	Category 2	Total
Normal	35	10	45
Not normal	20	35	55
Total	55	45	100

The result, with Kappa statistic,

$$\kappa = \frac{2[(35)(35)-(20(10)]}{[(45)(55)(55)(45)]}$$

$$= 0.406$$

indicates that the agreement is only barely acceptable.

It should also be pointed out that

(1) Kappa statistic, as a measure for agreement, can also be used when there are more than two categories for classification,

$$\kappa = \frac{\sum_i p_{ii} - \sum_i p_{i+}p_{+i}}{1 - \sum_i p_{i+}p_{+i}}$$

(2) We can form *category-specific Kappa statistics*; for example, with two categories, we have two statistics, one for each category

$$\kappa_1 = \frac{p_{11} - p_{1+}p_{+1}}{1 - p_{1+}p_{+1}}$$

$$\kappa_2 = \frac{p_{22} - p_{2+}p_{+2}}{1 - p_{2+}p_{+2}}$$

(3) The major problem with Kappa is that it approaches zero (even with high degree of agreement) if the prevalence is near 0 or near 1.

3.2. THE NORMAL DISTRIBUTION

3.2.1. Shape of the Normal Curve

The histogram of Figure 2.1 is reproduced here as Figure 3.1 (for numerical details, see Table 2.1). A close examination shows that, in general, the relative frequencies (or densities) are greatest in the vicinity of the intervals 20–29, 30–39, and 40–49 and decrease as we go toward both extremes of the range of the measurements.

Figure 3.1 shows a distribution based on a total of 57 patients; the frequency distribution consists of intervals with a width of 10 lb. Now imagine that we increase the number of children to 50,000 and decrease the width of the intervals to .01 lb. The histogram would now look more like the one in the following Figure 3.2. In this figure, the step to go from one rectangular bar to the next is very small. Finally, suppose we increase the number of children to 10 million and decrease the width of the interval to .00001 lb. You can now imagine a histogram with bars having practically no widths and the steps have all but disappeared. And if we continue to increase the size of the data set

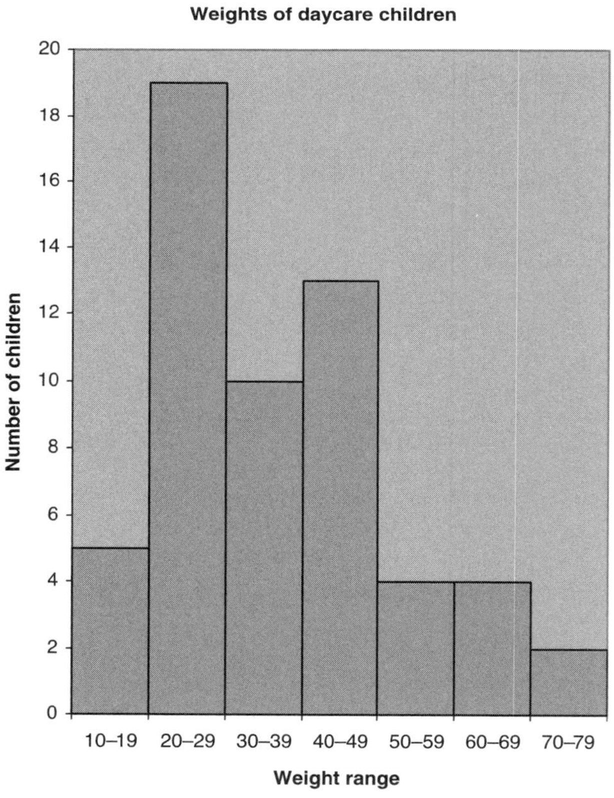

Figure 3.1. Distribution of weights of 57 children.

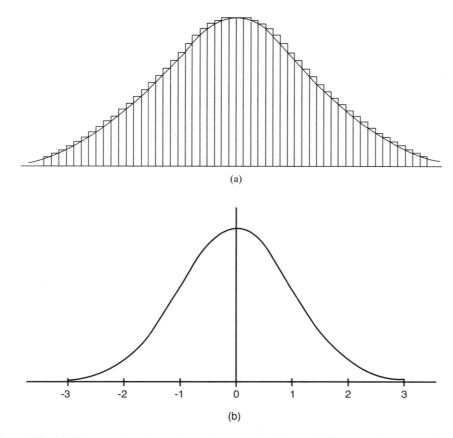

Figure 3.2. (a) Histogram based on a large data set of weights and (b) the standard normal curve.

and decrease the interval width, we eventually arrive at a smooth *curve* that is superimposed on the histogram of Figure 3.2. It is called a *density curve*. You may have already heard about the normal distribution before you took a course in statistics; it is described as a bell-shaped distribution, sort of like a handlebar moustache, similar to that in Figure 3.2. The name may suggest that most distributions in nature are normal. Strictly speaking, this is false. Even more strictly speaking, they cannot be exactly normal. Some, such as heights of adults of a particular sex and race, are amazingly close to normal, but never exactly.

The *normal distribution* is extremely useful in statistics, but for a very different reason—not because it occurs in nature. Mathematicians proved that, for samples that are "big enough," values of their sample means (including sample proportions as a special case) are approximately distributed as normal, even if the samples are taken from really strangely shaped distributions. This important result was called the *central limit theorem*. It is as important to statistics as the understanding of germs is to the understanding of disease. Keep in mind that "normal" is just a name for this curve; if an attribute is not distributed normally, it does not imply that it is "abnormal." Many statistics texts provide statistical procedures for finding out whether a distribution is normal, but they are beyond the level of this text.

A sample is a subgroup of a target population; we already briefly learned and random sampling and random samples. From now on, to distinguish samples from populations, we adopt the following set of notations. Quantities in the second column are parameters representing numerical properties of populations (μ, σ, σ^2, π). Quantities in the first column are statistics representing summarized information from samples (x-bar, s, s^2, and p).

	Notation	
Quantity	Sample	Population
Mean	x-bar	μ (mu)
Variance	s^2	σ^2 (sigma squared)
Standard deviation	s	σ (sigma)
Proportion	p	π

Parameters are fixed (constants) but unknown, and each *statistic* can be used as an estimate for the parameter listed in the same row of the above table. For example, the sample mean x-bar is used as an estimate of the population mean, μ; this topic will be discussed with more details in Chapter 4. A major problem in dealing with statistics, such as x-bar and p, is that if we take a different sample—even using the same sample size— values of a statistic change from sample to sample. The central limit theorem tells us that if sample sizes are fairly large, values of x-bar (or p) in repeated sampling have a very nearly normal distribution. Therefore, to handle variability due to chance so as to be able to declare—for example—that a certain observed difference is more than would occur by chance but is real, we first have to learn how to calculate probabilities associated with normal curves.

The term normal curve, in fact, refers not to one curve but to a family of many curves, each characterized by a mean μ and a variance σ^2. In the special case where $\mu = 0$ and $\sigma^2 = 1$, we have the *standard normal curve*. For a given μ and a given σ^2, the curve is bell shaped with the tails dipping down to the baseline. In theory, the tails get closer and closer to the baseline but never touch it, proceeding to infinity in either direction. In practice, we ignore that and work within practical limits.

The peak of the curve occurs at the mean μ (which for this special distribution is also median and mode), and the height of the curve at the peak depends, inversely, on the variance σ^2. Figure 3.3 shows some of these curves.

3.2.2. Areas Under the Standard Normal Curve

A variable that has a normal distribution with mean $\mu = 0$ and variance $\sigma^2 = 1$ is called the standard normal variate and is commonly designated by the letter Z. As with any continuous variable, probability calculations here are always concerned with finding the probability that the variable assumes any value in an interval between two specific points "a" and "b". The probability that a continuous variable assumes a value between two points a and b is the area under the graph of the density curve between point a and point b;

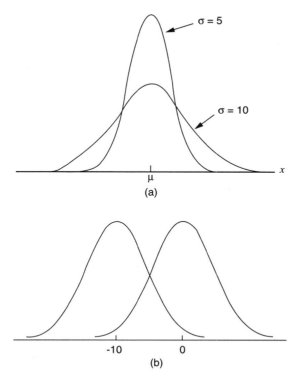

Figure 3.3. (a) Two normal distributions with the same mean but different variances and (b) two normal distributions with the same variance but different means.

the vertical axis of the graph represents the densities as defined in Chapter 2. The total area under any such curve is unity (or 100%), and Figure 3.4 shows the standard normal curve with some important divisions. For example, about 68% of the area is contained within ± 1 and about 95% within ± 2, that is,

$$Pr(-1 < Z < +1) = .6826$$
$$Pr(-2 < Z < +2) = .9545$$
$$Pr(-3 < Z < +3) = .9974$$

Almost 100% of all possible values of Z (99.74% to be exact) are in the interval $(-3, +3)$.

Areas under the standard normal curve have been computed and are available in tables, one of which is our Appendix B. The entries in the table of Appendix B give the area under the standard normal curve between the mean ($z = 0$) and a specified positive value of z. Graphically, it is represented by the shaded region of the following graph (Figure 3.5).

Using the table of Appendix B and the symmetric property of the standard normal curve, we will show how some other areas are computed (with access to some computer packaged program, these can be easily obtained, see Section 3.5; however, we believe that some of these practices do add to the learning even they may be no longer needed).

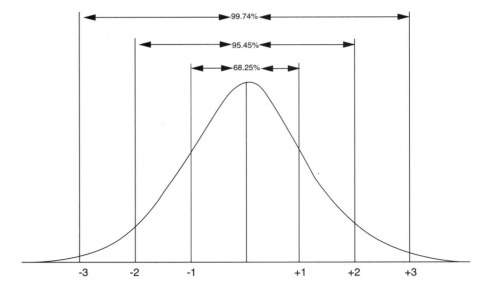

Figure 3.4. The standard normal curve and some important divisions.

How to Read the Table

The entries in the table, Appendix B, give the area under the standard normal curve between zero and a positive value of Z. Suppose we are interested in the area between $Z = 0$ and $Z = 1.35$ (numbers are first rounded off to two decimal places). To do this, first find the row marked with 1.3 in the left-hand column of the table and then find the column marked with .05 in the top row of the table $(1.35 = 1.30 + .05)$. Then looking in the body of the table, we find that the "1.30 row" and the ".05 column" intersect at the value .4115. This number, .4115, is the desired area between $Z = 0$ and $Z = 1.35$. A portion of Appendix B relating to these steps is shown below.

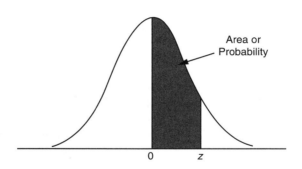

Figure 3.5. The area under standard normal curve as in Appendix B.

Value Z	0.00	0.01	0.02	0.03	0.04	0.05	0.06	0.07	0.08	0.09
0.0										
0.1										
0.2										
. . .										
. . .										
1.3						0.4115				
. . .										
. . .										

Another example: The area between $Z = 0$ and $Z = 1.23$ is .3907; this value is found at the intersection of the "1.2" row and the ".03" column of the table.

Inversely, given the area between zero and some positive value "z", we can find Z. Suppose we want a z-value so that the area between zero and z is .20. To find this z-value, we look into the body of the table and find .2019. This number is found at the intersection of the ".5" row and the ".03" column. Therefore, the desired Z value is .53 (.53 = .50 + .03).

Example 3.2

What is the probability of obtaining a z-value between -1 and 1? We have

$$\Pr(-1 \leq Z \leq 1) = \Pr(-1 \leq Z \leq 0) + \Pr(0 \leq Z \leq 1)$$
$$= 2x\Pr(0 \leq Z \leq 1)$$
$$= (2)(.3413)$$
$$= .6828$$

this confirms the number in Figure 3.4. This area is shown as follows:

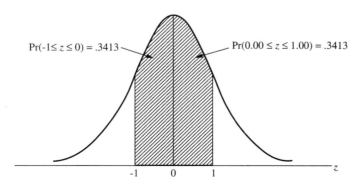

$\Pr(-1 \leq z \leq 0) = .3413$ $\Pr(0.00 \leq z \leq 1.00) = .3413$

Example 3.3

What is the probability of obtaining a *z*-value of at least 1.58? We have

$$\Pr(Z \geq 1.58) = .5 - \Pr(0 \leq Z \leq 1.58)$$
$$= .5 - .4429$$
$$= .0571$$

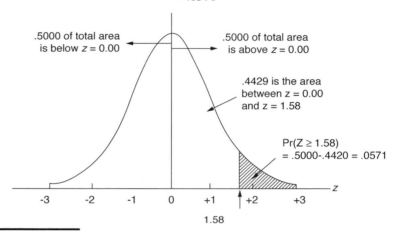

.5000 of total area is below *z* = 0.00

.5000 of total area is above *z* = 0.00

.4429 is the area between *z* = 0.00 and *z* = 1.58

Pr(Z ≥ 1.58) = .5000-.4420 = .0571

-3 -2 -1 0 +1 +2 +3   *z*

1.58

Example 3.4

What is the probability of obtaining a *z*-value of $(-.5)$ or larger? We have

$$\Pr(Z \geq -.50) = \Pr(-.50 \leq Z \leq 0) + \Pr(0 \leq Z)$$
$$= \Pr(0 \leq Z \leq .50) + \Pr(0 \leq Z)$$
$$= .1915 + .5$$
$$= .6915$$

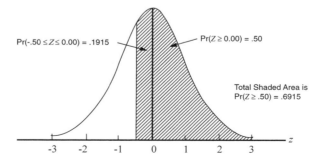

Pr(-.50 ≤ Z ≤ 0.00) = .1915

Pr(Z ≥ 0.00) = .50

Total Shaded Area is Pr(Z ≥ .50) = .6915

-3 -2 -1 0 1 2 3   *z*

Example 3.5

What is the probability of obtaining a z-value between 1.0 and 1.58? We have

$$\Pr(1.0 \leq Z \leq 1.58) = \Pr(0 \leq Z \leq 1.58) - \Pr(0 \leq Z \leq 1.0)$$
$$= .4429 - .3413$$
$$= .1058$$

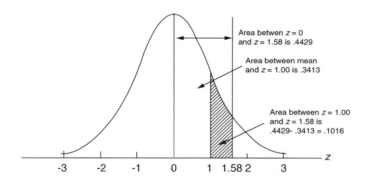

Example 3.6

Find a Z value such that the probability of obtaining a larger Z value is only .10. We have

$$\Pr(Z \geq ?) = 0.10$$

Scanning the table in Appendix B, we find .3997 (area between 0 and 1.28), so that

$$\Pr(Z \geq 1.28) = .5 - \Pr(0 \leq Z \leq 1.28)$$
$$= .5 - .3997$$
$$= .1003$$

In terms of the question asked, there is approximately a .1 or 10% probability of obtaining a *z* value 1.28 or larger.

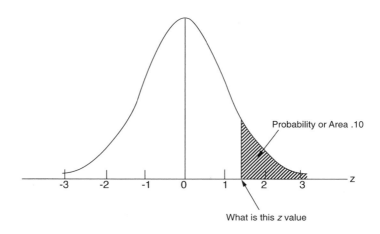

3.2.3. The Normal as a Probability Model

The reason we have been discussing the standard normal distribution so extensively with many examples is that probabilities for all normal distributions are computed using the standard normal distribution. That is, when we have a normal distribution with a given mean μ and a given standard deviation σ (or variance σ^2), we answer probability questions about the distribution by first converting to the standard normal, namely,

$$Z = \frac{X - \mu}{\sigma}$$

We say that we *standardize* the X value; and we interpret the *z*-value (or *z*-score) as the number of standard deviations from the mean.

Example 3.7

If the total cholesterol values for a certain target population are approximately normally distributed with a mean of 200 (mg/100 ml) and a standard deviation of 20 (mg/100 ml), then the probability that an individual picked at random from this population will have a cholesterol value greater than 240 (mg/100 ml) is

$$\Pr(X \geq 240) = \Pr\left(\frac{X-200}{20} \geq \frac{240-200}{20}\right)$$

$$= \Pr(Z \geq 2.0).5 - \Pr(Z \leq 2.0)$$

$$= .5 - .4772$$

$$= .0228 \text{ or } 2.28\%$$

Example 3.8

The following is a model for hypertension and hypotension (Journal of the American Medical Association, 1964). This is presented here as a simple illustration on the use of the normal distribution; the acceptance of the model itself is not universal.

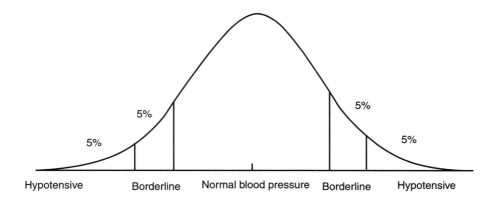

Data from a population of males were collected by age as shown in the table. We have, for example,

(1) For men between the ages of 20 and 24, the average SBP is 123.9 mmHg with a standard deviation of 13.74 mmHg.
(2) For men between the ages of 55 and 64, the average SBP is 139.8 mmHg with a standard deviation of 19.99, and as compared to men between the ages of 20 and 24, the mean SBP increases by 13%.

Table 3.1. Means and Standard Deviation of Systolic Blood Pressure for Males by Age Groups

Age (in years)	Mean (in mmHg)	Standard Deviation (mmHg)
16	118.4	12.17
17	121.0	12.88
18	119.8	11.95
19	121.8	14.99
20–24	123.9	13.74
25–29	125.1	12.58
30–34	126.1	13.61
35–39	127.1	14.2
40–44	129.0	15.07
45–54	132.3	18.11
55–64	139.8	19.99

From Table 3.1, and using the same table of Appendix B, systolic blood pressure limits for each group can be calculated as follows:

For example, the highest healthy limit, say (?), for the 20–24 years group is obtained as follows:

$$\Pr(X \geq (?)) = .10$$

$$= \Pr\left(\frac{X - 123.9}{13.74} \geq \frac{(?) - 123.9}{13.74}\right)$$

Then we have, from the result of Example 3.6,

$$\frac{(?) - 123.9}{13.74} = 1.28$$

Leading to the number needed on the third column in Table 3.2:

$$(?) = 123.9 + (1.28)(13.74) = 141$$

3.3. PROBABILITY MODELS

In Section 3.2, we treated the family of normal curves very informally because it was intended to reach more students and readers for whom mathematical formulas may not be very relevant. This section is aimed to provide some supplement that may be desirable for those who may be more interested in some more details of the fundamentals of biostatistical inference.

Table 3.2. Means and Standard Deviation of Systolic Blood Pressure for Males by Age Groups

Age	Hypotension if below	Lowest health	Highest health	Hypertension if above
16	98	103	134	139
17	100	105	138	142
18	100	104	135	139
19	97	103	141	147
20–24	?	?	(?)	?
25–29	?	?	?	?
30–34	104	109	144	149
35–39	104	109	145	151
40–44	104	110	148	154
45–54	102	109	155	162
55–64	107	114	165	173

3.3.1. Variables and Distributions

A class of measurements or a characteristic on which individual observations or measurements are made, or any rule that associates with each outcome of an experiment a corresponding number, is called a *variable*. The number that a variable associates with a particular outcome is called the *value* of the variable for that outcome or that characteristic. If values of a variable may lie only at a few isolated points, we have a discrete variable, and the examples include race, sex, or some sort of artificial grading. If values of a variable may theoretically lie anywhere on the numerical scale, we have a continuous variable, and the examples include weight, height, blood pressure, among others.

Suppose we have a discrete variable X, then a list of possible values of the variable, together with their corresponding probabilities, is called the *distribution* of the variable. For example, let us conduct a simple "experiment" in which two students are selected at random from a college. Consider, among others, a simple variable X that counts the number of females in the sample; possible values of X are 0, 1, and 2. To determine the distribution of X, we need to know the proportion of female students of that college. Suppose 60% of students are women, then

(1) $\Pr(X=0) = (.4)(.4) = .16$
(2) $\Pr(X=2) = (.6)(.6) = .36$
(3) $\Pr(X=1) = 1 - .16 - .36 = .48$

3.3.2. Probability Models For Discrete Data

Again, a class of measurements or a characteristic on which individual observations or measurements are made is called a variable. If values of a variable may lie only at a few isolated points, we have a discrete variable, and the examples include race, sex, or some sort of artificial grading. Topics introduced in this section, which are needed in subsequent chapters, will involve two of these discrete distributions: the Binomial distribution and the Poisson distribution.

The Binomial Distribution

In Chapter 1, we discussed cases with dichotomous outcomes such as Male–Female, Survived–Not survived, Infected–Not infected, White–Nonwhite, or simply Positive–Negative. We have seen that such data can be summarized into proportions, rates, and ratios. In this section, we are concerned with the probability for the occurrence of events.

Let us focus on a "trial" with binary outcome, for example, the gender of a student selected at random, or the opinion (approved, not approved) of a resident selected at random from certain city on a new piece of legislation. Suppose the experiment consists of repeating the above trial n times independently, for example, asking the opinion of n persons in a survey, and then we "count" the number of people who approve that piece of legislation. Let X be the number of "approvals" from the survey, X is said to have a *binomial distribution*; various probabilities associated with this variable X are often of interest. In another health science example, if a certain drug is known to cause a side effect 10% of the time and if four patients are given this drug, then what is the probability that two or more experience the side effect?

In general, let us denote the two possible outcome of a binary trial by S (for Success) and F (for Failure). The number X of successes from n independent trials has what we call a binomial distribution. Possible values of X are 0, 1, 2,..., n; the probability associated with each value depends on n and the probability of getting a success in a single trial, let us call this probability π, is $B(n,\pi)$. For example, we considered a simple experiment of counting the number X of females between two students selected at random from college. In that example, the Binomial distribution was $B(2,.60)$. The two assumptions here are

(i) The n trials are all independent,
(ii) The parameter π is the same for each trial.

And the question is: When it is more complicated, say a larger value of n, how do we find the probability associated with each value of X?

Let us start with this simple counting experiment: How many different ways to select two courses from among four electives that are offered this term? You could call the four courses a, b, c, and d, and you could list all possible pairs: ab, ac, ad, bc, bd, cd. There are six ways to form your program. What if you need three courses from a list of eight offered? This is needed because in a binomial distribution, we need to know how many ways to obtain k successes out of n trials ($k = 1, 2, ..., n$). The number of ways to select k things out of a group of n is

$$\binom{n}{k} = \frac{n!}{(n-k)!k!}$$

In the above formula, the symbol "!" signifies "factorial," for example, "3!" is "3 factorial" denoting the product of that number and all whole numbers less than this all the way down to 1, for example, $3! = (3)(2)(1) = 6$. As an example, the number of ways to select two courses out of four is

$$\binom{4}{2} = \frac{4!}{(4-2)!2!} = \frac{4!}{2!2!} = \frac{(4)(3)(2)(1)}{[(2)(1)][(2)(1)]} = 6$$

Back to the binomial distribution $B(n,p)$, we have

$$\Pr(X = k) = \binom{n}{k} p^k (1-p)^{n-k}$$

Example: Let X be the number of females when two students are selected at random from a college with 60% women, we have

$$\Pr(X = 1) = \binom{2}{1}(.6)^1(1-.6)^{2-1} = \frac{2!}{1!1!}(.6)(.4) = .48$$

This confirms the earlier result from direct calculation.

The mean of binomial distribution and variance of binomial distribution are

$$\mu = n\pi$$
$$\sigma^2 = n\pi(1-\pi)$$

and when the number of trials n is from moderate to large ($n > 25$, say), we approximate the binomial distribution by a normal distribution and answer probability questions by first converting to the standard normal score

$$z = \frac{x - n\pi}{\sqrt{n\pi(1-\pi)}}$$

where, again, n is the number of trial and π is the probability of having a positive outcome from a single trial. For example, for $\pi = 10$ and $n = 30$, we have

$$\mu = (30)(.10)$$
$$= 3$$
$$\sigma^2 = (30(.10)9.90)$$
$$= 2.7$$

so that

$$\Pr(X \geq 7) = \Pr(Z \geq \frac{7-3}{\sqrt{2.7}})$$
$$\Pr(Z \geq 2.43)$$
$$= .007$$

In other words, if the true probability for having the side effect is 10%, then the probability of having 7 or more of 30 patients with the side effect is less than 1% (= .0075).

The Poisson Distribution

The next discrete distribution that we consider is the Poisson distribution, named after a French mathematician. This distribution has been used extensively in health science to model the distribution of the number of occurrences X of some random event in an interval of time or space, or some volume of matter. For example, a hospital administrator has been studying daily emergency admissions over a period of several months and has found that admissions have averaged three per day. He/she is then interested in finding the probability that no emergency admissions will occur on a particular day.

The *Poisson distribution* is characterized by its "probability density function":

$$\Pr(X = x) = \frac{\theta^x e^{-\theta}}{x!}$$

In the above formula, the symbol "e" represents a mathematical operation called *exponentiation*; it is the inverse of the process of taking *natural logarithm* (log of base "e", "e" is a constant value approximately 2.72. It turns out, interestingly, that for a Poisson distribution the *variance* is equal to the *mean*, the above parameter θ. Therefore, we can answer probability questions by using the above formula for the Poisson density more difficult) or by converting the number of occurrences X to the standard normal score (easier), provided $\theta \geq 10$:

$$z = \frac{x - \theta}{\sqrt{\theta}}$$

In other words, we can approximate a Poisson distribution by a normal distribution with mean θ if θ is at least 10; even for smaller values of the mean, this normal approximation works very well and much easier than an exact calculation.

The following is another example involving the Poisson distribution. The infant mortality rate (IMR) is defined as

$$IMR = \frac{d}{N}$$

for a certain target population during a given year where d is the number of deaths during the first year of life and N is the total number of live births. In the studies of IMRs, N is conventionally assumed as fixed and d to follow a Poisson distribution.

Example 3.9

For the year 1981, we have the following data for the New England states (Connecticut, Maine, Massachusetts, New Hampshire, Rhode Island, and Vermont):

$$d = 1585$$
$$N = 164,200$$

year where d is the number of deaths during the first year of life and N is the total number of live births. For the same year, the national infant mortality rate was 11.9 (per 1000 live births). If we apply national IMR to the New England states, that is, to "assume" that New England states have the (national) average infant mortality, then we would have

$$\theta = (11.9)(164.2)$$
$$= 1954 \text{ infant deaths}$$

Then, assuming that the region has an average infant mortality, the event of having as few as 1585 infant deaths would occur with a probability of

$$\Pr(d \leq 1585) = \Pr\left(\frac{d-1954}{\sqrt{1954}} \leq \frac{1585-1954}{\sqrt{1954}}\right)$$
$$= \Pr(Z \leq -8.35)$$
$$\cong 0.0$$

The conclusion is clear: either we observed an extremely improbable event, or the infant mortality of New England states is lower than the national average. The observed rate for New England states was 9.7 deaths per 1000 live births.

3.3.3. Probability Models For Continuous Data

As it can be seen from Section 3.2, each continuous variable is characterized by a smooth density curve. Mathematically, a curve can be characterized by an equation of the form $y = f(x)$, called probability density function, which includes one or several (unknown) parameters. The probability that the variable assumes any value in an interval between two specific points a and b is given by

$$\Pr(a \leq X \leq b) = \int_{a}^{b} f(x) dx$$

The Normal Distributions

The probability density function for the family of normal curves, sometimes also referred to as the *Gaussian distribution*, is given by

$$f(x) = \frac{1}{\sqrt{2\pi}} \exp\left[-\frac{1}{2}\left(\frac{x-\mu}{\sigma}\right)^2\right]$$

for $-\infty < x < \infty$. In the above formula, the symbol "e" represents the same exponentiation as in the probability density function of the Poisson distribution, just a different way to write when term to be exponentiated is long and complicated. The meaning and significance of the parameters μ and σ^2 have been discussed in section 3.2; μ is the mean, σ^2 is the variance, and σ is the standard deviation. When $\mu = 0$ and $\sigma = 1$, we have the standard normal distribution. The numerical values listed in our Appendix B are those of

$$\Pr(0 \leq Z \leq z) = \int_0^z \frac{1}{\sqrt{2\pi}} \exp\left[-\frac{1}{2}x^2\right] dx$$

The normal distribution plays an important role in statistical inference because

(1) Many real-life distributions are approximately normal;
(2) Many other distributions can be almost normalized by appropriate data transformations, for example, taking log. When $\log X$ has a normal distribution, X is said to have a lognormal distribution;
(3) As a sample size increases, the means of samples drawn from a population of any distribution will approach the normal distribution. This theorem, when rigorously stated, is known as the central limit theorem (more details in Chapter 4).

Other Continuous Distributions

In addition to the normal distribution (Appendix B), topics introduced in subsequent chapters will involve three other continuous distributions:

(1) The "t" distribution (Appendix C)
(2) The chi-square distribution (Appendix D)
(3) The "F" distribution (Appendix E)

The *t distribution* is similar to the standard normal distribution in that it is unimodal, bell shaped, and symmetrical, extends infinitely in either direction, and the mean is zero. This is a family of curves, each indexed by a number called the degrees of *freedom* (abbreviated as "df"). Given a sample of continuous data, the degrees of freedom measure the quantity of information available in a data set that can be used for estimating the population variance σ^2, that is, $(n-1)$, the denominator of s^2. The t curves have "thicker" tails compared to the standard normal curve, and their variance is slightly greater than 1 (it is equal to $df/(df-2)$, almost 1 for larger degrees of freedom); however, the area under each curve is still equal to unity (or 100%). Areas under a curve from the right tail, shown by the shaded region, are listed in Appendix C; the t distribution for infinite degrees of freedom is precisely equal to the standard normal distribution. This equality is readily seen by examining the column marked with, say, area $= .025$. The last row (infinite df) shows a value of 1.96, which can be verified using the table in Appendix B.

Unlike the normal and the t distributions, the *chi-square* and the F distributions are concerned with nonnegative attributes and will be used only for certain "tests" in Chapter 6 (chi-square distribution) and Chapter 7 (F distribution). Similar to the case of the t distribution, the formulas for the probability distribution functions of the chi-square and the F distributions are rather mathematically complicated and are not presented here. Each chi-square distribution is indexed by a number called the degrees of freedom r. We will refer to it as "the chi-square distribution with r degrees of freedom"; its mean and variance are r and $2r$, respectively. An F *distribution* is indexed by *two* degrees of freedom.

3.4. COMPUTATIONAL AIDS

Sections 1.4 and 2.4 covered basic techniques for Microsoft's Excel, topics such as how to open or to form a new spreadsheet, save it, retrieve it, and perform certain descriptive statistical tasks. Topics included data entry steps, such as select and drag, use of formula bar, bar and pie charts, histograms, calculations of descriptive statistics such as mean and standard deviation, and calculation of a coefficient of correlation. This section focuses on probability models focusing on the calculation of areas under density curves, especially the normal curves and the t curves.

3.4.1. Normal Curves

The first two steps are the same as in obtaining descriptive statistics (but no data are needed now): (1) click the *paste function icon*, f*, and (2) click *Statistical*. Among the many functions available, two are related to the normal curves: *NORMDIST* and *NORMINV*. Excel provides needed information for any normal distribution, not just the standard normal distribution as in Appendix B. Upon selecting either one of the above two function, a box appears asking you to provide

(1) The mean
(2) The standard deviation and
(3) In the last row, marked with "cumulative," enter "*TRUE*" (there is a choice "FALSE," but you do not need that). The answer will appear in a preselected cell.

Normdist

NORMDIST gives the area under the normal curve (with mean and variance provided) all the way from the far left side (minus infinity) to the value "x" that you have to specify. For example, if you specify $\mu = 0$ and $\sigma = 1$, the return is the area under the standard normal curve up to the specified point (which is the same as the number from Appendix B plus .5).

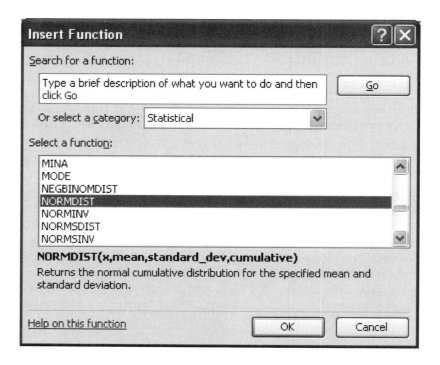

Norminv

NORMINV performs the inverse process where you provide the area under the normal curve (a number between 0 and 1), together with mean μ and standard deviation σ, and request the point x on the horizontal axis so that the area under that normal curve from the far left side (minus infinity) to the value x is equal to the provided number between 0 and 1. For example, if you put in $\mu = 0$ and $\sigma = 1$, and probability $= .975$, the return is 1.96; unlike Appendix B, if you want some number in right tail of the curve, the input probability should be a number greater than .5.

3.4.2. The "t" Curves

We want to learn how to find the areas under the normal curves so that we can determine the p-values for statistical tests (a topic starting in Chapter 5). Another popular family in this category is the t distributions. After the same first two steps, (1) click the paste function icon, f*, and (2) click Statistical, among functions available, two are related to the t distributions are *TDIST* and *TINV*. Similar to the case of NORMDIST and NORMINV, TDIST gives the area under a t curve and TINV performs the inverse process where you provide the area under the curve and request for the point x on the horizontal axis. In each case, you have to provide the degree of freedom. In addition, (3) in the last row, marked with "tails", enter

(1) (Tails=) "1" if you do a *one-sided test*, and

(2) (Tails =) "2" if you do a *two-sided test*.

(more details on the concepts of one-sided and two-sided areas are in Chapter 5). For example, using TINV, we obtain the following results in Example 3.10:

Example 3.10

(1) If you enter (i) ($x=$) 2.73, (ii) (deg freedom=) 18, and (iii) (Tails=) 1, You are requesting the area under a *t* curve with 18 degrees of freedom and to the right of 2.73 (i.e., right tail); the answer is .00687.

(2) If you enter (i) ($x=$) 2.73, (ii) (deg freedom=) 18, and (iii) (Tails=) 2, You are requesting the area under a *t* curve with 18 degrees of freedom and to the right of 2.73 and to the left of (-2.73) (i.e., both right and left tails); the answer is .01374, which is twice the previous answer of .00687.

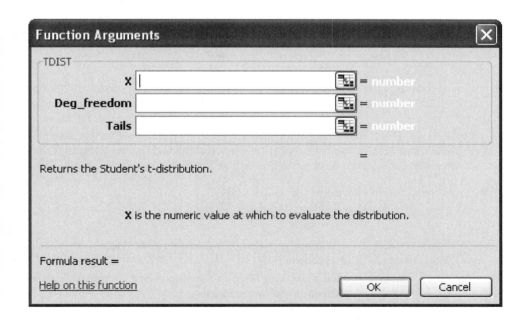

EXERCISES

3.1. Although cervical cancer is not a leading cause of death among American women, it has been suggested that virtually all such deaths are preventable (5166 American women died from cervical cancer in 1977). In an effort to find out who is being or not being screened for cervical cancer (Pap testing), the following data were collected from a certain community:

Pap Test	White	Black	Total
No	5,244	785	6,029
Yes	25,117	2,348	27,465
Total	30,361	3,133	33,494

Is there a statistical relationship here? (*Hint*: Try calculating the odds ratio; even finding a few different methods such a comparison of conditional probabilities).

3.2. In a study of intraobserver variability in assessing cervical smears, 3325 slides were screened for the presence or absence of abnormal squamous cells. Each slide was screened by a particular observer and then rescreened 6 ∼ months later by the same observer. The results are as follows:

First Screening	Second Screening		
	Present	Absent	Total
Present	1,763	489	2,252
Absent	403	670	1,073
Total	2,166	1,159	3,325

Is there a statistical relationship between first screening and second screening? (Try a few different methods as in the previous exercise.)

3.3. From the above intraobserver variability study, find
   (a) The probability that abnormal squamous cells were found to be absent in both screenings.
   (b) The probability of an absence in the second screening given that abnormal cells were found in the first screening.
   (c) The probability of an abnormal presence in the second screening given that no abnormal cells were found in the first screening.
   (d) The probability that the screenings disagree.

3.4. Given the screening test of Example 1.4, where
   Sensitivity = .406,
   Specificity = .985,

calculate the positive predictive values when the test is applied to the following populations:

Population A: 80% prevalence

Population B: 25% prevalence.

3.5. Consider the following data on the use of X-ray as a screening test for tuberculosis.

X-ray	Tuberculosis	
	No	Yes
Negative	1739	8
Positive	51	22
Total	1790	30

(a) Calculate the sensitivity and specificity.

(b) Find the disease prevalence.

(c) Calculate the positive predictive value, both directly and indirectly, using Bayes' theorem.

3.6. From the sensitivity and specificity of X-rays found in Exercise 3.55, compute the positive predictive value corresponding to these prevalences: .2, .4, .6, .7, .8, and .9. Can we find a prevalence when the positive predictive value is preset at .80 or 80%?

3.7. Refer to the standard normal distribution. What is the probability of obtaining a z-value:

(a) at least 1.25?

(b) at least $(-.84)$?

(*Hint*: In this and in the following problems, try to use Appendix B and Excel).

3.8. Refer to the standard normal distribution. What is the probability of obtaining a z-value

(a) between (-1.96) and 1.96?

(b) between 1.22 and 1.85?

(c) between $(-.84)$ and 1.28?

3.9. Refer to the standard normal distribution. What is the probability of obtaining z-value

(a) less than 1.72?

(b) less than (-1.25)?

3.10. Refer to the standard normal distribution. Find a Z-value such that the probability of obtaining a larger z-value is

(a) .05

(b) .025

(c) .20.

3.11. Verify the numbers in the first two rows of Table 3.2; for example, show that the lowest healthy systolic blood pressure for 16-year-old boys is 102.8.

3.12. Complete Table 3.2 at the question marks.

3.13. Medical research has concluded that individuals experience a common cold roughly two times per year. Assume that the time between colds is normally distributed with a mean of 160 days and a standard deviation of 40 days.

(a) What is the probability of going 200 or more days between colds? Of going 365 or more days?

(b) What is the probability of getting a cold within 80 days of a previous cold?

3.14. Assume that the test scores for a large class are normally distributed with a mean of 74 and a standard deviation of 10.

(a) Suppose you receive a score of 88. What percent of the class received scores higher than yours?

(b) Suppose the teacher wants to limit the number of A grades in the class to no more than 20%. What would be the lowest score for an A?

3.15. Intelligence test scores, referred to as intelligence quotient or IQ scores, are based on characteristics such as verbal skills, abstract reasoning power, numerical ability, and spatial visualization. If plotted on a graph, the distribution of IQ scores approximates a normal curve with a mean of about 100. An IQ score above 115 is considered superior. Studies of "intellectually gifted" children have generally defined the lower limit of their IQ scores at 140; approximately 1% of the population have IQ scores above this limit. (Based on "Your Intelligence Quotient" by Tom Biracree in *How You Rate*, New York: Dell Publishing Co. Inc., 1984).

(a) Find the standard deviation of this distribution.

(b) What percent are in the "superior" range of 115 or above?

(c) What percent of the population have IQ scores of 70 or below?

3.16. IQ scores for college graduates are normally distributed with a mean of 120 (compared to 100 for the general population) with a standard deviation of 12. What is the probability of randomly selecting a graduate student with an IQ score

(a) between 110 and 130?

(b) above 140?

(c) below 100?

3.17. Suppose it is known that the probability of recovery for a certain disease is .4. If 35 people are stricken with the disease, what is the probability that

(a) 25 or more will recover?

(b) fewer than 5 will recover?

(*Hint*: Use the normal approximation to the Binomial distribution)

3.18. A study found that for 60% of the couples who have been married 10 years or less, both spouses work. A sample of 30 couples who have been married 10 years or less are selected from marital records available at a local courthouse. We are interested in the number of couples in this sample in which both spouses work. What is the probability that this number is

(a) 20 or more?

(b) 25 or more?

(c) 10 or fewer?

3.19. Many samples of water, all of the same size, are taken from a river suspected of having been polluted by irresponsible operators at a sewage treatment plant. The number of coliform organisms in each sample was counted; the average number of organisms per sample was ~15. Assuming the number of organisms to be Poisson distributed, find the probability that

(a) the next sample will contain at least 20 organisms.

(b) the next sample will contain no more than five organisms.

3.20. For the year 1981 (see Example 3.8), we also have the following data for the South Atlantic states (Delaware, Florida, Georgia, Maryland, North and South Carolina, Virginia, and West Virginia, and the District of Columbia):

$d = 7643$ infant deaths,

$N = 550,300$ live births

Find the infant mortality rate and compare it to the national average using the method of Example 3.9.

3.21. For the t curve with 20 dfs, find the areas

(a) to the left of 2.086 and of 2.845;

(b) to the right of 1.725 and of 2.528;

(c) beyond ± 2.086 and beyond ± 2.845.

3.22. For the chi-square distribution with two dfs, find the areas

(a) to the right of 5.991 and of 9.210;

(b) to the right of 6.348;

(c) between 5.991 and 9.210.

3.23. For the F distribution with 2 numerator dfs and 30 denominator dfs, find the areas

(a) to the right of 3.32 and of 5.39;

(b) to the right of 2.61;

(c) between 3.32 and 5.39.

3.24. In a study of intraobserver variability in assessing cervical smears, 3325 slides were screened for the presence or absence of abnormal squamous cells. Each slide was screened by a particular observer and then rescreened 6 months later by the same observer. The results are as in Exercise 3.2. Calculate the kappa statistic representing the agreement between the two screenings.

3.25. Ninety-eight heterosexual couples, at least one of whom was HIV infected, were enrolled in an HIV transmission study and interviewed about sexual behavior. The following table provides a summary of condom use reported by heterosexual partners:

Woman	Man Ever	Never	Total
Ever	45	6	51
Never	7	40	47
Total	52	46	98

How strongly do the couples agree?

CHAPTER

4

Confidence Estimation

The whole process of statistical design and analysis can be described briefly as follows. The target of a scientist's investigation is a population with certain characteristics of interest; for example, a man's systolic blood pressure or his cholesterol level or whether a leukemia patient is responding to certain investigative drug. A numerical characteristic of a target population is called a *parameter*; for example, the population mean μ (average SBP) or the population proportion π (a drug's response rate). Most of the times it would be too time-consuming or too costly to obtain the totality of population information to learn about the parameter(s) of interest. For example, there are millions of men in a target population to survey, and the value of the information may not justify the high cost. Sometimes the population does not even exist. For example, in the case of an investigative drug for leukemia, we are interested in *future* patients as well as present patients. To deal with the problem, the researcher may decide to take a sample or to conduct a small phase-II clinical trial. Chapters 1 and 2 provide methods by which we can learn about data from the sample or samples. We learned how to organize data, how to summarize data, and how to present them. The topic of probability in Chapter 3 sets the framework for dealing with uncertainties. By this point, the researcher is ready to draw inferences about the population of his interest based on what he or she learned from his/her sample(s). Depending on the research objectives, we can classify inferences into two categories: one in which we want to estimate the value of a parameter, for example, the response rate of a leukemia investigative drug, and the other in which we want to compare the parameters for two subpopulations using statistical tests of significance. For example, we want to know whether men have higher cholesterol level, on average, than women. This chapter deals with the first category and the statistical procedure called *estimation* or *parameter estimation.* It is extremely useful, one of the most useful procedures of statistics. The word "estimate" actually has a language problem, the opposite of the language problem of statistical "tests" (the topic of Chapter 5). The colloquial meaning of the word "test" makes one think that statistical tests are especially objective, no-nonsense procedures that reveal the truth. Conversely, the colloquial meaning

Health and Numbers: A Problems-Based Introduction to Biostatistics, Third Edition, by Chap T. Le
Copyright © 2009 John Wiley & Sons, Inc.

of the word "estimate" is guessing, perhaps off the top of the head and uninformed, not to be taken too seriously. It is used by car body repair shops, which "estimate" how much it will cost to fix your car after an accident. The *estimate* in that case is actually a bid of a for-profit business establishment seeking your trade. In our case, the word *estimation* is used in the usual sense that provides a "substitute" for an unknown truth, but it isn't that bad a choice of word, once you understand *how* to do it. But it is important to make it clear that statistical estimation is no less objective than any other formal statistical procedure; statistical estimation requires calculations and tables just as statistical testing does. In addition it is very important to differentiate formal statistical estimation from ordinary guessing. In formal statistical estimation, we can determine the *amount of uncertainty* (and so the error) in the estimate. How often have you heard of someone making a guess and then giving you a number measuring the "margin of error" of the guess? That is what statistical estimation does. It gives you the best guess and then tells you how "wrong" the guess could be, in quite precise terms. Certain media, sophisticated newspapers in particular have started to educate the public about statistical estimation. They do it when they report the results of polls. They say things like, "74% of the voters disagree with the governor's budget proposal," and then go on to say that the margin error is plus or minus 3%. What they are saying is that whoever conducted the poll is claiming to have polled about 1,000 people chosen at random, and that statistical estimation theory tells us to be 95% certain that *if all the voters* were polled their disagreement percentage would be discovered to be within 3% of 74%. In other words, it is very unlikely that the 74% is off the mark by more than 3%; the truth is almost certainly between 71 and 77%. In subsequent sections of this chapter, we will introduce the strict interpretation of these so-called *confidence intervals*.

4.1. BASIC CONCEPTS

A class of measurements or a characteristic on which individual observations or measurements are made is called a *variable* or *random variable*. The value of a random variable varies from subject to subject; examples include weight, height, blood pressure, or the presence or absence of a certain habit or practice, such as smoking or use of drugs. The distribution of a random variable is often assumed to belong to a certain family of distributions such as binomial, Poisson, or normal. This assumed family of distributions is specified or indexed by one or several parameters such as a population mean μ or a population proportion π. It is usually either impossible, too costly, or too time-consuming to obtain the entire population data on any variable in order to learn about a parameter involved in its distribution. Decisions in health science are thus often made using a small sample of a population. The problem for a decision maker is to decide on the basis of data the estimated value of a parameter, such as the population mean, as well as to provide certain ideas concerning errors associated with that estimate.

4.1.1. Statistics as Variables

A *parameter* is a numerical property of a population; examples include population mean μ and population proportion π. The corresponding quantity obtained from a sample is called a *statistic*; examples of statistics include the sample mean $\bar{x}$ and sample proportion p. Statistics help us draw *inferences* or conclusions about population parameters. After a sample has already been obtained, the value of a statistic – for example, the sample mean $\bar{x}$ – is known and fixed; however, if we take a different sample we almost certainly have a different numerical value for that same statistic. In this repeated sampling context, a statistic is looked upon as a variable that takes different values from sample to sample.

4.1.2. Sampling Distributions

The distribution of values of a statistic obtained from repeated samples of the same size from a given population is called the sampling distribution of that statistic.

Example 4.1

Consider a population consisting of six subjects (this small size is impractical but we need something small enough to use as an illustration here); the following table gives the subject names (for identification) and values of a variable under investigation (for example, 1 for a smoker and 0 for a nonsmoker):

Subject	Value
A	1
B	1
C	1
D	0
E	0
F	0

In this case the population mean μ (also population proportion π for this very special dichotomous variable) is .5 (=3/6).

We now consider all possible samples, without replacement, of size 3; none or some or all subjects in each sample have value 1, the remaining 0. The following table represents the sampling distribution of the sample mean:

Samples	Number of Samples	Sample Mean
(D,E,F)	1	0
(A,D,E), (A,D,F), (A,E,F) (B,D,E), (B,D,F), (B,E,F) (C,D,E), (C,D,F), (C,E,F)	9	1/3
(A,B,D), (A,B,E), (A,B,F) (A,C,D), (A,C,E), (A,C,F) (B,C,D), (B,C,E), (B,C,F)	9	2/3
(A,B,C)	1	1
All possible samples	20	

This sampling distribution gives us a few interesting properties:

(i) Its mean, that is, the mean of all possible sample means, is

$$\frac{(1)(0) + (9)(1/3) + (9)(2/3) + (1)(1)}{20} = .50$$

which is the same as the mean of the original distribution. Because of this we say that the sample mean (sample proportion) is an "unbiased estimator" for the population mean (population proportion). In other words, if we use the sample mean (sample proportion) to estimate the population mean (population proportion), we are "correct on the average."

(ii) If we form a bar graph for this *sampling distribution*, it shows a shape somewhat similar to that of a symmetric, bell-shaped normal curve. This resemblance is much clearer with real populations and larger sample sizes.

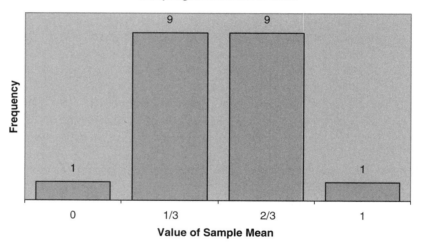

Sampling Distribution of Mean

We now consider the same population and all possible samples of size $n = 4$. The following table represents the new sampling distribution:

Samples	Number of Samples	Sample Mean
(A,D,E,F), (B,D,E,F), (C,D,E,F)	3	0.25
(A,B,D,E), (A,B,D,F), (A,B,E,F) (A,C,D,E), (A,C,D,F), (A,C,E,F) (B,C,D,E), (B,C,D,F), (B,C,E,F)	9	0.50
(A,B,C,D), (A,B,C,E), (A,B,C,F)	3	0.75
All possible samples	15	

It can be seen that we have a different sampling distribution because the sample size is different ($n = 4$ versus $n = 3$). However, we still have both above-mentioned properties:

(i) The unbiasedness of the sample mean

$$\frac{(3)(.25) + (9)(.50) + (3)(.75)}{15} = .50$$

(ii) The normal shape of the sampling distribution (bar graph)

Sampling Distribution of Mean

In addition, we can see that

(iii) The variance of the new distribution is smaller. The two faraway values of $\bar{x}$, 0 and 1, are no longer possible; new values .25 and .75 are closer to the mean .5 and the majority (nine samples) have values that are right at the sampling distribution mean. The major reason for this is that the new sampling distribution is associated with a larger sample size ($n = 4$), compared to ($n = 3$) of the previous sampling distribution.

4.1.3. Introduction to Confidence Estimation

Statistical inference is the procedure whereby inferences about a population are made on the basis of the results obtained from a sample drawn from that population.

Professionals in health science are often interested in a *parameter* of a certain population. For example, a health professional may be interested in knowing what proportion of a certain type of individual, treated with a particular drug, suffers undesirable side effects. The process of *estimation* entails calculating, from the data of a sample, some statistic that is offered as an estimate of the corresponding parameter of the population from which the sample was drawn.

A *point estimate* is a single numerical value used to estimate the corresponding population parameter. For example, the sample mean is a point estimate for the population mean and the sample proportion is a point estimate for the population proportion. However, having access to the data of a sample and knowledge of statistical theory, we can do more than just provide a point estimate. The sampling distribution of a statistic, if available, would provide information on:

(i) Biasedness/unbiasedness several statistics, such as $\bar{x}$, p, and s^2 are unbiased;
(ii) Variance.

Variance is important; a small variance for a sampling distribution indicates that most possible values for the statistic are close to each other so that a particular value is more likely to be reproduced. In other words, the variance of a sampling distribution of a statistic can be used as a measure of precision or *reproducibility* of that statistic; the smaller this quantity the better the statistic as an estimate of the corresponding parameter. The square root of this variance is called the "standard error" of the statistic; for example, we will have the standard error of the sample mean, or $SE(\bar{x})$, standard error of the sample proportion, $SE(p)$, and so on. It is the same quantity, but we use the term *standard deviation* (SD) for measurements and the term *standard error* when we refer to the standard deviation of a statistic. In the next few sections, we will introduce a process whereby the point estimate and its standard error are combined to form an interval estimate or a *confidence interval*. A confidence interval consists of two numerical values defining an interval that, with a specified *degree of confidence*, we believe, includes the parameter being estimated.

4.2. ESTIMATION OF A POPULATION MEAN

The results of Example 4.1 are not coincidences but are examples of the characteristics of sampling distributions in general. The key tool here is the *Central Limit Theorem* introduced in Section 3.2.1, which may be summarized as follows:

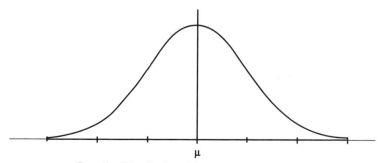

Sampling Distribution of Sample Mean for larger n

Given any population with mean μ and variance σ^2, the sampling distribution of $\bar{x}$ will be approximately normal with mean μ and variance σ^2/n when the sample size n is large. In other words, when the sample size is realistically larger, say $n > 30$ instead of $(n = 3)$ or $(n = 4)$, the sampling distribution of the sample mean is almost perfectly normal (of course, the larger the sample size the better the approximation; in practice, an $n = 30$ or more could be considered adequately large). In addition, we always have the two properties concerning the mean and the variance of this sampling distribution:

$$\mu_{\bar{x}} = \mu$$

$$\sigma_{\bar{x}}^2 = \frac{\sigma^2}{n}$$

The following example will show how good the sample mean is as an estimate for the population μ even if the sample size is as small as 25 (of course, it is used only as an illustration; in practice, the population mean μ and variance σ^2 are almost always unknown).

Example 4.2

Birth weights obtained from deliveries over a long period of time at certain hospital show a mean μ of 112 ounces and a standard deviation σ of 20.6 ounces. Suppose we want to compute the probability that the mean birth weight from a sample of 25 infants will fall between 107 and 117 ounces (i.e., the estimate is off the mark by no more than 5 ounces).

The Central Limit Theorem is applied and it indicates that $\bar{x}$ follows a normal distribution with mean

$$\mu_{\bar{x}} = 112$$

and variance

$$\sigma_{\bar{x}}^2 = (20.6)^2/25$$
$$= (4.12)^2$$

or standard error

$$SE(\bar{x}) = 4.12$$

It follows that

$$Pr(107 \leq \bar{X} \leq 117) = Pr\left(\frac{107-112}{4.12} \leq Z \leq \frac{117-112}{4.12}\right)$$
$$= Pr(-1.21 \leq Z \leq 1.21)$$
$$= (2)(.3869)$$
$$= .7738$$

In other words, if we use the mean of a sample of size $n = 25$ to estimate the population mean, about 80% (77.38% to be exact) of the times, we are correct within 5 ounces; this figure would be 98.5% if the sample size is $n = 100$ instead of $n = 25$.

4.2.1. Confidence Intervals for a Population Mean

Similar to what was done in Example 4.2 we can write, for example,

$$\Pr\left[-1.96 \le \frac{\bar{x}-\mu}{s/\sqrt{n}} \le 1.96\right] = (2)\Pr\left[0 \le \frac{\bar{x}-\mu}{s/\sqrt{n}} \le 1.96\right]$$
$$= (2)(.475)$$
$$= .95$$

This statement is a consequence of the Central Limit Theorem, which indicates that, for a large sample size n, the sample mean $\bar{X}$ is a random variable (in the context of repeated sampling) with a normal sampling distribution with mean μ and variance σ^2/n. The quantity inside the square bracket of the above equation is equivalent to:

$$\left[-1.96 \le \frac{\bar{x}-\mu}{s/\sqrt{n}} \le 1.96\right] \Leftrightarrow \left[\bar{x}-1.96\frac{s}{\sqrt{n}} \le \mu \le \bar{x}+1.96\frac{s}{\sqrt{n}}\right]$$

All we need to do now is to select a random sample, calculate the numerical value of the sample mean and its standard error with σ replaced by sample standard deviation "s", and then substitute these values to form the end points "a" and "b" of the interval,

$$a = \bar{x}-1.96\frac{s}{\sqrt{n}} \le \mu \le b = \bar{x}+1.96\frac{s}{\sqrt{n}}$$

and we have an interval for parameter μ: $a \le \mu \le b$.

But here we run into a logical problem. We are sampling from a fixed population. We are examining values of a random variable obtained by selecting a random sample from that fixed population. The random variable has a distribution with mean μ that we wish to estimate. Since the population and the distribution of the random variable we are investigating are fixed, it follows that the parameter μ is fixed. The three quantities μ, "a," and "b" are all fixed (after the sample has been obtained); then we cannot assert the *probability* that μ lies between "a" and "b" is .95. It only involves probability when it's *uncertain*; nothing is uncertain here. In fact, either μ lies in the interval (a, b) or it does not, and it is not correct to assign a probability to a *sure* statement (even the truth remains unknown).

The difficulty here arises at the point of substitution of the observed numerical values for $\bar{x}$ and its standard error. The random variation in $\bar{x}$ is variation from sample to sample in the context of repeated sampling. When we substitute $\bar{x}$ and its standard error, $s/\sqrt{n}$, by their numerical values resulting in interval (a, b), it is understood that the repeated sampling process could produce many different intervals of the same form:

$$\bar{x} \pm 1.96s/\sqrt{n}$$

About 95% of these intervals would actually include the population mean μ and 5% of them would not. Since we have only one of these possible intervals, that is, the interval (a, b) from our sample, we say we are 95% confident that μ lies between these limits. The interval (a, b) is called *a 95% confidence interval* for the population mean μ and the figure "95" is called the *degree of confidence* or confidence level.

In forming confidence intervals, the degree of confidence is determined by the investigator of a research project. Different investigators may prefer different confidence intervals; the coefficient to be multiplied with the standard error of the mean should be determined accordingly. Here are a few typical choices; 95% is the most conventional:

Degree of Confidence	Coefficient
99%	2.576
95%	1.96
90%	1.645
80%	1.282

Finally, it should be noted that since the standard error is

$$\mathrm{SE}(\bar{x}) = \frac{s}{\sqrt{n}}$$

It is obvious that the width of a confidence interval becomes narrower as sample size increases, and the above process is applicable only to large samples (say, $n > 30$). The next section will show how to handle smaller samples (there is nothing magic about $n > 30$ or $n > 25$; see the note at the end of Section, 4.2.2).

Example 4.3

For the data on percentage saturation of bile for 31 male patients of Example 2.4, 40, 86, 111, 86, 106, 66, 123, 90, 112, 52, 88, 137, 88, 88, 65, 79, 87, 56, 110, 106, 110, 78, 80, 47, 74, 58, 88, 73, 118, 67, and 57, we have

$$\bar{x} = 84.65$$
$$s = 24.00$$
$$n = 31$$

leading to a standard error of the mean

$$\mathrm{SE}(\bar{x}) = 24.0/\sqrt{31}$$
$$= 4.31$$

and a 95% confidence interval for the population mean

$$84.65 \pm (1.96)(4.31) = (76.2, 93.1)$$

(The resulting interval is wide due to a large standard deviation as observed from the sample, $s = 24.0$, reflecting heterogeneity of sample subjects.)

4.2.2. Use of Small Samples

The procedure in previous section for confidence intervals is applicable only to large samples (say, $n > 30$). For smaller samples, the results are still valid if the population variance σ^2 is known and standard error is expressed as $\sigma/\sqrt{n}$. However, σ^2 is almost always unknown. When σ is unknown, we can estimate it by "s" but the procedure has to be modified by changing the coefficient to be multiplied by the standard error to accommodate the error in estimating σ by s; how much larger the coefficient is depends on how much information we have in estimating σ, that is, the sample size n. Therefore, instead of taking coefficients from the standard normal distribution table (numbers such as 2.58, 1.96, 1.65, and 1.28 for degrees of confidence 99%, 95%, 90%, and 80%, respectively), we will use corresponding numbers from the t-curve where the quantity of information is indexed by the *degree of freedom* (df $= n - 1$). The figures needed are listed in Appendix C; the column to read is the one with the correct normal coefficient on the bottom row (marked with df $= \infty$). For example, if the degree of confidence is .95, we have

Degree of Freedom (df)	t-Coefficient
5	2.571
10	2.228
15	2.231
20	2.086
24	2.064
∞	1.960

(It is important to note that for better results, it is a good practice to always use the t-table regardless of sample size because coefficients such as 1.96 are only for very large sample sizes).

Example 4.4

In an attempt to assess the physical condition of joggers, a sample of $n = 25$ joggers was selected and maximum volume oxygen (VO_2) uptake was measured with the following results:

$$\bar{x} = 47.5 \, \text{ml/kg}$$

$$s = 4.8 \, \text{ml/kg}$$

$$SE(\bar{x}) = \frac{4.8}{\sqrt{25}}$$

$$= .96$$

From Appendix C we find that the t-coefficient with 24 df for use with a 95% confidence interval is 2.064, leading to a 95% confidence interval for the population mean μ (this is the population of joggers' VO_2 uptake) of

$$47.5 \pm (2.064)(.96) = (45.5, 49.5)$$

Example 4.5

In addition to the data in Example 4.4, we have data from a second sample consisting of $n = 26$ nonjoggers that were summarized into these statistics:

$$\bar{x} = 37.5 \, \text{ml/kg}$$
$$s = 5.1 \, \text{ml/kg}$$
$$SE(\bar{x}) = \frac{5.1}{\sqrt{26}}$$
$$= 1.0$$

From Appendix C we find that the t-coefficient with 25 df for use with a 95% confidence interval is 2.060, leading to a 95% confidence interval for the population mean μ (this is the population of joggers' VO_2 uptake) of

$$37.5 \pm (2.060)(1.0) = (35.4, 39.6)$$

It can be seen that the mean volume oxygen uptake for population of nonjoggers is much lower than that for the population of joggers, (35.4, 39.6) versus (45.5, 49.5). The mean volume oxygen uptake for population of nonjoggers is less likely to be above 39.6 ml/kg and the mean volume oxygen uptake for population of joggers is less likely to be below 45.5.

4.2.3. Evaluation of Interventions

In efforts to determine the effect of a risk factor or an *intervention*, we may want to estimate the *difference of means*; say between the population of cases and the population of controls. However, we choose not to present the methodology with all the details at this level with one exception, the case of a *matched design* or *before-and-after intervention* where each experimental unit serves as its own control. This design makes it possible to control for confounding variables that are difficult to measure, for example, environmental exposure, and therefore difficult to adjust at the analysis stage. The main reason to include this method here, however, because we treat the data as one sample and the aim is still estimating the (population) mean. That is, data from matched or before-and-after experiments *should not* be considered as coming from two independent samples. The procedure is to reduce the data to a *one-sample problem* by computing before-and-after (or control-and-case) differences for each subject (or pairs of matched subjects). By doing this with paired observations, we get a set of differences that can be handled as in a problem with one sample. The mean to be estimated, using the sample of differences, represents the effects of the intervention (or the effects of the disease) under investigation. This method applies to the analysis of pair-matched case–control studies, a very popular type of study design in the field of epidemiology.

Example 4.6

The systolic blood pressures of 12 women between 20 and 35 years of age were measured before and after administration of a newly developed oral contraceptive; the data are

Table 4.1. Systolic Blood Pressure in mmHg

Subject	Before	After	After–Before Difference (d)	(d^2)
1	122	127	5	25
2	126	128	2	4
3	132	140	8	64
4	120	119	−1	1
5	142	145	3	9
6	130	130	0	0
7	142	148	6	36
8	137	135	−2	4
9	128	129	1	1
10	132	137	5	25
11	128	128	0	0
12	129	133	4	16

Given the data in Table 4.1, we have the following summarized figures from the last column

$$n = 12$$

$$\sum d = 31$$

$$\sum d^2 = 185$$

These lead to

$$\bar{d} = \text{Average after–before difference}$$
$$= 31/12$$
$$= 2.58 \text{ mmHg}$$
$$s^2 = \frac{185-(31)^2/12}{11}$$
$$= 9.54$$
$$s = 3.09$$
$$\text{SE}(\bar{d}) = 3.09/\sqrt{12}$$
$$= .89$$

With a degree of confidence of .95, the t-coefficient from Appendix C is 2.201, for 11 degrees of freedom, so that a 95% confidence interval for the mean difference is

$$2.58 \pm (2.201)(.89) = (.62, 4.54)$$

That means the "after" mean is larger, an increase of between .62 and 4.54.

In many other interventions, or in studies to determine possible effects of a risk factor, it may not be possible to employ matched design. The comparison of means is based on data from two independent samples. The process of estimating the *difference of means* is more difficult but can be briefly summarized as follows:

(i) Data are summarized separately to obtain:

$$\text{Sample \# 1} : n_1, \bar{x}_1, s_1$$
$$\text{Sample \# 2} : n_2, \bar{x}_2, s_2$$

(ii) Standard error of the difference of means is given by

$$\text{SE}(\bar{x}_2 - \bar{x}_1) = \sqrt{\frac{s_1^2}{n_1} + \frac{s_2^2}{n_2}}$$

(iii) Finally, a 95% confidence interval for the difference of population means, $(\mu_2 - \mu_1)$, can be calculated by using the following formula

$$(\bar{x}_2 - \bar{x}) \pm (\text{coefficient})\text{SE}(\bar{x}_2 - \bar{x}_1)$$

where the "coefficient" is 1.96 if $(n_1 + n_2)$ is large; otherwise a t-coefficient is used with a degree of freedom of approximately $(n_1 + n_2)$.

4.3. ESTIMATION OF A POPULATION PROPORTION

The sample proportion is defined as in Chapter 1,

$$p = \frac{x}{n}$$

where x is the number of positive outcomes and n is the sample size. However, it can also be expressed as

$$p = \frac{\sum x_i}{n}$$

where x_i is 1 if the ith outcome is positive and zero otherwise. In other words, a sample proportion can be viewed as a sample mean where data are coded as 0/1. Because of this, the Central Limit Theorem applies: the sampling distribution of p will be approximately normal when the sample size n is large. In this context, although the proportion viewed as a sample mean, its standard error is still derived using the same process:

$$SE(p) = \frac{s}{\sqrt{n}}$$

with a standard deviation s to be determined. First, we can write out s using the following short-cut formula of Chapter 2 but with denominator n instead of $(n-1)$ (this would make little difference because we always deal with *large* samples of binary data):

$$s = \sqrt{\frac{\sum x^2 - (\sum x^2)/n}{n}}$$

Since x is binary, coded as 1 if the ith outcome is positive and zero otherwise, we have $(x^2 = x)$ and, therefore,

$$s = \sqrt{\frac{\sum x^2 - (\sum x^2)/n}{n}}$$
$$= \sqrt{\frac{\sum x - (\sum x^2)/n}{n}}$$
$$= \sqrt{\frac{\sum x}{n}\left(1 - \frac{\sum x}{n}\right)}$$
$$== \sqrt{p(1-p)}$$

In other words, the *standard error* of the sample proportion is calculated from

$$SE(p) = \sqrt{\frac{p(1-p)}{n}}$$

To state it more formally, the Central Limit Theorem implies that the sampling distribution of p will be approximately normal when the sample size n is large; the mean and variance of this sampling distribution are as follows where π is the population proportion that we want to estimate:

$$\mu_p = \pi$$

$$\sigma_p^2 = \frac{\pi(1-\pi)}{n}$$

From this sampling distribution of the sample proportion, in the context of repeated sampling, we have an approximate 95% confidence interval for a population proportion π:

$$p \pm 1.96 \, SE(p)$$

where, again, the standard error of the sample proportion, $SE(p)$, is calculated as above.

There are no easy ways for small samples; this is applicable only to larger samples ($n > 30$), n should be much larger for a narrow interval (procedures for small samples are very complicated and are not covered in this book).

Example 4.7

Suppose the true proportion of smokers in a community is known to be in the vicinity of π, and we want to estimate it using a sample of size ($n = 100$), and suppose we want our estimate to be correct within $\pm 3\%$.

The Central Limit Theorem indicates that p follows a normal distribution with mean .40 and standard deviation:

$$\sqrt{\frac{(.4)(.6)}{100}} = .049$$

It follows that

$$\Pr(.37 \le p \le .43) = \Pr\left(\frac{.37 - .40}{.049} \le Z \le \frac{.43 - .40}{.049}\right)$$

$$= \Pr(-.61 \le Z \le .61)$$

$$= (2)(.2291)$$

$$= .4582, \quad \text{or approximately } 46\%$$

That means if we use the proportion of smokers from a sample of ($n = 100$) to estimate the true proportion of smokers, only about 46% of the time we are correct within $\pm 3\%$; this figure would be 95.5% if the sample size is raised to ($n = 1,000$). What we learn from this example is that, compared to the case of continuous data in Example 4.2, it may take a much larger sample to have a good estimate of a proportion such as disease prevalence or a drug side effect.

Example 4.8

Consider the problem of estimating the prevalence of malignant melanoma in 45–54-year-old women in the United States. Suppose a random sample of ($n = 5000$) women is selected from this age group and ($x = 28$) are found to have the disease. Our point estimate for the prevalence of this disease is 0056 (=28/5000), its standard error is

$$\mathrm{SE}(p) = \sqrt{\frac{(.0056)(1-.0056)}{5000}}$$
$$= .0011$$

Therefore, a 95% confidence interval for the prevalence π of malignant melanoma in 45–54-year-old women in the United States is given by

$$.0056 \pm (1.96)(.0011) = (.0034, .0078), \text{ or } (.34\%, .78\%)$$

Example 4.9

A public health official wishes to know how effective health education efforts are regarding smoking. Of ($n = 100$) males sampled in 1965 at the time of the release of the Surgeon General's Report on the health consequences of smoking, ($x = 51$) were found to be smokers. In 1980, a second random sample of ($n = 100$) males, similarly gathered, indicated that ($x = 43$) were smokers. Application of the above method yields the following 95% confidence intervals for the smoking rates in those two years:

(1) For the data obtained in 1965, we have:

$$p = \frac{51}{100}$$
$$= .51$$
$$\mathrm{SE}(p) = \sqrt{\frac{(.51)(.49)}{100}}$$
$$= .05$$

This leads to a 95% confidence interval of $.51 \pm (1.96)\,(.05) = (.41, .61)$.

(2) For the data obtained in 1980, we have:

$$p = \frac{51}{100}$$
$$= .51$$

$$SE(p) = \sqrt{\frac{(.51)(.49)}{100}}$$
$$= .05$$

This leads to a 95% confidence interval of $.43 \pm (1.96)(.05) = (.33, .53)$.

It can be seen that the two confidence intervals, one for 1965 and the other for 1980, are both quite long and overlapped, even though the estimated rates show a decrease of 8% in smoking rate, because the sample sizes are rather small. The smoking rate in 1965 could be as high as 41% and the smoking rate in 1980 could be as high as 53%. For practical applications, one should employ much larger sample sizes to have narrower intervals. Opinion surveys, for example, use $n = 1200$–1400 to achieve a margin of error of $\pm 3\%$.

Example 4.10

A study was conducted to look at the effects of oral contraceptives (OCs) on heart condition in women 40–44 years of age. It was found that among ($n = 5000$) current OC users, 13 developed a myocardial infarction (MI) over a 3-year period, while among ($n = 10,000$) non-OC users, 7 developed MI over a 3-year period. Application of the above method yields the following 95% confidence intervals for the MI rates:

(1) For the data from OC users, we have:

$$p = \frac{13}{5000}$$
$$= .0026$$

$$SE(p) = \sqrt{\frac{(.0026)(1-.0026)}{5000}}$$
$$= .0007$$

This leads to a 95% confidence interval of $.0026 \pm (1.96)(.0007) = (.0012, 0040)$.

(2) For the data from non-OC users, we have:

$$p = \frac{7}{10,000}$$
$$= .0007$$

$$SE(p) = \sqrt{\frac{(.0007)(1-.0007)}{100}}$$
$$= .0003$$

This leads to a 95% confidence interval of $.0007 \pm (1.96) (.0003) = (.0001, .0013)$. It can be seen that the two confidence intervals, one for the OC users and the other for the non-OC users, very small rates do not overlap, a strong indication that the two population MI rates are likely not the same.

_____

In many trials for interventions, or in studies to determine possible effects of a risk factor, the comparison of proportions is based on data from two independent samples. However, the process of constructing two confidence intervals separately, one from each sample, as briefly mentioned at the end of the last few examples is not efficient. The reason is that the *overall confidence level* may no longer be, say, 95% as intended because the process involves two separate inferences; possible errors may add up. The estimation of the *difference of proportions* should be formed using the following formula (for a 95% confidence interval):

$$(p_2 - p_1) \pm (1.96) \, \text{SE} \, (p_2 - p_1)$$

where

$$\text{SE}(p_2 - p_1) = \sqrt{\frac{p_1(1-p_1)}{n_1} + \frac{p_2(1-p_2)}{n_2}}$$

4.4. ESTIMATION OF A POPULATION ODDS RATIO

So far we have relied heavily on the Central Limit Theorem in forming confidence intervals for a population mean (Section 4.2) and a population proportion (Section 4.3). The theorem stipulates that, as a sample size increases, the mean values of samples drawn from a population of any distribution will approach the normal distribution, and a sample proportion can be seen as a special case of the sample means. Even when the sample sizes are not large, since many real-life distributions are approximately normal, we still can form confidence intervals for the mean values (see subsection 4.2.2 on the use of small samples).

Besides the mean and the proportion, we have had two other statistics of interest, the *odds ratio* (OR) and the (Pearson's) *coefficient of correlation*. However the method used to form confidence intervals for the mean and the proportion does not directly apply to the case of these two new parameters. The sole reason is that they do not have the backing of the Central Limit Theorem. The sampling distribution of the (sample) odds ratio and the (sample) coefficient of correlation are positively skewed. Fortunately, these sampling distributions can be almost normalized by an appropriate data transformation; in these cases, by taking the logarithm. Therefore, we will learn to form confidence intervals on the log scale; then taking antilog (a process that is also referred to as *exponentiation*) of the two end points, a method has been used in Chapter 2 to obtain the *geometric mean*. In this section, we present in detail such a method for the calculation of *confidence intervals for a population odds ratio*.

Data from a case–control study, for example, may be summarized in a 2 × 2 table,

Exposure	Cases	Controls
Exposed	a	b
Unexposed	c	d

We have:

(i) The odds that a case was exposed are

$$\text{Odds for cases} = \frac{a}{b}$$

(ii) The odds that a control was exposed are

$$\text{Odds for controls} = \frac{c}{d}$$

Therefore, the (observed) odds ratio from the samples is

$$OR = \frac{a/b}{c/d}$$
$$= \frac{ad}{bc}$$

Confidence intervals are derived from the normal approximation to the sampling distribution of the odds ratio on the log scale, ln(OR), with variance:

$$\text{Variance}[\ln(OR)] = \frac{1}{a} + \frac{1}{b} + \frac{1}{c} + \frac{1}{d}$$

Consequently, an approximate 95% confidence interval, on the log scale, for odds ratio is given by

$$\ln\left(\frac{ad}{bc}\right) \pm (1.96)\sqrt{\frac{1}{a} + \frac{1}{b} + \frac{1}{c} + \frac{1}{d}}$$

(again, "ln" is logarithm to base e, also called the "natural" logarithm). A 95% confidence interval for the odds ratio under investigation is obtained by "exponentiating" (the reverse log operation or antilog) the two end points, one with the minus sign and the other with the plus sign.

Example 4.11

The role of smoking in the etiology of pancreatitis has been recognized for many years. To provide estimates of the quantitative significance of these factors, a hospital-based study was carried out in eastern Massachusetts and Rhode Island between 1975 and 1979. Ninety-eight patients who had a hospital discharge diagnosis of pancreatitis were included in this unmatched case–control study. The control group consisted of 451 patients admitted for diseases other than those of the pancreas and biliary tract. Risk factor information was obtained from a standardized interview with each subject, conducted by a trained interviewer.

The following are some data for the males:

Use of Cigarettes	Cases	Controls
Never	2	56
Ex-smokers	13	80
Current smokers	38	81
Total	53	217

We have from the data in the table above

(i) For ex-smokers, compared to those who never smoked,

$$OR = \frac{(13)(56)}{(80)(2)}$$

$$= 4.55$$

and a 95% confidence interval for the population odds ratio on the log scale is from

$$\ln(4.55) - 1.96\sqrt{\frac{1}{13} + \frac{1}{56} + \frac{1}{80} + \frac{1}{2}} = -.01 \text{ to } \ln(4.55) + 1.96\sqrt{\frac{1}{13} + \frac{1}{56} + \frac{1}{80} + \frac{1}{2}} = 3.04$$

and, hence, the corresponding 95% confidence interval for the population odds ratio is (.99, 20.96).

(ii) For current smokers, compared to those who never smoked,

$$OR = \frac{(38)(56)}{(81)(2)}$$

$$= 13.14$$

and a 95% confidence interval for the population odds ratio on the log scale is from

$$\ln(13.14) - 1.96\sqrt{\frac{1}{38} + \frac{1}{56} + \frac{1}{81} + \frac{1}{2}} = 1.11 \text{ to } \ln(4.55) + 1.96\sqrt{\frac{1}{38} + \frac{1}{56} + \frac{1}{81} + \frac{1}{2}} = 4.04$$

and, hence, the corresponding 95% confidence interval for the population odds ratio is (3.04, 56.70).

The result for ex-smokers is "inconclusive," with the confidence interval (.99, 20.96) showing a slim possibility that the odds ratio could be "1.0," due to a small cell frequency: only two cases who never smoked. Unlike data on continuous scale, we need to have all four frequencies larger to have a narrow confidence interval; a total large sample size is not enough.

Example 4.12

Toxic shock syndrome (TSS) is a disease that was first recognized in the 1980s, characterized by sudden onset of high fever (over 102 °F), vomiting, diarrhea, rapid progression to hypotension, and, in most cases, shock. Because of its striking association with menses, several studies have been conducted to look at various practices associated with the menstrual cycle. In a study by the Center for Disease Control, 30 of the 40 TSS cases and 30 of the 114 controls, who used a single brand of tampons, "Rely." Data are presented in the following table:

Brand	Cases	Controls
Rely	30	30
Others	10	84
Total	40	114

We have:

$$OR = \frac{(30)(84)}{(10)(30)}$$

$$= 8.4$$

and a 95% confidence interval for the population odds ratio on the log scale is from

$$\ln(8.4) - 1.96\sqrt{\frac{1}{30} + \frac{1}{10} + \frac{1}{30} + \frac{1}{84}} = 1.30 \quad \text{to} \quad \ln(8.4) + 1.96\sqrt{\frac{1}{30} + \frac{1}{10} + \frac{1}{30} + \frac{1}{84}} = 2.96$$

and hence the corresponding 95% confidence interval for the population odds ratio is (3.67, 19.30), indicating a very high risk elevation for Rely users.

4.5. ESTIMATION OF A POPULATION CORRELATION COEFFICIENT

Similar to the odds ratio, the sampling distribution of the (Pearson's) coefficient of correlation is positively skewed. After completing our descriptive analysis (Section 2.4 of

Chapter 2), information about a possible relationship between two continuous factors is sufficiently contained in two statistics: the number of pairs of data n (sample size) and the (Pearson's) coefficient of correlation r (which is a number between 0 and 1). Confidence intervals are then derived from the normal approximation to the sampling distribution of

$$z = \frac{1}{2}\ln\left\{\frac{(1+r)}{(1-r)}\right\}$$

with variance of approximately,

$$\text{Variance }(z) = \frac{1}{n-3}$$

Consequently, an approximate 95% confidence interval for correlation coefficient interval, on this newly transformed scale, for the Pearson's correlation coefficient is given by

$$(z_L, z_U) = z \pm 1.96\sqrt{\frac{1}{n-3}}$$

A 95% confidence interval (r_L, r_U) for the coefficient of correlation under investigation is obtained by transforming the two end points z_L and z_U:

$$r_L = \frac{\exp(2z_L)-1}{\exp(2z_L)+1}$$

And

$$r_U = \frac{\exp(2z_U)-1}{\exp(2z_U)+1}$$

Example 4.13

The following data represent systolic blood pressure readings on 15 women:

Age (x)	SBP (y)	Age (x)	SBP (y)
42	130	85	162
46	115	72	158
42	148	64	155
71	100	1	160
80	156	41	125
74	162	61	150
70	151	75	165
80	156		

The descriptive analysis in Example 2.12 yields $r = .566$ and we have:

$$z = \frac{1}{2}\ln\left\{\frac{(1+.566)}{(1-.566)}\right\}$$

$$= .642$$

$$(z_L, z_U) = .642 \pm 1.96\sqrt{\frac{1}{12}}$$

$$= (.076, 1.207)$$

or a 95% confidence interval for the population coefficient of correlation of (.076, .836)

Example 4.14

The following table gives the values for the birth weight (x) and the increase in weight between 70th and 100th days of life, expressed as a percentage of the birth weight (y) for $(n = 12)$ infants:

Birth Weight, x (oz)	Percent Increase, y
112	63
111	66
107	72
119	52
92	75
80	118
81	120
84	114
118	42
106	72
103	90
94	91

The descriptive analysis in Example 2.11 yields $r = -.946$ and we have:

$$z = \frac{1}{2}\ln\left\{\frac{(1-.946)}{1+.946)}\right\} = -1.972$$

$$(z_L, z_U) = -1.792 \pm 1.96\sqrt{\frac{1}{9}} = (-2.446, -1.139)$$

A conversion of these two end points leads to a 95% confidence interval for the population coefficient of correlation of $(-.985, -.814)$:

$$r_L = \frac{\exp[(2)(-2.446)-1]}{\exp[(2)(-2.446)+1]} = -.985$$

$$r_L = \frac{\exp[(2)(-1.139)-1]}{\exp[(2)(-1.139)+1]} = -.814$$

This indicates a very strong negative association between a baby's birth weight and his or her increase in weight between 70th and 100th days of life; that is, smaller babies are likely to growth faster during that period (that may be why most babies look the same size at three months).

4.6. A NOTE ON COMPUTATION

All the computations for confidence intervals can be put together by using a calculator, even though some are quite tedious, especially the confidence intervals for odds ratios and coefficients of correlation. Descriptive statistics, such as sample mean and sample standard deviation, can be obtained with the help of Excel (see Section 2.4), so can be standard, normal, and t-coefficients (see Section 3.4). If you try the first two usual steps: (1) click *the paste function icon*, f*, and (2) click *Statistical*; among the functions available, you will find CONFIDENCE that is intended for forming confidence intervals. But it is not worth the effort; that process is only for 95% confidence interval for the mean using very large sample (with coefficient 1.96), and you still need to enter sample mean, standard deviation, and sample size.

EXERCISES

4.1. Consider a population consisting of four subjects, A, B, C, and D, with the following values for a random variable X under investigation:

Subject	Value
A	1
B	1
C	0
D	0

Form the sampling distribution for the sample mean of size $(n = 2)$ and verify that the mean of all possible sample mean values is equal to the population mean μ; then repeat the process with sample size of $(n = 3)$.

4.2. The body mass index (kg/m^2) is calculated by dividing a person's weight by the square of his/her height and is used as a measure of the extent to which the individual is overweight. Suppose the distribution of the body mass index for men has a standard deviation of $\sigma = 3 \, kg/m^2$ and we wish to estimate the mean μ using a sample of size $(n = 49)$. Find the probability that we would be correct within $1 \, kg/m^2$.

4.3. Self-reported injuries among left-handed and right-handed people were compared in a survey of 1,896 college students in British Columbia, Canada.

Ninety-three of the 180 left-handed students reported at least one injury and 619 of the 1716 right-handed students reported at least one injury in the same period. Calculate the 95% confidence interval for the proportion of students with at least one injury for each of the two subpopulations, left-handed students and right-handed students.

4.4. A study was conducted to evaluate the hypothesis that tea consumption and premenstrual syndrome are associated. One hundred and eighty-eight nursing students and 64 tea factory workers were given questionnaires. The prevalence of premenstrual syndrome was 39% among the nursing students and 77% among the tea factory workers. Calculate the 95% confidence interval for the prevalence of premenstrual syndrome for each of the two populations, nursing students and tea factory workers.

4.5. A study was conducted to investigate drinking problems among college students. In 1983, a group of students was asked whether they had ever driven an automobile while drunk. In 1987, after the legal drinking age was raised, a different group of college students was asked the same question. The results are as follows:

Drove While Drunk	Year of Survey		
	1983	1987	Total
Yes	1250	991	2241
No	1387	1666	3053
Total	2637	2657	5294

Calculate, separately for 1983 and 1987, the 95% confidence interval for the proportion of students who had driven an automobile while drunk.

4.6. In August 1976, tuberculosis was diagnosed in a high school student (Index case) in Corinth, Mississippi. Laboratory studies revealed that the disease was caused by drug-resistant *Tubercule bacilli*. An epidemiologic investigation was conducted at the high school.

The following table gives the rate of positive tuberculin reactions, determined for various groups of students according to the degree of exposure to the index case.

Exposure Level	Number Tested	Number Positive
High	129	63
Low	325	36

Calculate the 95% confidence interval for the rate of positive tuberculin reaction separately for each of the two subpopulations, those with high exposure and those with low exposure.

4.7. The prevalence rates of hypertension among adult (ages 18–74) white and black Americans were measured in the second in the second National Health and Nutrition

Examination Survey, 1976–80. Prevalence estimates (and their standard errors) for women are given below:

Race	$p(\%)$	$SE(p)$
Whites	25.3	0.9
Blacks	38.6	1.8

Calculate and compare the 95% confidence intervals for the proportions of the two groups, blacks and whites, and draw appropriate conclusion. Do you need the sample sizes, or any other numbers, to do your calculations? Why or why not?

4.8. Consider the following data:

	Tuberculosis		
X-Ray	No	Yes	Total
Negative	1739	8	1747
positive	51	22	73
Total	1790	30	1820

Calculate the 95% confidence intervals for the sensitivity and specificity of X-ray as a screening test for tuberculosis.

4.9. Sera from a human T-lymphotropic virus type 1 (HTLV-I) risk group (women prostitutes) were tested with two commercial "research" enzyme-linked immuno-sorbent assays (ELISAs) for HTLV-I antibodies. These results were compared with a gold standard and the outcomes are shown below.

	Dupont's ELISA		Cellular Product's ELISA	
Truth	Positive	Negative	Positive	Negative
Positive	15	1	16	0
Negative	2	164	7	179

Calculate the 95% confidence intervals for the sensitivity and specificity separately for the two ELISAs.

4.10. In a seroepidemiologic survey of health workers representing a spectrum of exposure to blood and patients with hepatitis B virus (HBV), it was found that infection increased as a function of contact. The following table provides data for hospital workers with uniform socioeconomic status at an urban teaching hospital in Boston, Massachusetts.

Personnel	Exposure	No. tested	HBV Positive
Physicians	Frequent	81	17
	Infrequent	89	7
Nurses	Frequent	104	22
	Infrequent	126	11

Calculate the 95% confidence intervals for the proportions of HBV positive workers in each subpopulation and at each level of exposure.

4.11. Consider the data taken from a study that attempts to determine whether the use of electronic fetal monitoring (EFM) during labor affects the frequency of caesarean section deliveries. Of the 5,824 infants included in the study, 2,850 were electronically monitored and 2,974 were not. The outcomes are as follows:

	EFM Exposure		
Caesarean Delivery	Yes	No	Total
Yes	358	229	587
No	2492	2745	5237
Total	2850	2974	5824

(a) Use the data from the group without EFM exposure, calculate the 95% confidence interval for the proportion of caesarean delivery.

(b) Calculate the 95% confidence interval for the odds ratio representing the relationship between EFM exposure and caesarean delivery.

4.12. A study was conducted to investigate the effectiveness of bicycle safety helmets in preventing head injury. The data consist of a random sample of 793 individuals who were involved in bicycle accidents during a 1-year period.

	Wearing Helmet		
Head Injury	Yes	No	Total
Yes	17	218	237
No	130	428	558
Total	147	646	793

(a) Use the data from the group without helmets, calculate the 95% confidence interval for the proportion of head injury.

(b) Calculate the 95% confidence interval for the odds ratio representing the relationship between use (or nonuse) of helmet and head injury.

4.13. A case–control study was conducted in Auckland, New Zealand, to investigate the effects of alcohol consumption on both nonfatal myocardial infarction and coronary death in 24 h after drinking, among regular drinkers. Data were tabulated separately for men and women.

(1) Data for Men

Drink in the Last 24 h	Myocardial Infarction		Coronary Death	
	Controls	Cases	Controls	Cases
No	197	142	135	103
Yes	201	136	159	69

(2) Data for Women

Drink in the Last 24 h	Myocardial Infarction		Coronary Death	
	Controls	Cases	Controls	Cases
No	144	41	89	12
Yes	122	19	76	4

(a) Refer to myocardial infarction (the middle columns of the tables), calculate the 95% confidence interval for the odds ratio associated with drinking, separately for men and women.

(b) Refer to coronary deaths (the columns on the right), calculate the 95% confidence interval for the odds ratio associated with drinking, separately for men and women.

(c) From the results in (a) and/or (b), is there any indication that gender may act as an effect modifier?

4.14. Adult male residents of 13 counties of western Washington State, in whom testicular cancer had been diagnosed during the years 1977–1983, were interviewed over the telephone regarding their history of genital tract conditions, including vasectomy. For comparison, the same interview was given to a sample of men selected from the population of these counties by dialing telephone numbers at random. The following data are tabulated by religious background.

Religion	Vasectomy	Cases	Controls
Protestant	Yes	24	56
	No	205	239
Catholic	Yes	10	6
	No	32	90
Others	Yes	18	39
	No	56	96

Calculate the 95% confidence interval for the odds ratio associated with vasectomy for each religious group. Is there any evidence of an effect modification?

4.15. A case–control study was conducted relating to the epidemiology of breast cancer and the possible involvement of dietary fats, along with other vitamins and nutrients. It included 2024 breast cancer cases, who were admitted to Roswell Park Memorial Institute, Erie County, New York, from 1958 to 1965. A control group of 1463 was chosen from the patients having no neoplasm and no pathology of gastrointestinal or reproductive systems. The primary factors being investigated were vitamins A and E (measured in international units per month). Data for 1,500 women over 54 years of age are as follows:

Vitamin A (IU/mo)	Cases	Controls
<150,500	893	392
>150,500	132	83
Total	1025	475

(a) Calculate the 95% confidence interval for the proportion among the controls who consumed at least 150,500 international units of Vitamin A per month.

(b) Calculate the 95% confidence interval for the odds ratio associated with Vitamin A deficiency.

4.16. A study was undertaken to investigate the roles of blood-borne environmental exposures on ovarian cancer from assessment of consumption of coffee, tobacco, and alcohol. The study enrolled 188 women in the San Francisco Bay area with epithelial ovarian cancers diagnosed in 1983–1985 and 539 control women. Of the 539 controls, 280 were hospitalized without overt cancer and 259 were chosen from the general population by random telephone dialing. Data for coffee consumption are summarized as follows:

Coffee Drinkers	Cases	Hospital Controls	Population Controls
No	11	31	26
Yes	177	249	233

Calculate the odds ratio and its 95% confidence interval for

(a) Cases versus hospital controls;

(b) Cases versus population controls.

4.17. Postneonatal mortality due to respiratory illnesses is known to be inversely related to maternal age, but the role of young motherhood as a risk factor for respiratory morbidity in infants has not been thoroughly explored. A study was conducted in Tucson, Arizona, aimed at the incidence of lower respiratory tract illnesses (LRI) during the first year of life. In this study, over 1,200 infants were enrolled at birth between 1980 and 1984 and the following data are concerned with wheezing lower respiratory tract illnesses (wheezing LRI: No/Yes).

Maternal Age (years)	Boys		Girls	
	No	Yes	No	Yes
<21	19	8	20	7
21–25	98	40	128	36
26–30	160	45	148	42
Over 30	110	20	116	25

Using "Over 30" as the baseline, calculate the odds ratio and its 95% confidence interval for each other maternal age group.

4.18. Data were collected from 2,197 white ovarian cancer patients and 8,893 white controls in 12 different U.S. case–control studies conducted by various investigators in the period 1956–1986. These were used to evaluate the relationship of invasive epithelial ovarian cancer with reproductive and menstrual characteristics, exogenous estrogen use, and prior pelvic surgeries. The following are parts of the data related to unprotected intercourse and to history of infertility.

Duration of Unprotected Intercourse (years)	Cases	Controls
Below 2	237	477
2–9	166	354
10–14	47	91
15 and over	133	174

History of Infertility	Cases	Controls
No	526	966
Yes; No drug use	76	124
Yes; Drug use	20	11

(a) For the unprotected intercourse, using "Below 2" as the baseline, calculate the odds ratio and its 95% confidence interval for each other level of exposure.

(b) Using "No history of infertility" as the baseline, calculate the odds ratio and its 95% confidence interval for each group with a history of infertility.

4.19. Consider this data taken from a study that examines the response to ozone and sulfur dioxide among adolescents suffering from asthma. The following are measurements of forced expiratory volume (liters) for 10 subjects:

$$\{3.50, 2.60, 2.75, 2.82, 4.05, 2.25, 2.68, 3.00, 4.02, 2.85\}.$$

Calculate the 95% confidence interval for the (population) mean of forced expiratory volume.

4.20. The percentage of ideal body weight was determined for 18 randomly selected insulin-dependent diabetics. The outcomes (%) are

{107, 119, 99, 114, 120, 104, 124, 88, 114, 116, 101, 121, 152, 125, 100, 114, 95, 117}.

Calculate the 95% confidence interval for the (population) mean of the percentage of ideal body weight.

4.21. A study on birth weight provided the following data (in ounces) for 12 newborns:

{112, 111, 107, 119, 92, 80, 81, 84, 118, 106, 103, 94}.

Calculate the 95% confidence interval for the (population) mean of the birth weight.

4.22. The ages (in days) at the time of death for samples of 11 girls and 16 boys who died of sudden infant death syndrome are shown below:

Girls : {53, 56, 60, 60, 78, 87, 102, 117, 134, 160, 277}

Boys : {46, 52, 58, 59, 77, 78, 80, 81, 84, 103, 114, 115, 133, 134, 175, 175}.

Calculate, separately for boys and girls, the 95% confidence interval for the (population) mean of age (in days) at the time of death.

4.23. A study was conducted to investigate whether oat bran cereal helps to lower serum cholesterol in men with high cholesterol levels. Fourteen men were randomly placed on a diet that included either oat bran or corn flakes; after two weeks, their low-density lipoprotein cholesterol levels were recorded. Each man was then switched to the alternative diet. After a second two-week period, the LDL cholesterol level of each individual was again recorded. The data were:

Subject	LDL (mmol/l)	
	Corn Lakes	Oat Bran
1.00	4.61	3.84
2.00	6.42	5.57
3.00	5.40	5.85
4.00	4.54	4.84
5.00	3.98	3.68
6.00	3.82	2.96
7.00	5.01	4.41
8.00	4.34	3.72
9.00	3.80	3.49
10.00	4.56	3.84
11.00	5.35	5.26
12.00	3.89	3.73
13.00	2.25	1.84
14.00	4.24	4.14

Calculate the 95% confidence interval for the (population) mean difference of the low-density lipoprotein cholesterol level LDL (mmol/l; Corn flake–Oat bran).

4.24. An experiment was conducted at the University of California at Berkeley to study the psychological environment effect on the anatomy of the brain. A group of 19 rats was randomly divided into two groups. Twelve animals in the treatment group lived together in a large cage, furnished with playthings that were changed daily, while animals in the control group lived in isolation with no toys. After a month, the experimental animals were killed and dissected. The following table gives the cortex weights (the thinking part of the brain) in milligrams:

Treatment : $\{707, 740, 745, 652, 649, 676, 699, 696, 712, 708, 749, 690\}$

Control : $\{669, 650, 651, 627, 656, 642, 698\}$

Calculate, separately for each treatment, the 95% confidence interval for the (population) mean of the cortex weight. How do the mean values compare?

4.25. The systolic blood pressures (in mmHg) of 12 women between the ages of 20 and 35 were measured before and after the administration of a newly developed oral contraceptive.

Subject	Before	After	After–Before Difference, d
1	122	127	5
2	126	128	2
3	132	140	8
4	120	119	−1
5	142	145	3
6	130	130	0
7	142	148	6
8	137	135	−2
9	128	129	1
10	132	137	5
11	128	128	0
12	129	133	4

(a) Calculate the 95% confidence interval for the mean systolic blood pressure *change*. Does the oral contraceptive seem to change the mean systolic blood pressure?

(b) Calculate a 95% confidence interval for the Pearson's correlation coefficient representing a possible relationship between systolic blood pressures measured before and after the administration of oral contraceptive.

4.26. Suppose that we are interested in studying patients with systemic cancer who subsequently develop a brain metastasis; our ultimate goal is to prolong their lives by controlling the disease. A sample of 23 such patients, all of whom were treated with radiotherapy, was followed from the first day of their treatment until recurrence of the original tumor. Recurrence is defined as the reappearance of a metastasis at exactly the same site or, in the case of patients whose tumor never completely disappeared, enlargement of the original lesion. Times to recurrence (in weeks) for the 23 patients were

$$\{2, 2, 2, 3, 4, 5, 5, 6, 7, 8, 9, 10, 14, 14, 18, 19, 20, 22, 22, 31, 33, 39, 195\}.$$

First, calculate the 95% confidence interval for the mean time to recurrence on the log scale, then convert – by exponentiating – the end points to week.

4.27. An experimental study was conducted with 136 five-year-old children in four Quebec schools to investigate the impact of simulation games designed to teach children to obey certain traffic safety rules. The transfer of learning was measured by observing children's reactions to a quasireal-life model of traffic risks. The scores of the two groups are summarized below:

Summarized Data	Control	Simulation Game
Sample Size	30	33
Mean	7.9	10.1
Standard Deviation	3.7	2.3

Find and compare the 95% confidence intervals for the mean of the two groups.

4.28. The body mass index is calculated by dividing a person's weight by the square of his/her height (it is used as a measure of the extent to which the individual is overweight). A sample of 58 men, selected (retrospectively) from a large group of middle-aged men who later developed diabetes mellitus, yields:

$$\bar{x} = 25.0 \, \text{kg/m2}$$
$$S = 2.7 \, \text{kg/m2}$$

(a) Calculate a 95% confidence interval for the mean of this subpopulation.

(b) If it is known that the average body mass index for middle-aged men who do not develop diabetes is $24.0 \, \text{kg/m}^2$, what can you say about the relationship between body mass index and diabetes in middle-aged men?

4.29. A study was undertaken to clarify the relationship between heart disease and occupational carbon disulphide exposure along with another important factor, elevated diastolic blood pressure (DBP), in a data set obtained from a 10-year prospective follow-up of two cohorts of over 340 male industrial workers in Finland. Carbon disulphide is an industrial solvent that is used all over the world to produce viscose rayon fibers. The following table gives the mean and standard deviation of serum cholesterol (mg/100 ml) among exposed and nonexposed cohorts, by diastolic blood pressure.

DBP (mmHg)	Exposed			Nonexposed		
	n	Mean	SD	n	Mean	SD
Below 100	205	220	50	271	221	42
95–100	92	227	57	53	236	46
Over 100	20	233	41	10	216	48

Compare serum cholesterol levels between exposed and nonexposed cohorts at each level of DBP by calculating the two 95% confidence intervals for the mean (exposed and nonexposed groups).

4.30. Refer to the data on prostate cancer in Exercise 2.33, calculate the 95% confidence interval for the (Pearson's) correlation between age and level of serum acid phosphatase.

4.31. The following data give the net food supply (x, that is the number of calories per person per day) and the infant mortality rate (y) for certain selected countries before World War II.

Country	x	y	Country	x	y
Argentina	2730	98.8	Iceland	3160	42.4
Australia	3300	39.1	India	1970	161.6
Austria	2990	87.4	Ireland	3390	69.6
Belgium	3000	83.6	Italy	2510	102.7
Burma	1080	202.1	Japan	2180	60.6
Canada	3070	67.4	New Zealand	3260	32.2
Chile	2240	240.8	Netherlands	3010	37.4
Cuba	2610	116.8	Sweden	3210	43.3
Egypt	2450	162.9	England	3100	53.3
France	2880	66.1	USA	3150	53.2
Germany	2960	63.3	Uraguay	2380	94.1

Calculate the 95% confidence interval for the (Pearson's) correlation coefficient between the net food supply and the infant mortality rate.

4.32. In an assay of heparin, a standard preparation is compared with a test preparation by observing the log clotting times (y, in seconds) of the blood containing different doses of heparin (x is log dose, replicate readings are made at each dose level):

Log Clotting Times				
Standard		Test		Log(Dose)
1.81	1.76	1.80	1.76	0.72
1.85	1.79	1.83	1.83	0.87
1.95	1.93	1.90	1.88	1.02
2.12	2.00	1.97	1.98	1.17
2.26	2.16	2.14	2.10	1.32

Calculate, separately for the standard preparation and the test preparation, the 95% confidence interval for the (Pearson's) correlation coefficient between the log clotting times and log dose.

4.33. There have been times the city of London experienced periods of dense fog. The following table shows such data for a 15-day very severe period that include the number of deaths in each day (Y), the mean atmospheric smoke (X_1, in mg/m^3), and the mean atmospheric sulfur dioxide content (X_2, in parts/million):

Y	X1	X2
112	0.30	0.09
140	0.49	0.16
143	0.61	0.22
120	0.49	0.14
196	2.64	0.75
294	3.45	0.86
513	4.46	1.34
518	4.46	1.34
430	1.22	0.47
274	1.22	0.47
255	0.32	0.22
236	0.29	0.23
256	0.50	0.26
222	0.32	0.16
213	0.32	0.16

Calculate the 95% confidence interval for the (Pearson's) correlation coefficient between the number of deaths (Y) and the mean atmospheric smoke (X_1, in mg/m^3) and between the number of deaths (y) and the mean atmospheric sulfur dioxide content (X_2, in parts/million), respectively.

4.34. The following are the heights (measured to the nearest 2 cm) and the weights (measured to the nearest kilogram) of 10 men and 10 women.

Men

Height:	162	168	174	176	180	180	182	184	186	186
Weight:	65	65	84	63	75	76	82	65	80	81

Women

Height:	152	156	158	160	162	162	164	164	166	166
Weight:	52	50	47	48	52	55	55	56	60	60

Calculate, separately for men and women, the 95% confidence interval for the (Pearson's) correlation coefficient between height and weight. Is there any indication of an effect modification?

4.35. Data are shown below for two groups of patients who died of acute myelogenous leukemia. Patients were classified into the two groups according to the presence or the absence of a morphologic characteristic of white cells. Patients termed "AG-positive" were identified by the presence of Auer rods and/or significant granulature of the leukemic cells in the bone marrow at diagnosis. For the AG-negative patients these factors were absent. Leukemia is a cancer characterized by an over-proliferation of white blood cells; the higher the white blood count (WBC) the more severe the disease.

AG-Positive, $n = 17$		AG-Negative, $n = 16$	
White Blood Count (WBC)	Survival Time (weeks)	White Blood Count (WBC)	Survival Time (weeks)
2300	65	4400	56
750	156	3000	65
4300	100	4000	17
2600	134	1500	7
6000	16	9000	16
10,500	108	5300	22
10,000	121	10,000	3
17,000	4	19,000	4
5400	39	27,000	2
7000	143	28,000	3
9400	56	31,000	8
32,000	26	26,000	4
35,000	22	21,000	3
100,000	1	79,000	30
100,000	1	100,000	4
52,000	5	100,000	43
100,000	65		

Calculate, separately for the AG-positive patients and AG-negative patients, the 95% confidence interval for the Pearson's correlation coefficient between survival time and white blood count (both on log scale). Is there any indication of an effect modification?

5

Introduction to Hypothesis Testing

This chapter covers the most used and yet most misunderstood statistical procedures, called tests of significance of hypothesis tests. The reason for the misunderstanding is simple: language. The colloquial meaning of the word "test" is one of no-nonsense objectivity. Students take tests in school, hospitals draw blood to be sent to laboratories for tests, and automobiles are tested by the manufacturer for performance and safety. It is thus natural to think that statistical tests are the "objective" procedures to use on data. The truth is that statistical tests are no more or less objective than any other statistical procedure such as confidence estimation of Chapter 4.

Statisticians have made the problem worse by using the word "significance". Significance is another word that has a powerful meaning in ordinary, colloquial language: importance. Statistical tests that result in "significance" are naturally misunderstood by the public to mean that the findings or results are important. That is not what statisticians mean; it only means that, for example, the difference they hypothesized was *real*.

Statistical tests are commonly and seriously misinterpreted by nonstatisticians, but the misinterpretations are very natural. It is very natural to look at data and ask whether there is "anything going on", or whether it is just a bunch of meaningless numbers that cannot be interpreted. Statistical tests appeal to investigators and readers of research for a reason in addition to the aforementioned reasons of language confusion. Statistical tests are appealing because they seem to make a decision; they are attractive because they say "yes" or "no". There is comfort in using a procedure that gives definitive answers from confusing data.

One way of explaining statistical tests is to use criminal court procedures as a metaphor. In criminal court, the accused is "presumed innocent" until "proven guilty beyond all reasonable doubt". This framework of presumed innocence has nothing whatsoever to do with anyone's personal belief as to the innocence or guilt of the defendant. Sometimes everybody in their right mind, including the jury, the judge, and even the defendant's attorney think the defendant is guilty as sin. The rules and procedures of criminal court, however, must be followed. There may be a mistrial, or a hung jury, or the arresting officer forgot to read the defendant his or her rights. Any number of things can happen to save the guilty from a conviction. On the other hand, an innocent defendant is sometimes convicted by overwhelming circumstantial evidence. Criminal courts occasionally make mistakes, sometimes releasing the guilty and sometimes convicting the innocent. Statistical tests are like that. Sometimes statistical significance is attained when nothing is going on and sometimes no statistical significance is attained when something very important is going on.

Just as in the court room, everyone would like statistical tests to make mistakes as infrequently as possible. Actually, the mistake rate of one of two possible mistakes made by statistical tests has usually been (arbitrarily) chosen to be 5 or 1%. The kind of mistake referred to here is the mistake of attaining statistical significance when there is actually nothing going on, just as the mistake of convicting the innocent in a trial by jury. This mistake is called a Type I mistake or Type I error. Statistical tests are often constructed so that Type I errors occur 5 or 1% of the time. There is no custom regarding the rate of Type II errors, however. A Type II error is the mistake of not getting statistical significance when there is something going on, just as the mistake of releasing the guilty in a trial by jury. The rate of Type II mistakes is dependent on several factors. One of the factors is how much is going on, just as the severity of the crime in a trial by jury. If there is a lot going on, one is less likely to make Type II errors. Another factor is the amount of variability ("noise") there is in the data, just as the quality of collected evidence in a trial by jury. A lot of variability makes Type II errors more likely. Yet another factor is the size of the study, just as the amount of collected evidence in a trial by jury. There are more Type II errors in small studies than there are in big ones. Type II errors are rare in really huge studies, but quite common in small studies.

There is a very important, subtle aspect of statistical tests, based on the aforementioned three things that make Type II errors very improbable. Since really huge studies virtually guarantee getting statistical significance if there is even the slightest amount going on, such studies result in statistical significance when the amount that is going on is of no practical importance. In this case, statistical significance is attained in the face of no practical significance. On the contrary, small studies can result in statistical nonsignificance when something of great practical importance is going on. The conclusion is that the attainment of statistical significance in a study is just as affected by extraneous factors as it is by practical importance. It is essential to learn that statistical significance is not synonymous with practical importance.

5.1. BASIC CONCEPTS

From the introduction of sampling distributions in Chapter 4, it was clear that the value of a sample mean is influenced by

(i) The population mean μ, because, by The Central Limit Theorem, the mean of all possible sample means is equal to μ.

(ii) Chance; the sample mean and the population mean are almost never identical. The variance of the sampling distribution is

$$\text{Variance}(\bar{x}) = \frac{\sigma^2}{n}$$

which represents a combined effect of the natural variation in the population, through its variance, and the sample size n.

Therefore, when an observed value of the sample mean is far from a hypothesized value of μ (e.g., mean high blood pressures for a group of oral contraceptive users as compared to a typical average for women in the same age group), a natural question would be "Was it just due to chance, or something else?" To deal with questions such as this, statisticians have invented the concept of hypothesis tests and these tests have become widely used statistical techniques in the health sciences. In fact, it is almost impossible to read a research article in public health or medical sciences without running across hypothesis tests!

5.1.1. Hypothesis Tests

When a health investigator seeks to understand or explain something, for example the effect of a toxin or a drug, he/she usually formulates his/her research question in the form of a hypothesis. In the statistical context, a hypothesis is a statement about a distribution (e.g., "the distribution is normal") or its underlying parameter(s) (e.g., "$\mu = 10$"), or a statement about the relationship between probability distributions (e.g., "there is no statistical relationship"), or its parameters (e.g., "$\mu_1 = \mu_2$", that is equality of two population means). The hypothesis to be tested is called the null hypothesis and will be denoted by "H_0"; it is usually stated in the "null" form indicating *no difference* or *no relationship* between distributions or parameters, just as the constitutional guarantee that the accused is presumed innocent until proven guilty. In other words, under the null hypothesis, an observed difference (like the one between sample means for sample 1 and sample 2, respectively) just reflects chance variation. A hypothesis test, is a decision-making process, which examines a set or sets of data and, on the basis of expectation under H_0, leads to a decision on whether or not to reject H_0. An alternative hypothesis, which we denote by H_A, is a hypothesis that in some sense contradicts the null hypothesis H_0, just as the charge by the prosecution in a trial by jury. Under H_A, the difference is real, because $\mu_1 \neq \mu_2$, not by chance. A null hypothesis is rejected if and only if there is sufficiently strong evidence from the data to support its alternative—the names are somewhat unsettling, because the "alternative hypothesis" is, for a health investigator, the one he/she usually wants to prove (the null hypothesis is just a dull explanation of the findings—in terms of chance variation!). However, these are entrenched statistical terms and will be used as standard terms for the rest of this book.

Why is hypothesis testing important? Because in many circumstances we merely wish to know whether a certain proposition is true or false. The process of hypothesis tests provides a framework for making decisions on an objective basis, by weighing the relative merits of different hypotheses, rather than a subjective basis by simply looking at the numbers. Different people can form different opinions by looking at data (confounded by chance variation or sampling errors), but a hypothesis test provides a standardized decision-making process that will be consistent for all people. The mechanics of the tests vary with the hypotheses and measurement scales (Chapters 6–8), but the general philosophy and foundation is common and will be discussed with some details in this chapter.

5.1.2. Statistical Evidence

A null hypothesis is often concerned with a parameter or parameters of population(s). However, it is often either impossible, or too costly or time-consuming, to obtain the entire population data on any variable in order to see whether or not a null hypothesis is true. Decisions are thus made using sample data. Sample data are summarized into a statistic or statistics, which are used to estimate the parameter(s) involved in the null hypothesis. For example, if a null hypothesis is about μ (e.g., H_0: $\mu = 10$), then a good place to look for information about population mean μ is the sample mean. In that context, the statistic is called a test statistic; a test statistic can be used to measure the difference between the data (i.e., the numerical value of the mean obtained from the sample) and what is expected if the null hypothesis is true (i.e., "$\mu = 10$"). However, this evidence is statistical evidence; it varies from sample to sample (in the context of repeated sampling). It is a variable with a specific sampling distribution. The observed value is thus usually converted to a standard unit: the number of standard errors away from a hypothesized value. At this point, the logic of the test can be seen more clearly. It is an argument by contradiction, designed to show that the null hypothesis will lead to a less acceptable conclusion (an almost impossible event—some event which occurs with near zero probability) and must therefore be rejected. In other words, the difference between the data and what is expected on the null hypothesis would be very difficult—even absurd—to explain as a chance variation; it makes you want to abandon (or reject) the null hypothesis and believe in the alternative hypothesis because it is more plausible.

5.1.3. Errors

Since a null hypothesis H_0 may be true or false and our possible decisions are whether to reject or not to reject it, there are four possible outcomes or combinations. Two of the four outcomes are correct decisions:

(i) Not rejecting a true H_0
(ii) Rejecting a false H_0

but there are also two possible ways to commit an error:

(i) Type I error: a true null hypothesis H_0 is rejected
(ii) Type II error: a false null hypothesis H_0 is not rejected

These possibilities are shown as follows:

Truth	Decision by the Test	
	H_0 is not Rejected	H_0 is Rejected
H_0 is true	Correct decision	Type I error
H_0 is false	Type II error	Correct decision

The general aim in hypothesis testing is to keep "alpha" (α) and "beta" (β), the probabilities—in the context of repeated sampling—of Type I and Type II errors, respectively, as small as possible. However, if resources are limited, this goal requires a compromise because these actions are contradictory; for example, a decision to decrease the size of α will increase the size of β, and vice versa. Conventionally, we fix α at some specific conventional level, say $\alpha = .05$ or $\alpha = .01$, and β is controlled through the use of sample size(s).

Example 5.1

Suppose the national smoking rate among men is 25% and we want to study the smoking rate among men in the New England states. Let π be the proportion of New England men who smoke. The null hypothesis that the smoking prevalence in New England is the same as the national rate is expressed as:

$$H_0 : \pi = .25$$

Suppose we plan to take a sample of size ($n = 100$) and use this decision-making rule based on the sample proportion p:

$$\text{"If } p \leq .20, \quad \text{then } H_0 \text{ is rejected,"}$$

Then we have:

(i) Alpha (α) is defined as the probability of wrongly rejecting a true null hypothesis, that is,

$$\alpha = \Pr(p \leq .20; \quad \text{given that } \pi = .25)$$

Since ($n = 100$) is large enough for the Central Limit Theorem to apply, the sampling distribution of p is approximately normal with mean and variance, under H_0, given by

$$\text{Mean}(p) = .25$$

$$\text{Variance}(p) = \frac{(.25)(1-.25)}{100}$$

$$= (.043)^2$$

respectively. Therefore, for this decision-making rule,

$$\alpha = \Pr(p \le .20)$$

$$= \Pr\left(\frac{p - .25}{.043} \le \frac{.20 - .25}{.043}\right)$$

$$= \Pr(Z \le -1.16)$$

$$= .123$$

Of course, we can make this smaller (as small as we wish) by changing the decision-making rule; however, that will increase the value of β (the probability of a Type II error).

(ii) Suppose that the truth is

$$H_A : \pi = .15$$

Beta (β) is defined as the probability of not rejecting a false H_0, that is,

$$\beta = \Pr(p > .20; \quad \text{given that } \pi = .15)$$

Again, an application of the Central Limit Theorem indicates that the sampling distribution of p, under H_A, is approximately normal with mean and variance

$$\text{Mean}(p) = .15$$

$$\text{Variance}(p) = \frac{(.15)(1 - .15)}{100}$$

$$= (.036)^2$$

Therefore

$$\alpha = \Pr(p > .20)$$

$$= \Pr\left(\frac{p - .15}{.036} > \frac{.20 - .15}{.036}\right)$$

$$= \Pr(Z > 1.39)$$

$$= .082$$

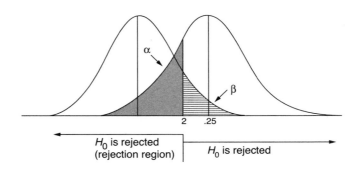

It can be seen that the probability of a Type II error, β, depends on a specific alternative (e.g., β is larger for H_A: $\pi = .17$ or any alternative hypothesis that specifies a value of π that is nearer to .25 than for H_A: $= .15$) and if we change the decision-making rule by using a smaller "cut point" then we would decrease α but increase β.

5.2. ANALOGIES

To reinforce some of the definitions or terms we have encountered, we consider in this section two analogies: trials by jury and medical screening tests.

5.2.1. Trials by Jury

Statisticians and statistics users may find a lot in common between a court trial and a statistical test of significance. In a criminal court, the jury's duty is to evaluate the evidence of the prosecution and the defense to determine whether a defendant is guilty or innocent. By use of the judge's instructions, which provide guidelines for their reaching a decision, the members of the jury can arrive at one of two verdicts: guilty or not guilty. Their decision may be correct or they could make one of two possible errors: convict an innocent person or free a criminal. The analogy between statistics and trials by jury goes as follows:

$$\text{Test of significance} \Longleftrightarrow \text{Court trial}$$

$$\text{Null hypothesis} \Longleftrightarrow \text{``Every defendant is innocent until proven guilty''}$$

$$\text{Research design} \Longleftrightarrow \text{Police investigation}$$

$$\text{Data and test statistics} \Longleftrightarrow \text{Evidence and exhibits}$$

$$\text{Statistical principles} \Longleftrightarrow \text{Judge's instruction}$$

$$\text{Statistical decision} \Longleftrightarrow \text{Verdict}$$

$$\text{Type I error} \Longleftrightarrow \text{Conviction of an innocent defendant}$$

$$\text{Type II error} \Longleftrightarrow \text{Acquittal of a criminal}$$

This analogy clarifies a very important concept: when a null hypothesis is not rejected it does not necessarily lead to its acceptance, because a "not guilty" verdict is just an indication of "lack of evidence" and "innocence" is one of the possibilities. That is, when a difference is not statistically significant, there are still two possibilities:

(i) The null hypothesis is true.
(ii) The null hypothesis is false, but there is not enough evidence from sample data to support its rejection (i.e., sample size is too small).

5.2.2. Medical Screening Tests

Another analogy of hypothesis testing can be found in the application of screening tests or diagnostic procedures. Following these procedures, clinical observations or laboratory techniques, individuals are classified as healthy or as having a disease. Of course, these tests are imperfect: healthy individuals will occasionally be classified wrongly as being ill while some individuals who are ill may fail to be detected. The analogy between statistical tests and screening tests goes briefly as follows:

$$\text{Type I error} \Longleftrightarrow \text{False positive}$$

$$\text{Type II error} \Longleftrightarrow \text{False negative}$$

so that:

$$\text{Alpha} = 1 - \text{Specificity}$$

$$\text{Beta} = 1 - \text{Sensitivity}$$

5.2.3. Common Expectations

The medical care system, with its high visibility and remarkable history of achievements, has been perceived somewhat naively by the general public as a perfect remedy factory. Medical tests are expected to correctly diagnose any disease (and physicians are expected to effectively treat and cure all diseases!). Another common misconception is the assumption that all tests, regardless of the disease being tested for, are equally accurate. People are shocked to learn that a test result is wrong (of course, the psychological effects could be devastating). Another analogy between tests of significance and screening tests exists here: statistical tests are also wrongly expected to always provide a correct decision!

In some medical cases such as infections, the presence or absence of bacteria and viruses are easier to confirm correctly. In other cases, such as the diagnosis of diabetes by a blood sugar test, the story is different. One very simple model for these situations would be to assume that the variable "X" (e.g., sugar level in blood) on which the test is based is distributed with different means for the healthy and diseased sub-populations:

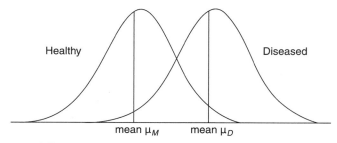

Difference between healthy and diseased subpopulations.

It can be seen from the figure that errors are unavoidable, especially when the two means of the two sub-populations, those healthy and those with the disease, μ_H and μ_D are close. The same is true for statistical tests of significance; when the null hypothesis H_0 is not true, it could be wrong a little or it could be very wrong. For example, for

$$H_0 : \mu = 10$$

the truth could be "$\mu = 12$" or "$\mu = 50$". If ($\mu = 50$), a Type II error would be less likely than if the truth is ($\mu = 12$) for which a Type II error is more likely.

5.3. SUMMARIES AND CONCLUSIONS

To perform a hypothesis test we take the following steps:

(1) Formulate a null hypothesis and an alternative hypothesis (this would follow our research question; the idea resulting from our research question would form our alternative hypothesis).

(2) From our research question forms our alternative hypothesis.

(3) Design the experiment and obtain data.

(4) Choose a test statistic (this choice depends on the null hypothesis and measurement scale).

(5) Summarize findings and state appropriate conclusions.

This section involves the last step of the above process.

5.3.1. Rejection Region

The most common approach is the formation of a *decision rule*. All possible values of the chosen test statistic (in the repeated sampling context) are divided into two regions. The region consisting of values of the test statistic for which the null hypothesis H_0 is rejected is called the *rejection region*. The values of the test statistic comprising the rejection region are those values that are *less likely to occur* if the null hypothesis is true, and the decision rule tells us to reject H_0 if the value of the test statistic that we compute from our sample(s) is one of the values in this region. For example, if a null hypothesis is about the population mean μ, say

$$H_0 : \mu = 10$$

then a good place to look for a test statistic for H_0 is the sample mean, and it is obvious that H_0 should be rejected if the observed value of the sample mean is far away from "10"— the hypothesized value of the population mean μ. Before we proceed, a number of related concepts should be made clear:

One-Sided Versus Two-Sided Tests

In the above example with (H_0: $\mu = 10$), a vital question is "Are we interested in the deviation of the sample mean from 10 in one or both directions?" If we are interested in determining whether μ is significantly *different* from 10, we would perform a *two-sided test* and the rejection region would consist of values of the sample mean in both direction: we reject H_0 if the observed value of the sample mean is too small (compared to "10") and we also reject H_0 if the observed value of the sample mean is too large. On the contrary, if we are interested in whether μ is significantly *larger* than 10, we would perform a *one-sided test* and the rejection region would consist of only larger values of the sample mean. A one-sided test is indicated for research questions like these: Is a new drug *superior* to a standard drug? Does the air pollution *exceed* safe limits? Has the death rate been *reduced* for those who quit smoking? A two-sided test is indicated for research questions like these: Is there a *difference* between cholesterol levels of men and women? Does the mean age of a target population *differ* from that of the general population? In other words, a *key word* or two in the research question whether a one-sided test or a two-sided test is appropriate.

Level of Significance

The decision as to which values of the test statistic go into the rejection region, or where is the cut point, is made on the basis of the desired level of Type I error α (also called the *size* of the test). A computed value of the test statistic that falls in the rejection region is said to be *statistically significant*. Common choices for α, the level of significance, are .01, .05, and .10; the .05 or 5% level is especially popular.

Reproducibility

Here we aim to clarify another misconception about hypothesis tests. A very simple and common situation for hypothesis tests is that the test statistic, for example, the sample mean, is normally distributed with different means under the null hypothesis H_0 and alternative hypothesis H_A. A one-tailed test could be graphically represented as follows:

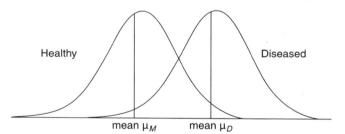

Difference between healthy and diseased subpopulations.

It should now be clear that a statistical conclusion is not guaranteed to be reproducible. For example if the alternative hypothesis is true and the mean of the distribution of the test statistic (see graph above) is right at the cut point then the probability would be 50% to obtain a test statistic inside the rejection region.

p-Values

Instead of saying that an observed value of the test statistic is significant (i.e., falling into the rejection region for a given choice of α) or is not significant, many writers in the research literature prefer to report findings in terms of *p*-values. The *p-value* is the probability of getting values of the test statistic as extreme as, or more extreme than, that observed if the null hypothesis is true. For the above example of

$$H_0 : \mu = 10$$

if the test is a one-sided test, we would have

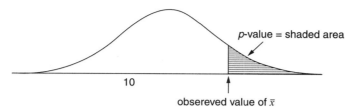

and if the test is a two-sided test then we have

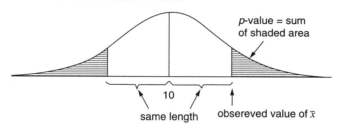

The curve in these graphs represents the sampling distribution of the *test statistic,* the sample mean, if the null hypothesis is true.

As compared to the approach of choosing a level of significance and formulating a decision rule, the use of the *p*-value criterion would be as follows:

(i) If *p*-value is less than a chosen α, the null hypothesis is rejected.

(ii) If *p*-value is greater than a chosen α, the null hypothesis is not rejected.

However, the reporting of *p*-values as part of the results of an investigation is more informative to the readers than such statements as "the null hypothesis is rejected at the .05 level of significance" or "the results were not significant at the .05 level". Reporting the *p-value* associated with a test lets the reader know how common or how rare is the computed value of the test statistic given that the null hypothesis is true. In other words, the *p*-value can be used as a *measure* of the *compatibility* between the data (reality) and a null hypothesis (theory); the smaller the *p*-value, the less compatible the theory and the reality. A compromise between the two approaches would be to report both in statements such as "the difference is statistically significant (*p*-value < .05)".

In the reporting of *p*-values as in the above statement "the difference is statistically significant (*p*-value < .05)", researchers generally agree on the following conventional terms:

$$p\text{-value} > .10 \leftrightarrow \text{Result is not significant}$$

$$.05 < p\text{-value} < .10 \leftrightarrow \text{Result is marginally significant}$$

$$.01 < p\text{-value} < .05 \leftrightarrow \text{Result is significant}$$

$$p\text{-value} < .01 \leftrightarrow \text{Result is highly significant}$$

Finally, it should be noted that the difference, between means for example, although statistically significant may be so small that it has little health consequence. In other words, the result may be *statistically significant* but may not be *practically significant*.

Example 5.2

Suppose the national smoking rate among men is 25% and we want to study the smoking rate among men in the New England states. The null hypothesis under investigation is

$$H_0 : \pi = .25$$

Of $(n = 100)$ males sampled, $(x = 15)$ were found to be smokers. Does the proportion π of smokers in New England states *differ* from that of the nation?

Since $(n = 100)$ is large enough for the Central Limit Theorem to apply it indicates that the sampling distribution of the sample proportion p, under the null hypothesis, is approximately normal with mean and variance:

$$\text{Mean } (p) = .25$$
$$\text{Variance } (p) = \frac{(.25)(1-.25)}{100}$$
$$= (.043)^2$$

The observed value of p from our sample is .15 (=15/100) representing a difference of .10 from the hypothesized value of .25. The p-value is defined as the probability of getting a value of the test statistic as extreme as, or more extreme than, that observed if the null hypothesis is true. We have

$$p\text{-value} = \Pr(p \le .15 \quad \text{or } p \ge .35)$$
$$= (2)\Pr(p \ge .35)$$
$$= (2)\Pr(Z \ge \frac{.35-.25}{.043} = 2.33)$$
$$= (2)\Pr(.5-.4901)$$
$$\cong .02$$

In other words, with the data given, the difference between the national smoking rate and the smoking rate of New England states is statistically significant $(p < .05)$.

5.3.2. Relationship to Confidence Intervals

Suppose we consider a hypothesis of the form

$$H_0 : \mu = \mu_0$$

where μ_0 is a known hypothesized value, say "10". A two-sided hypothesis test for H_0 is related to confidence intervals as follows:

(1) If μ_0 is not included in the 95% confidence interval for μ, the null hypothesis H_0 should be rejected at the .05 level.
(2) If μ_0 is included in the 95% confidence interval for μ, the null hypothesis H_0 should not be rejected at the .05 level.

Example 5.3

Consider the hypothetical data set in Example 5.2. Our point estimate of smoking prevalence in New England is .16 ($p = 15/100$); its standard error is

$$SE(p) = \sqrt{\frac{(.15)(1-.15)}{100}}$$
$$= .036$$

Therefore, a 95% confidence interval for the New England states smoking rate π is given by

$$.15 \pm (1.96)(.036) = (.079, .221)$$

It is noted that the national rate of .25 is *not included* in that confidence interval; the result agrees with that of Example 5.2.

EXERCISES

5.1 For each part, state the null H_0 and alternative H_A hypotheses:
   (a) Has the average community level of suspended particulates for the month of August exceeded $30 \, mcg/m^3$?
   (b) Does mean age of onset of a certain acute disease for school children differ from 11.5?
   (c) A psychologist claims that the average IQ of a sample of 60 children is significantly above the normal IQ of 100.
   (d) Is the average cross-sectional area of the lumen of coronary arteries for men, ages 40–59, less than 31.5% of the total arterial cross section?
   (e) Is the mean hemoglobin level of a group of high-altitude workers different from 16 g/cc?
   (f) Does the average speed of 50 cars as checked by radar on a particular highway differ from 55 mph?

5.2 The distribution of diastolic blood pressures for the population of female diabetics between the ages of 30 and 34 has an unknown mean μ and a standard deviation of $\sigma = 9$ mmHg. It may be useful to physicians to know whether the mean μ of this population is equal to the mean diastolic blood pressure of the general population of females of this age group, which is 74.5 mmHg. What is the null hypothesis and what is the alternative hypothesis for this test?

5.3 E. canis infection is a tick-borne disease of dogs that is sometimes contracted by humans. Among infected humans, the distribution of white blood cell counts has an unknown mean μ and a standard deviation σ. In the general population, the mean white blood count is 7250/mm^3. It is believed that persons infected with E. canis must on average have a lower white blood cell count. What is the null hypothesis for the test? Is this a one-sided or two-sided alternative?

5.4 It is feared that the smoking rate in young females has increased in the last several years. In 1985, 38% of the females in the 17–24 years age group were smokers. An experiment is to be conducted to gain evidence to support the increase contention. Set up the appropriate null and alternative hypotheses. Explain in a practical sense what, if anything, has occurred if a Type I or Type II error has been committed.

5.5 A group of investigators wishes to explore the relationship between the use of hair dyes and the development of breast cancer in females. A group of 1000 beauticians 40–49 years of age is identified and followed for 5 years. After 5 years, 20 new cases of breast cancer have occurred. Assume that breast cancer incidence over this time period for average American women in this age group is 7/1000. We wish to test the hypothesis that using hair dyes increases the risk of breast cancer. Is a one-sided or a two-sided test appropriate here? Compute the p-value for your choice.

5.6 Height and weight are often used in epidemiological studies as possible predictors of disease outcomes. If the people in the study are assessed in a clinic, then heights and weights are usually measured directly. However, if the people are interviewed at home or by mail, then a person's self-reported height and weight are often used instead. Suppose we conduct a study on 10 people to test the comparability of these two methods. Data from these 10 people were obtained using both methods on each person. What is the criterion for the comparison? What is the null hypothesis? Should a two-sided or a one-sided test be used here?

5.7 Suppose that 28 cancer deaths are noted among workers exposed to asbestos in a building materials plant from 1981 to 1985. Only 20.5 cancer deaths are expected from statewide mortality rates. Suppose we want to know if there is a significant excess of cancer deaths among these workers. What is the null hypothesis? Is a one-sided or two-sided test appropriate here?

5.8 A food frequency questionnaire was mailed to 20 subjects to assess the intake of various food groups. The sample standard deviation of vitamin C intake over the 20 subjects was 15 (exclusive of vitamin C supplements). Suppose we know from using an in-person diet interview method in a large previous study that the standard deviation is 20. Formulate the null and alternative hypotheses if we want to test for any differences between the standard deviations of the two methods.

5.9 In Example 5.1, it was assumed that the national smoking rate among men is 25%. A study is to be conducted for New England states using a sample size ($n = 100$) and the decision rule:

"If $p \leq .20$, H_0 is rejected"

where the null hypothesis H_0 is:

$$H_0 : \pi = .25$$

where π and p are population and sample proportions, respectively, for New England states. Is this a one-tailed or two-tailed test?

5.10 In Example 5.1, with the rule

"If $p \leq .20$, H_0 is rejected"

it was found that the probabilities of Type I and Type II errors are $\alpha = .123$ and $\beta = .082$ for the alternative hypothesis H_A: $\pi = .15$. Find the probabilities of Type I and Type II errors α and β if the rule is changed to

"If $p \leq .18$, H_0 is rejected"

5.11 Answer the questions in Exercise 10 above for the decision rule

"If $p \leq .22$, H_0 is rejected"

5.12 Recalculate the p-value in Example 5.2, it was found that 18 (instead of 15) men in a sample of ($n = 100$) are smokers.

Comparison of Population Proportions

If each element of a data set may lie only at a few isolated points, we have a *discrete* or *categorical data* set; examples include sex, race, or some sort of artificial grading used as outcomes. For discrete data, the basic *statistics* representing the outcomes is the *sample proportion* that is an estimate of the corresponding *population proportion*. If each element of a data set may lie anywhere on the numerical scale, we have a *continuous* data set; examples include blood pressure, cholesterol level, or time of a certain event. For continuous data, the basic *statistic* representing the outcomes is the *sample mean*, which is an estimate of the corresponding *population mean*. This chapter presents basic inferential methods for categorical data starting with the most simple case of the one-sample problem with binary data.

6.1. ONE-SAMPLE PROBLEM WITH BINARY DATA

In this type of problem, we have a *sample of binary data* (n, x) with n being an adequately large sample size and x the number of positive outcomes among the n observations, and we consider the null hypothesis:

$$H_0 : \pi = \pi_0$$

where π is a fixed and known number between 0 and 1; for example,

$$H_0 : \pi = .25$$

π_0 is often a *standardized* or *referenced figure*, for example, the effect of a standard drug or therapy or the national smoking rate (where the national sample is often large enough so as to produce negligible sampling error in π_0). Or, we could be concerned with a research question like "Does the side effect (of a certain drug) exceed regulated limit π_0?" In Exercise 5.2, we tried to compare the incidence of breast cancer among female beauticians

Health and Numbers: A Problems-Based Introduction to Biostatistics, Third Edition, by Chap T. Le
Copyright © 2009 John Wiley & Sons, Inc.

(who are frequently exposed to the use of hair dyes) versus a standard level of 7/1000 (for 5 years) for "average American women." The figure 7/1000 is π_0 for that example.

In a typical situation, the null hypothesis of a statistical test is concerned with a parameter; the parameter in this case is the proportion π. Sample data are summarized into a statistic that is used to estimate the parameter under investigation. Since the parameter under investigation is the proportion π, our focus in this case is the sample proportion p. In general, a statistic is itself a variable with a specific sampling distribution (in the context of repeated sampling). Our statistic in this case is the sample proportion p, the corresponding sampling distribution is easily obtained by invoking the *Central Limit Theorem*. With large sample size and assuming that the null hypothesis H_0 is true, it is the normal distribution with mean and variance given by

$$\mu_p = \pi_0$$

$$\sigma_p^2 = \frac{\pi_0(1-\pi_0)}{n}$$

respectively. From this sampling distribution, the observed value of the sample proportion can be converted into standard unit: the number of standard errors away from the hypothesized value of π_0. In other words, to perform a test of significance for H_0, we proceed with the following steps:

(1) Decide whether a *one-sided* test or a *two-sided* test is appropriate.
(2) Choose a *level of significance* alpha (α), a common choice being .05.
(3) Calculate the z-*score*

$$z = \frac{p-\pi_0}{\sqrt{\dfrac{\pi_0(1-\pi_0)}{n}}}$$

(4) From the table for the standard normal distribution (Appendix B) and the choice of α, a common choice is $\alpha = .05$, the *rejection region* is determined by

(a) For a one-sided test,

$$z < -1.65 \quad \text{for} \quad H_A : \pi < p_0$$
$$z > +1.65 \quad \text{for} \quad H_A : \pi > p_0$$

(b) For a two-sided test or $H_A : \pi \neq \pi_0$

$$z < -1.96 \quad \text{or} \quad z > +1.96$$

Example 6.1

A group of investigators wishes to explore the relationship between the use of hair dyes and the development of breast cancer in women. A sample of ($n = 1000$) female beauticians 40–49 years of age is identified and followed for 5 years. After 5 years, ($x = 20$) new cases of breast cancer have occurred. It is known that breast cancer incidence over this time period for average American women in this age group is $\pi_0 = 7/1000$. We wish to test the hypothesis that using hair dyes *increases* the risk of breast cancer (a *one-sided* alternative). We have the following:

(1) A one-sided test with

$$H_A : \pi > 7/1000$$

(2) Using the conventional choice of $\alpha = .05$ leads to the rejection region: $z > 1.65$

(3) From the data,

$$p = \frac{20}{1000}$$
$$= .02$$

an observed sample proportion leading to

$$z = \frac{.02 - .007}{\sqrt{\dfrac{(.007)(1 - .007)}{1000}}}$$
$$= 4.93$$

that is, the observed proportion p is 4.93 standard errors away from the hypothesized value of $\pi_0 = .007$

(4) Since the computed z-score falls into the rejection region ($4.93 > 1.65$), the null hypothesis is rejected at the chosen .05 level. In fact, the difference is very highly significant ($p < .001$).

6.2. ANALYSIS OF PAIR-MATCHED BINARY DATA

The method presented in this section applies to cases where each subject or member of a group is observed twice for the presence or absence of a certain characteristic (e.g., at admission to and discharge from a hospital), or matched pairs are observed for the presence or absence of the same characteristic. A popular application is an *epidemiological design* called a *pair-matched case–control study*. In case–control studies, cases of a specific disease are ascertained as they arise from population-based registers or lists of hospital admissions, and controls are sampled either as disease-free individuals from the population at risk or as hospitalized patients having a diagnosis other than the one under investigation. As a technique to control confounding factors, individual cases are matched, often one-to-one, to controls chosen to have similar values for confounding variables such as age, sex, race, and so on.

For *pair-matched data* with a single binary exposure (e.g., smoking versus nonsmoking), data can be represented by a 2×2 table, where $(+, -)$ denotes the (exposed, nonexposed) outcome, as follows:

Cases	Matching Control	
	Exposed	Nonexposed
Exposed	a	b
Nonexposed	c	d

In this 2×2 table, a denotes the number of pairs with two exposed members, b denotes the number of pairs where the case is exposed but the matched control is unexposed, c denotes the number of pairs where the case is unexposed but the matched control is exposed, and d denotes the number of pairs with two unexposed members. The analysis of pair-matched data with a single binary exposure can be seen, heuristically, as follows. What we really want to do is to compare the incidence of exposure among the cases with that of the controls; the parts of the data showing no difference, the number a of pairs with two exposed members and the number d of pairs with two unexposed members, would contribute nothing as evidence in such a comparison. The comparison, therefore, relies solely on two other frequencies, b and c; under the null hypothesis that the exposure has nothing to do with the disease, we *expect* $(b = c)$ or $(b)/(b + c) = .5$. In other words, the analysis of pair-matched data with a single binary exposure can be seen as a special case of the one-sample problem with binary of Section 6.1 with $(n = b + c)$, x is b, and $\pi_0 = .5$. Recall the form of the test statistic of the previous section, we have:

$$z = \frac{p - \pi_0}{\sqrt{\dfrac{\pi_0(1 - \pi_0)}{n}}}$$

$$= \frac{\dfrac{b}{b + c} - \dfrac{1}{2}}{\sqrt{\dfrac{\left(\dfrac{1}{2}\right)\left(\dfrac{1}{2}\right)}{b + c}}}$$

$$= \frac{b - c}{\sqrt{b + c}}$$

The decision is based on the standardized z-score and referring to the percentiles of the standard normal distribution or, in the two-sided form, the square of the above statistic, denoted by

$$X^2 = \frac{(b - c)^2}{b + c}$$

and the test is known as the McNemar's Chi-square test. (1) If the test is one-sided, z is used and the null hypothesis is rejected at the .05 level when $z > 1.65$; (2) If the test is two-sided, X^2 is used and the null hypothesis is rejected at the .05 level when $X^2 > 3.84$. It should be noted that $3.84 = (1.96)^2$, so that $X^2 > 3.84$ is equivalent to $z < -1.96$ or $z > +1.96$) and the McNemar's Chi-square test is equivalent to the two-sided "z-test" (comparing the computed value of the above z statistic to percentiles of the standard normal distribution).

Example 6.2

It has been noted that metalworkers have an increased risk of cancer of the internal nose and paranasal sinuses, perhaps as a result of exposure to cutting oils. Therefore, a study was conducted to see whether this particular exposure also increases the risk of squamous cell carcinoma of the scrotum.

Cases included all 45 squamous cell carcinomas of the scrotum diagnosed in Connecticut residents from 1955 to 1973, as obtained from the Connecticut Tumor Registry. Matched controls were selected for each case based on the age at death (within 8 years), year of death (within 3 years), and number of jobs as obtained from combined death certificate and Directory sources. An occupational indicator of metalworker (yes/no) was evaluated as the possible risk factor in this study; results are as follows:

	Matching Controls	
Cases	Yes	No
Yes	2	26
No	5	12

We have, for a one-tailed test,

$$z = \frac{26-5}{\sqrt{26+5}}$$
$$= 3.77$$

indicating a very highly significant increased risk associated with the exposure ($p < .001$).

Example 6.3

A study in Maryland identified 4032 white persons, enumerated in a nonofficial 1963 census, who became widowed between 1963 and 1974. These people were matched, one-to-one, to married persons on the basis of race, sex, year of birth, and geography of residence. The matched pairs were followed to a second census in 1975, and we have the following overall male mortality:

Widowed	Married Men	
Men	Died	Alive
Died	2	292
Alive	210	700

An application of the McNemar's Chi-square test yields

$$X^2 = \frac{(292-210)^2}{292+210}$$
$$= 13.39$$

It can be seen that the null hypothesis of equal mortality should be rejected at the .05 level $(13.39 > 3.84$; p-value $< .001$.

6.3. COMPARISON OF TWO PROPORTIONS

Perhaps the most common problem involving categorical data is the comparison of two proportions. In this type of problem, we have two independent samples of binary data (n_1, x_1) and (n_2, x_2) where the ns are adequately large sample sizes that may or may not be equal, the xs are the numbers of "positive" outcomes in the two samples, and we consider the null hypothesis:

$$H_0 : \pi_1 = \pi_2$$

expressing the equality of the two population proportions.

To perform a test of significance for H_0, we proceed with the following steps:

(1) Decide whether a one-sided test, say

$$H_A : \pi_1 > \pi_2$$

or a two-sided test,

$$H_A : \pi_1 \neq \pi_2$$

is appropriate.

(2) Choose a significance level alpha (α), a common choice being $\alpha = .05$.

(3) Calculate the z-score

$$z = \frac{p_2 - p_1}{\sqrt{p(1-p)\left(\frac{1}{n_1} + \frac{1}{n_2}\right)}}$$

where p (without a subscript) is the "pooled proportion," a proportion obtained by pooling the two samples together – an estimate of the common proportion under H_0; p is defined by

$$p = \frac{x_1 + x_2}{n_1 + n_2}$$

(4) Refer to the table for standard normal distribution (Appendix B) for selecting a cut point. For example, if the choice of α is .05, then the rejection region is determined by

(a) For the one-sided alternative $H_A: \pi_1 > \pi_2$, $z > +1.65$.
(b) For the one-sided alternative $H_A: \pi_1 < \pi_2$, $z < -1.65$.
(c) For the two-sided alternative $H_A: \pi_1 \neq \pi_2$, $z \leq -1.96$ or $z \geq 1.96$.

What we are doing here follows the same format used in the previous sections.

(1) The basic term of $(p_2 - p_1)$ measures the difference between the two samples,
(2) Its expected hypothesized value (i.e. under H_0) is zero.
(3) The denominator of z is the standard error of $(p_2 - p_1)$, a measure of how good $(p_2 - p_1)$ is as an estimate of $(\pi_2 - \pi_1)$; z measures how many standard errors $(p_2 - p_1)$ is from zero, its hypothesized value.
(4) The z-score measures the number of standard errors that $(p_2 - p_1)$, the evidence, is away from its hypothesized value.

In the two-sided form, the square of the z-score, denoted X^2 and called "Chi-squared," is used more often. The test is referred to as the *Chi-square test* and the null hypothesis is rejected at the .05 level when $X^2 > 3.84$ (since $3.84 = (1.96)^2$, the decision remains the same). With data arranged in the form of a 2×2 table, the test statistic can also be obtained using the short-cut formula with its denominator being the product of the four marginal totals.

Exposure	Sample #1	Sample #2	Total
Yes	a	c	$a + c$
No	b	d	$b + d$
Total	$a + b$	$c + d$	n

Test Statistic:

$$X^2 = \frac{n(ad - bc)^2}{(a+b)(c+d)(a+c)(b+d)}$$

Example 6.4

A study was conducted to see whether an important public health intervention would significantly reduce the smoking rate among men. Of ($n = 100$) males sampled in 1965 at the time of the release of the Surgeon General's report on the health consequences of smoking, ($x = 51$) were found to be smokers. In 1980, a second random sample of ($n = 100$) males, similarly gathered, indicated that ($x = 43$) were smokers.

An application of the above method yields:

$$p = \frac{51+43}{100+100}$$

$$= .47$$

$$z = \frac{.51-.43}{\sqrt{(.47)(.53)\left(\dfrac{1}{100}+\dfrac{1}{100}\right)}}$$

$$= 1.13$$

It can be seen that the observed rate was reduced from 51 to 43%, but the reduction is not statistically significant at the .05 level ($z = 1.13 < 1.65$; two-sided p-value $= .2585$).

Example 6.5

An investigation was made into fatal poisonings of children by two drugs that were among the leading causes of such deaths. In each case, an inquiry was made as to how the child had received the fatal overdose, and responsibility for the accident was assessed. Results were

	Drug A	Drug B
Child responsible	8	12
Child not responsible	31	19

We have the proportions of cases for which the child is responsible,

$$p_A = \frac{8}{8+31}$$

$$= .205$$

$$p_B = \frac{12}{12+19}$$

$$= .387$$

suggesting that they are not the same and that a child seems more prone to taking B (38.7%) than A (20.5%). However, the Chi-square statistic

$$X^2 = \frac{(39+31)[(8)(19)-(31)(12)]}{(39)(31)(20)(50)}$$

$$= 2.80$$

shows that the difference is not statistically significant at the .05 level (p-value $= .0943$).

Example 6.6

In Example mprb1.2, a case–control study was conducted to identify reasons for the exceptionally high rate of lung cancer among male residents of coastal Georgia. The primary risk factor under investigation was employment in shipyards during World War II, and the following table provides data for nonsmokers:

Shipbuilding	Cases	Controls
Yes	11	35
No	50	203
Total	51	238

With current smoking being the exposure, we have for the cases

$$p_2 = \frac{11}{58}$$
$$= .180$$

and for the controls

$$p_1 = \frac{35}{238}$$
$$= .147$$

An application of the procedure yields a pooled proportion of

$$p = \frac{11+35}{61+238}$$
$$= .154$$

leading to

$$z = \frac{.180-.147}{\sqrt{(.154)(.846)\left(\frac{1}{61} + \frac{1}{238}\right)}}$$
$$= .64$$

It can be seen that the rate of employment for the cases (18.0%) was higher than that for the controls (14.7%) but the difference is not statistically significant at the .05 level ($z = .64 < 1.65$; p-value $= .52218$).

Example 6.7

The role of smoking in the etiology of pancreatitis has been recognized for many years. To provide estimates of the quantitative significance of these factors, a hospital-based study was carried out in eastern Massachusetts and Rhode Island between 1975 and 1979. Ninety-eight patients who had a hospital discharge diagnosis of pancreatitis were included in this unmatched case–control study. The control group consisted of 451 patients admitted for diseases other than those of the pancreas and biliary tract. Risk factor information was obtained from a standardized interview with each subject, conducted by a trained interviewer. The following are some data for the males:

Use of Cigarettes	Cases	Controls
Never	2	56
Ex-smokers	13	80
Current smokers	38	81
Total	53	217

With current smoking being the exposure, we have for the cases

$$p_2 = \frac{38}{53}$$
$$= .717$$

and for the controls

$$p_1 = \frac{81}{217}$$
$$= .373$$

An application of the procedure yields a pooled proportion of

$$p = \frac{38 + 81}{53 + 217}$$
$$= .441$$

leading to

$$z = \frac{.717 - .373}{\sqrt{(.441)(.559)\left(\frac{1}{53} + \frac{1}{217}\right)}}$$
$$= 4.52$$

It can be seen that the proportion of smokers among the cases (71.7%) was higher than that for the controls (37.7%) and the difference is highly statistically significant (p-value $< .001$).

6.4. THE MANTEL–HAENSZEL METHOD

We are often interested only in investigating the relationship between two binary variables, for example, a disease and an exposure; however, we have to control for confounders. A confounding variable is a variable that may be associated with either the disease or the exposure or both. For example, in Example 1.2, a case–control study was undertaken to investigate the relationship between lung cancer and employment in shipyards during World War II among male residents of coastal Georgia. In this case, smoking is a confounder; it has been found to be associated with lung cancer and it may be associated with employment because construction workers are likely to be smokers. Specifically, we want to know

(i) Among smokers, whether or not shipbuilding and lung cancer are related, and

(ii) Among nonsmokers, whether or not shipbuilding and lung cancer are related.

The underlying question concerns conditional independence between lung cancer and shipbuilding; however, we do not want to reach separate conclusions, one at each level of smoking. Assuming that the confounder, smoking, is not an effect modifier (i.e., smoking does not alter the relationship between lung cancer and shipbuilding), we want to pool data for a combined decision. When both the disease and the exposure are binary, a popular method to achieve this task is the *Mantel–Haenszel method*. The process can be summarized as follows:

(i) We form 2×2 tables, one at each level of the confounder.

(ii) At a level of the confounder, we have

Exposure	Disease Classification		
	Positive	Negative	Total
Yes	a	b	r_1
No	c	d	r_2
Total	c_1	c_2	n

Under the null hypothesis and fixed marginal totals, frequency of the upper left cell a is distributed with mean and variance:

$$E_0(a) = \frac{r_1 c_1}{n}$$

$$\mathrm{Var}_0(a) = \frac{r_1 r_2 c_1 c_2}{n^2(n-1)}$$

and the Mantel–Haenszel test is based on the z-statistic

$$z = \frac{\sum a - \sum \dfrac{r_1 c_1}{n}}{\sqrt{\sum \dfrac{r_1 r_2 c_1 c_2}{n^2(n-1)}}}$$

where the summation (Σ) is across levels of the confounder. Of course, one can use the square of the z-score, a Chi-square test at one degree of freedom, for two-sided alternatives. When the above test is statistically significant, the association between the disease and the exposure is *real*. Since we assume that the confounder is not an effect modifier, the odds ratio is constant across its levels. The odds ratio at each level is estimated by ad/bc; the Mantel–Haenszel procedure pools data across levels of the confounder to obtain a combined estimate:

$$\text{OR}_{\text{MH}} = \frac{\sum \dfrac{ad}{n}}{\sum \dfrac{bc}{n}}$$

Example 6.8

A case–control study was conducted to identify reasons for the exceptionally high rate of lung cancer among male residents of coastal Georgia as first presented in Example 1.2. The primary risk factor under investigation was employment in shipyards during World War II, and data are tabulated separately for three levels of smoking as follows:

Smoking	Shipbuilding	Cases	Controls
No	Yes	11	35
	No	50	203
Moderate	Yes	70	42
	No	217	220
Heavy	Yes	14	3
	No	96	50

There are three 2×2 tables, one for each level of smoking.

(1) We begin with the 2×2 table for *nonsmokers*:

Smoking	Shipbuilding	Cases	Controls	Total
No	Yes	11(a)	35(b)	46
	No	50(c)	203(d)	253
	Total	51	238	299(n)

we have, for the nonsmokers,
$$a = 11$$

$$\frac{r_1 c_1}{n} = \frac{(46)(61)}{299}$$

$$= 9.38$$

$$\frac{r_1 r_2 c_1 c_2}{n^2(n-1)} = \frac{(46)(253)(61)(238)}{(299)^2(298)}$$

$$= 6.34$$

$$\frac{ad}{n} = \frac{(11)(203)}{299}$$

$$= 7.47$$

$$\frac{bc}{n} = \frac{(35)(50)}{299}$$

$$= 5.85$$

The process is repeated for each of the other two smoking levels.
(2) For moderate smokers

Smoking	Shipbuilding	Cases	Controls	Total
Moderate	Yes	70(a)	42(b)	112
	No	217(c)	220(d)	437
	Total	287	262	549(n)

$$a = 70$$

$$\frac{r_1 c_1}{n} = \frac{(112)(287)}{549}$$

$$= 58.55$$

$$\frac{r_1 r_2 c_1 c_2}{n^2(n-1)} = \frac{(112)(437)(287)(262)}{(549)^2(548)}$$

$$= 22.28$$

$$\frac{ad}{n} = \frac{(70)(220)}{549}$$

$$= 28.05$$

$$\frac{bc}{n} = \frac{(42)(217)}{549}$$

$$= 16.60$$

(3) And for heavy smokers

Smoking	Shipbuilding	Cases	Controls	Total
Heavy	Yes	14(a)	3(b)	17
	No	96(c)	50(d)	146
	Total	110	53	163(n)

$$a = 14$$

$$\frac{r_1 c_1}{n} = \frac{(17)(110)}{163}$$

$$= 14.47$$

$$\frac{r_1 r_2 c_1 c_2}{n^2 (n-1)} = \frac{(17)(146)(110)(53)}{(163)^2 (162)}$$

$$= 3.36$$

$$\frac{ad}{n} = \frac{(14)(50)}{163}$$

$$= 4.29$$

$$\frac{bc}{n} = \frac{(3)(96)}{163}$$

$$= 1.77$$

The above results from the three levels of the confounder (smoking) are combined to obtain the z-score:

$$z = \frac{(11-9.38) + (70-58.55) + (14-11.47)}{\sqrt{6.34 + 22.28 + 3.36}}$$

$$= 2.76$$

and a z-score of 2.76 yields a one-sided p-value of .0029, which is beyond the 1% level. This result is stronger than those for tests at each level because it is based on more information where all data at all three smoking levels are used. The combined odds ratio estimate is

$$OR_{MH} = \frac{7.47 + 28.05 + 4.28}{5.85 + 16.60 + 1.77}$$

$$= 1.64$$

This combined estimate of the odds ratio, 1.64, represents an approximate increase of 64% in lung cancer risk for those employed in the shipbuilding industry.

The following is another similar example aiming at the possible effects of oral contraceptive use on myocardial infarction (MI).

Example 6.9

A case–control study was conducted to investigate the relationship between myocardial infarction and OC use. The data, stratified by cigarette smoking, were

Smoking	OC Use	Cases	Controls
No	Yes	4	52
	No	34	754
Yes	Yes	25	83
	No	171	853

There are two 2×2 tables, one for each level of smoking.

(1) We begin with the 2×2 table for *nonsmokers*:

Smoking	OC Use	Cases	Controls	Total
No	Yes	4(a)	52(b)	56
	No	34(c)	754(d)	788
	Total	38	806	844

$$a = 4$$

$$\frac{r_1 c_1}{n} = \frac{(56)(38)}{844}$$

$$= 2.52$$

$$\frac{r_1 r_2 c_1 c_2}{n^2(n-1)} = \frac{(56)(788)(38)(806)}{(844)^2(843)}$$

$$= 2.25$$

(2) And for smokers,

Smoking	OC Use	Cases	Controls	Total
Yes	Yes	25(a)	83(b)	108
	No	171(c)	853(d)	1024
	Total	196	936	1132

$$a = 25$$

$$\frac{r_1 c_1}{n} = \frac{(108)(196)}{1132}$$

$$= 18.70$$

$$\frac{r_1 r_2 c_1 c_2}{n^2(n-1)} = \frac{(108)(1024)(196)(936)}{(1132)^2(1131)}$$

$$= 14.00$$

The above results from the two levels of smoking are combined to obtain the z-score:

$$z = \frac{(4-2.52) + (25-18.70)}{\sqrt{2.25 + 14.00}}$$

$$= 1.93$$

and a z-score of 1.93 yields a one-sided p-value of .0268, which is beyond the 5% level. This result is stronger than those for tests at each level because it is based on more information where all data at all three smoking levels are used.

We have for nonsmokers

$$\frac{ad}{n} = \frac{(4)(754)}{844}$$

$$= 3.57$$

$$\frac{bc}{n} = \frac{(52)(34)}{845}$$

$$= 2.09$$

And for smokers

$$\frac{ad}{n} = \frac{(25)(853)}{1132}$$

$$= 18.84$$

$$\frac{bc}{n} = \frac{(83)(171)}{1132}$$

$$= 12.54$$

The above results from the two levels of the confounder (smoking) are combined to estimate the common odds ratio:

$$OR_{MH} = \frac{3.57 + 18.84}{2.09 + 12.54}$$

$$= 1.53$$

This combined estimate of the odds ratio, 1.53, represents an approximate increase of 53% in myocardial infarction risk for oral contraceptive users.

6.5. COMPUTATIONAL AIDS

All the computations in this chapter can be implemented easily using a calculator *provided* that data have summarized into the form of a *2 × 2 table*. Read Section 1.4 on how to use

Excel's *Pivot Table* procedure to form a 2×2 table from a raw data file. After value of a statistic has been obtained, you can use *NORMDIST* (Section 3.4) to obtain exact *p*-value associated with a *z*-score and/or *CHIDIST* to obtain exact *p*-value associated with a Chi-square statistic and McNemar Chi-square statistic; CHIDIST procedure can be used in the same way as the *TDIST* procedure (Section 3.5). The first two steps, same as in obtaining *p*-value from CHIDIST procedure, involve (1) clicking of the *paste function icon*, f*, and (2) clicking of *the Statistical*. Among the many functions available, you will find CHIDIST (see the following first picture of Excel's). The second figure shows an example where we enter the "Chi-square test statistic" value of 3.841 with 1 degree of freedom and obtain a *p*-value of approximately .05.

(1) Choosing the Chi-square distribution:

(2) Enter the Chi-square statistic and its degree of freedom:

EXERCISES

6.1. Consider a sample of ($n = 110$) women drawn randomly from the membership list of the National Organization for Women (NOW), ($x = 25$) of whom were found to smoke. Use the result of this sample to test whether the rate found is significantly *different* from the U.S. proportion of .30 for women.

6.2. In a case–control study, 317 patients suffering from endometrial carcinoma were individually matched with 317 other cancer patients in a hospital and the use of estrogen in the six months prior to diagnosis was determined. The results were

	Matching Controls	
Cases	Estrogen	No Estrogen
Estrogen	39	113
No Estrogen	15	150

Use McNemar's chi square test to investigate the significance of the association between estrogen use and endometrial carcinoma; state your null and alternative hypotheses.

6.3. A study in Maryland identified 4,032 white persons, enumerated in a nonofficial 1963 census, who became widowed between 1963 and 1974. These people were matched, one-to-one, to married persons on the basis of race, sex, year of birth, and geography of residence. The matched pairs were followed to a second census in 1975, and, in Example 6.3, we have analyzed the data for men so as to compare the mortality of widowed men versus married men. The data for 2828 matched pairs of *women* were as follows:

Widowed	Married Women	
Women	Died	Alive
Died	1	264
Alive	249	2314

Test to compare the mortality of widowed women versus married women; state your null and alternative hypotheses.

6.4. It has been noted that metalworkers have an increased risk for cancer of the internal nose and paranasal sinuses, perhaps as a result of exposure to cutting oils. Therefore, a study was conducted to see whether this particular exposure also increases the risk for squamous cell carcinoma of the scrotum. Cases included all 45 squamous cell carcinomas of the scrotum diagnosed in Connecticut residents from 1955 to 1973, as obtained from the Connecticut Tumor Registry. Matched controls were selected for each case based on the age at death (within 8 years), year of death (within 3 years), and number of jobs as obtained from combined death certificate and directory sources.

An occupational indicator of metalworker (yes/no) was evaluated as the possible risk factor in this study; results are

	Matching Controls	
Cases	Yes	No
Yes	2	26
No	5	12

Test to compare the cases versus the controls, state clearly your null and alternative hypotheses, and your choice of the test size.

6.5. A matched case–control study on endometrial cancer, where the exposure was "ever having taken any estrogen," yields the following data:

	Matching Controls	
Cases	Exposed	Nonexposed
Exposed	27	29
Nonexposed	3	4

Test to compare the cases versus the controls; state clearly your null and alternative hypotheses, and your choice of the test size.

6.6. Ninety-eight heterosexual couples, at least one of whom was HIV-infected, were enrolled in an HIV transmission study and interviewed about sexual behavior. The following table provides a summary of condom use reported by heterosexual partners:

	Men	
Women	Ever	Never
Ever	45	6
Never	7	40

Test to compare the men versus the women; state clearly your null and alternative hypotheses, and your choice of the test size.

6.7. A matched case–control study was conducted to evaluate the cumulative effects of acrylate and methacrylate vapors on olfactory function. Cases were defined as scoring at or below the 10th percentile on the UPSIT (University of Pennsylvania Smell Identification Test).

	Matching Controls	
Cases	Exposed	Nonexposed
Exposed	25	22
Nonexposed	9	21

Test to compare the cases versus the controls, state clearly your null and alternative hypotheses, and your choice of the test size.

6.8. Self-reported injuries among left-handed and right-handed people were compared in a survey of 1896 college students in British Columbia, Canada. Ninety-three of the 180 left-handed students reported at least one injury and 619 of the 1716 right-handed students reported at least one injury in the same period. Test to compare the proportions of students with injury, left-handed versus right-handed, state clearly your null and alternative hypotheses, and your choice of the' test size.

6.9. A study was conducted to evaluate the hypothesis that tea consumption and premenstrual syndrome are associated. One hundred and eighty-eight nursing students and 64 tea factory workers were given questionnaires. The prevalence of premenstrual syndrome was 39% among the nursing students and 77% among the tea factory workers. Test to compare the prevalences of premenstrual syndrome, tea factory workers versus nursing students; state clearly your null and alternative hypotheses, and your choice of the test size.

6.10. A study was conducted to investigate drinking problems among college students. In 1983, a group of students was asked whether they had ever driven an automobile while drunk. In 1987, after the legal drinking age was raised, a different group of college students was asked the same question. The results are as follows:

| Drove While Drinking | Year of Survey | | |
	1983	1987	Total
Yes	1250	991	2241
No	1387	1666	3053
Total	2637	2657	5294

Test to compare the proportions of students with drinking problem, 1987 versus 1983; state clearly your null and alternative hypotheses, and your choice of the test size.

6.11. In August 1976, tuberculosis was diagnosed in a high school student (Index case) in Corinth, Mississippi. Subsequent laboratory studies revealed the disease was caused by the drug-resistant *Tubercule bacilli*. An epidemiologic investigation was conducted at the high school. The following table gives the rate of positive tuberculin reactions, determined for various groups of students according to the degree of exposure to the index case.

Exposure Level	No. Tested	No. Positive
High	129	63
Low	325	36

Test to compare the proportions of students with infection, high exposure versus low exposure; state clearly your null and alternative hypotheses, and your choice of the test size.

6.12. Epidemic keratoconjunctivitis (EKC) or "shipyard eye" is an acute infectious disease of the eye. A case of EKC is defined as an illness:

(a) consisting of redness, tearing, and pain in one or both eyes for more than three days duration,

(b) having diagnosed as EKC by an ophthalmologist.

In late October, 1977, one of the two ophthalmologists (Physician A) providing the majority of specialized eye care to the residents of a central Georgia county (population 45,000) saw a 27-year-old nurse who had returned from a vacation in Korea with severe EKC. She received symptomatic therapy and was warned that her eye infection could spread to others; nevertheless, numerous cases of an illness similar to hers soon occurred in the patients and staff of the nursing home (Nursing Home A) where she worked (these individuals came to Physician A for diagnosis and treatment). The following table provides exposure history of 22 persons with EKC between October 27, 1977, and January 13, 1978 (when the outbreak stopped after proper control techniques were initiated). Nursing Home B, included in this table, is the only other area chronic-care facility.

Exposed Cohort	Number Exposed	Number Positive
Nursing Home A	64	16
Nursing Home B	238	6

Using an appropriate test, compare the proportions of cases from the two nursing homes. State clearly your null and alternative hypotheses, and your choice of the test size.

6.13. Consider the data taken from a study that attempts to determine whether the use of electronic fetal monitoring (EFM) during labor affects the frequency of caesarean section deliveries. Of the 5824 infants included in the study, 2850 were electronically monitored and 2974 were not. The outcomes are as follows:

| Caesarean Delivery | EFM Exposure | | |
	Yes	No	Total
Yes	358	229	587
No	2492	2745	5237
Total	2850	2974	5824

Test to compare the rates of caesarean section delivery, EFM-exposed versus nonexposed; state clearly your null and alternative hypotheses, and your choice of the test size.

6.14. A study was conducted to investigate the effectiveness of bicycle safety helmets in preventing head injury. The data consist of a random sample of 793 individuals who were involved in bicycle accidents during a 1-year period.

Head Injury	Wearing		
	Yes	No	Total
Yes	17	218	237
No	130	428	558
Total	147	646	793

Test to compare the proportions with head injury, those with helmets versus those without; state clearly your null and alternative hypotheses, and your choice of the test size.

6.15. A case–control study was conducted relating to the epidemiology of breast cancer and the possible involvement of dietary fats, along with other vitamins and nutrients. It included 2024 breast cancer patients who were admitted to Roswell Park Memorial Institute, Erie County, New York, from 1958 to 1965. A control group of 1463 was chosen from the patients having no neoplasms and no' pathology of gastrointestinal or reproductive systems. The primary factors being investigated were vitamins A and E (measured in international units per month). The following are data for 1500 women over 54 years of age.

Vitamin A (IU/mo)	Cases	Control
<150,500	893	392
>150,500	132	83
Total	1025	475

Test to compare the proportions of subjects who consumed less Vitamin A ($\leq 150,500$ IU/mo), cases versus controls; state clearly your null and alternative hypotheses, and your choice of the test size.

6.16. Adult male residents of 13 counties of western Washington State, in whom testicular cancer had been diagnosed during 1977–1983, were interviewed over the telephone regarding their history of genital tract conditions, including vasectomy. For comparison, the same interview was given to a sample of men selected from the population of these counties by dialing telephone numbers at random. The following data are tabulated by religious background.

Religion	Vasectomy	Cases	Controls
Protestant			
	Yes	24	56
	No	205	239
Catholic			
	Yes	10	6
	No	32	90
Others			
	Yes	18	39
	No	56	96

Compare the cases versus controls vasectomy for each religious group; state your null and alternative hypotheses. Is there any evidence of an effect modification?

6.17. In a trial of diabetic therapy, patients were either treated with Phenformin or with a placebo. The numbers of patients and deaths from cardiovascular causes were as follows:

Result	Phenformin	Placebo	Total
Cardiovascular death	26	2	28
Not a death	178	62	240
Total	204	64	268

Investigate the difference in cardiovascular mortality between the Phenformin and Placebo groups; state your null and alternative hypotheses.

6.18. In a seroepidemiologic survey of health workers representing a spectrum of exposure to blood and patients with hepatitis B virus (HBV), it was found that infection increased as a function of contact. The following table provides data for hospital workers with uniform socioeconomic status at an urban teaching hospital in Boston, Massachusetts.

Personnel	Exposure	No. Tested	HBV Positive
Physicians			
	Frequent	81	17
	Infrequent	89	7
Nurses			
	Frequent	104	22
	Infrequent	126	11

Test to compare the proportions of HBV infection between the two levels of exposure (frequent exposure, infrequent exposure); perform separate comparisons for groups of physicians and nurses. State clearly your null and alternative hypotheses, and your choice of the test size.

6.19. It has been hypothesized that dietary fiber decreases the risk of colon cancer, while meats and fats are thought to increase this risk. A large study was undertaken to confirm these hypotheses. Fiber and fat consumptions are classified as "low" or "high" and data are tabulated separately for males and females as follows ("low" means below median):

	Males		Females	
Diet	Cases	Controls	Cases	Controls
Low fat, high fiber	27	38	23	39
Low fat, low fiber	64	78	82	81
High fat, high fiber	78	61	83	76
High fat, low fiber	36	28	35	27

For each group (males and females), using "low fat, high fiber" as the baseline, test to investigate the "risk' of each other diet group (by comparing each of the three groups, low fat and low fiber, high fat and high fiber, high fat and low fiber versus the baseline). State clearly your null and alternative hypotheses, and your choice of the test size.

6.20. Risk factors of gallstone disease were investigated in male self-defense officials who received, between October 1986 and December 1990, a retirement health examination at the Self-Defense Forces Fukuoka Hospital, Fukuoka, Japan. The following table provides parts of the data relating to three variables: smoking, drinking, and body mass index (BMI, which is dichotomized into below and above 22.5).

		No. of Men Surveyed	
Factor	Level	Total	No. with Gallstone
Smoking			
	Never	621	11
	Yes	2108	50
Alcohol			
	Never	447	11
	Yes	2292	50
BMI (kg/m2)			
	Below 22.5	719	13
	Over 22.5	2020	48

For each of the three 2×2 tables, test to investigate the relationship between that criterion and gallstone disease. State clearly your null and alternative hypotheses, and your choice of the test size.

6.21. In 1979 the U.S. Veterans Administration conducted a health survey of 11,230 veterans. The advantages of this survey are that it includes a large random sample with a high interview response rate and it was done before the recent public controversy surrounding the issue of the health effects of possible exposure to Agent Orange. The following table shows data relating Vietnam service to eight post-traumatic stress disorder symptoms among the 1787 veterans who entered the military service between 1965 and 1975.

Symptom	Level	Service in Vietnam	
		Yes	No
Nightmares			
	Yes	197	85
	No	577	925
Sleep problems			
	Yes	173	160
	No	599	851
Troubled memories			
	Yes	220	105
	No	549	906
Depression			
	Yes	306	315
	No	465	699
Temper control problem			
	Yes	176	144
	No	595	868
Life goal association			
	Yes	231	225
	No	539	786
Omit feelings			
	Yes	188	191
	No	583	821
Confusion			
	Yes	163	148
	No	607	864

For each of the symptoms, compare the veterans who served in Vietnam and those who did not. State clearly your null and alternative hypotheses, and your choice of the test size.

6.22. A case–control study was conducted in Auckland, New Zealand, to investigate the effects of alcohol consumption on both nonfatal myocardial infarction and coronary death in 24 h after drinking, among regular drinkers. Data were tabulated separately for men and women.
For each group, men and women, and for each type of event, myocardial infarction and coronary death, test to compare cases versus controls. State, in each analysis, your null and alternative hypotheses, and your choice of the test size.

(1) Data for Men

Drink in the Last 24 h	Myocardial Infarction		Coronary Death	
	Controls	Cases	Controls	Cases
No	197	142	135	103
Yes	201	136	159	69

(2) Data for Women

Drink in the Last 24 h	Myocardial Infarction		Coronary Death	
	Controls	Cases	Controls	Cases
No	144	41	89	12
Yes	122	19	76	4

6.23. Refer to the data in previous Exercise 6.22, but assume that gender (male/female) may be a confounder but not an effect modifier. For each type of event, myocardial infarction and coronary death, use the Mantel–Haenszel method to investigate the effects of alcohol consumption. State, in each analysis, your null and alternative hypotheses, and your choice of the test size.

6.24. Since incidence rates of most cancers rise with age, this must always be considered a confounder. The following are stratified data for an unmatched case–control study; the disease was esophageal cancer among men and the risk factor was alcohol consumption.

Age	Sample	Daily Alcohol Consumption	
		80 + g	0–79 g
25–44	Cases	5	5
	Controls	35	270
45–64	Cases	67	55
	Controls	56	277
65 and over	Cases	24	44
	Controls	18	129

Use the Mantel–Haenszel procedure to compare the cases versus the controls. State your null hypothesis and choice of the test size.

6.25. Postmenopausal women who develop endometrial cancer are, on average, heavier than women who do not develop the disease. One possible explanation is that heavy women are more exposed to endogenous estrogens that are produced in postmenopausal women by conversion of steroid precursors to active estrogens in peripheral fat. In the face of varying levels of endogenous estrogen production, one might ask whether the carcinogenic potential of exogenous estrogens would be the same in all women. A case–control study has been conducted to examine the relation between weight, replacement estrogen therapy, and endometrial cancer; results are as follows:

Weight (kg)	Sample	Estrogen Replacement	
		Yes	No
<57	Cases	20	12
	Controls	61	183
57–75	Cases	37	45
	Controls	113	378
>75	Cases	9	42
	Controls	23	140

(a) Compare the cases versus the controls separately for the three weight groups. State your null hypothesis and choice of the test size.

(b) Use the Mantel–Haenszel procedure to compare the cases versus the controls. State your null hypothesis and choice of the test size.

6.26. Prematurity, which ranks as the major cause of neonatal morbidity and mortality, has traditionally been defined on the basis of a birth weight under 2500 g. But this definition encompasses two distinct types of infants: infants who are small because they are born early and infants who are born at or near term but are small because their growth was retarded. "Prematurity" has now been replaced by

(i) "low birth weight" to describe the second type

(ii) "preterm" to characterize the first type (babies born before 37 weeks of gestation)

A case–control study of the epidemiology of preterm delivery was undertaken at Yale-New Haven Hospital in Connecticut during 1977. The study population consisted of 175 mothers of singleton preterm infants and 303 mothers of singleton full-term infants. The following tables give the distributions of age (first table) and socioeconomic status (second table).

Age	Cases	Controls
14–17	15	16
18–19	22	25
20–24	47	62
25–29	56	122
30 or over	35	78

Socioeconomic Level	Cases	Controls
Upper	11	40
Upper Middle	14	45
Middle	33	64
Lower Middle	59	91
Lower	53	58
Unknown	5	5

(a) Refer to the age data (first table) and choose the "30 or over" group as baseline; then compare each other age group versus the chosen baseline. State your null hypothesis and choice of the test size. Is this true, in general, that the younger the mother the higher the risk?

(b) Refer to the socioeconomic data (second table) and choose the "lower" group as the baseline; then compare each other age group versus the chosen baseline. State your null hypothesis and choice of the test size. Is this true, in general, that the poorer the mother the higher the risk?

6.27. Postneonatal mortality due to respiratory illnesses is known to be inversely related to maternal age, but the role of young motherhood as a risk factor for respiratory morbidity in infants has not been thoroughly explored. A study was conducted in Tucson, Arizona, aimed at the incidence of lower respiratory tract illnesses (LRIs) during the first year of life. In this study, over 1200 infants were enrolled at birth between 1980 and 1984, and the following data are concerned with wheezing lower respiratory tract illnesses (wheezing LRI: No/Yes).

Maternal Age (years)	Boys		Girls	
	No	Yes	No	Yes
Below 30	277	113	296	85
Over 30	110	20	116	25

For each of the two groups, boys and girls, test to investigate the relationship between maternal age and respiratory illness. State clearly your null and alternative hypotheses, and your choice of the test size.

6.28. Data were collected from 2197 white ovarian cancer patients and 8893 white controls in 12 different U.S. case–control studies conducted by various investigators in the period 1956–1986. These were used to evaluate the relationship of invasive epithelial ovarian cancer to reproductive and menstrual characteristics, exogenous estrogen use, and prior pelvic surgeries. The following are parts of the data related to unprotected intercourse and history of infertility.

Duration of Unprotected Intercourse	Cases	Controls
Less than 2 years	237	477
2 years and over	346	619
History of Infertility	Cases	Controls
No	526	966
Yes	96	135

For each of the two criteria, the duration of unprotected intercourse and history of infertility, test to investigate the relationship between that criterion and ovarian cancer. State clearly your null and alternative hypotheses, and your choice of the test size.

6.29. When a patient is diagnosed as suffering from the cancer of the prostate, an important question in deciding the treatment strategy for the patient is whether or not the cancer has spread to the neighboring lymph nodes. The question is so critical in prognosis and treatment that it is customary to operate on the patient (i.e., perform a laparotomy) for the sole purpose of examining the nodes and removing tissue samples to examine under the microscope for evidence of cancer. However, certain variables that can be measured without surgery are predictive of the nodal involvement; and the purpose of the study presented here was to examine the data for 53 prostate cancer patients receiving surgery, to determine which of the 5 preoperative variables are predictive of nodal involvement. For each of the 53 patients, there are 2 continuous independent variables, age at diagnosis and level of serum acid phosphatase (multiplied by 100; called "acid"), and 3 binary variables, X-ray reading, pathology reading (grade) of a biopsy of the tumor obtained by needle before surgery, and a rough measure of the size and the location of the tumor (stage) obtained by palpation with the fingers via the rectum. For these three binary independent variables, a value of one signifies a positive or more serious state and a zero denotes a negative or less serious finding. In addition, the sixth column presents the finding at surgery – the primary outcome of interest, which is binary, a value of one denoting nodal involvement and a value of zero denoting no nodal involvement found at surgery. In this exercise, again, we investigate the effects of the three binary preoperative variables (X-ray, grade, and stage). In Exercise 1.46, we calculated the odds ratio representing the strength of the relationship between each of these three factors and nodal involvement. In this exercise, test to see if the relationship between each factor and nodal involvement is "real"; state clearly your null and alternative hypotheses, and your choice of the test size.

7

Comparison of Population Means

If each element of a data set may lie only at a few isolated points, we have a *discrete* or *categorical data* set; examples include sex, race, or some sort of artificial grading used as outcomes. For discrete data, the basic *statistic* representing the outcomes is the *sample proportion*, which is an estimate of the corresponding *population proportion*. If each element of a data set may lie anywhere on the numerical scale, we have a *continuous* data set; examples include blood pressure, cholesterol level, or time to a certain event. For continuous data, the basic *statistic* representing the outcomes is the *sample mean* which is an estimate of the corresponding *population mean*. Chapter 6 deals with the comparison of population proportions. This chapter is focused on continuous measurements, especially the comparisons of population means. We will follow the same layout, starting with the simplest case, the one-sample problem.

7.1. ONE-SAMPLE PROBLEM WITH CONTINUOUS DATA

In this type of problem, we have a sample of continuous measurements of size n and we consider the null hypothesis

$$H_0 : \mu = \mu_0$$

where μ_0 is a fixed and known number. It is often a standardized or referenced figure; for example, the average blood pressure of men in certain age group (this figure may come from a sample itself, but referenced sample is often large enough so as to produce negligible sampling error in μ_0). Or, we could be concerned with a question like "Is the average birth weight for boys for this particular sub-population below normal average μ_0; say 7.5 lb?" In Exercise 7.1, we had tried to decide whether air quality on certain given day in a particular city exceeds regulated limit μ_0 set by a federal agency.

Health and Numbers: A Problems-Based Introduction to Biostatistics, Third Edition, by Chap T. Le
Copyright © 2009 John Wiley & Sons, Inc.

In a typical situation, the null hypothesis of a statistical test is concerned with a parameter; the parameter in this case, with continuous data, is the mean μ. Sample data are summarized into a statistic, which is used to estimate the parameter under investigation. Since the parameter under investigation is the proportion μ, our focus in this case is the sample mean. In general, a statistic is itself a variable with a specific sampling distribution (in the context of repeated sampling). Our statistic in this case is the sample mean, the corresponding sampling distribution is easily obtained by invoking the *Central Limit Theorem*. With large sample size and assuming that the null hypothesis H_0 is true, it is the normal distribution with mean and variance given by

$$\mu_{\bar{x}} = \mu_0$$

$$\sigma_{\bar{x}}^2 = \frac{\sigma^2}{n}$$

respectively. The extra needed parameter, the population variance σ^2 has to be estimated from our data by the sample variance s^2. From this sampling distribution, the observed value of the sample proportion can be converted to standard unit: the number of standard errors away from the hypothesized value of μ_0. In other words, to perform a test of significance for H_0, we proceed with the following steps:

(1) Decide whether a *one-sided* test or a *two-sided* test is appropriate.
(2) Choose a *level of significance* alpha (α), a common choice being .05.
(3) Calculate the *t-statistic*

$$t = \frac{\bar{x} - \mu_0}{s/\sqrt{n}}.$$

(4) From the table for the standard normal distribution (Appendix C) with $(n-1)$ degree of freedom and the choice of α, for example, $\alpha = .05$, the *rejection region* is determined by

(a) For a one-sided test,

$$t < (-\text{tabulated one-sided } t\text{-value}) \quad \text{for } H_A : \mu < \mu_0$$
$$t > (+\text{tabulated one-sided } t\text{-value}) \quad \text{for } H_A : \mu > \mu_0$$

(b) For a two-sided test or $H_A : \mu \neq \mu_0$

$$t < (-\text{tabulate two-sided } t\text{-value}) \quad \text{or} \quad t > (+\text{tabulated two-sided } t\text{-value})$$

This test is referred to as the *one-sample t-test*.

Example 7.1

Boys of a certain age have a mean weight of 85 lb. An observation was made that in a city neighborhood, children were underfed. As evidence, all 25 boys in the neighborhood of that age were weighed and found to have a mean of 80.94 lb and a standard deviation (SD) of 11.60 lb. An application of the above procedure yields

$$SE(\bar{x}) = \frac{s}{\sqrt{n}}$$
$$= \frac{11.60}{\sqrt{25}}$$
$$= 2.32$$

leading to

$$t = \frac{80.94 - 85}{2.32}$$
$$= -1.75$$

The underfeeding complaint corresponds to the one-sided alternative

$$H_A : \mu < 85$$

so that we would reject the null hypothesis if

$$t < (-\text{tabulated one-sided } t\text{-value})$$

From Appendix C, and with 24 degrees of freedom (df) $(n - 1)$, we find:

$$\text{tabulated one-sided } t\text{-value} = 1.71$$

under the column corresponding to .05 upper tail area; the null hypothesis is rejected at the .05 level $(-1.75 < -1.71)$. In other words, there is enough evidence to support the underfeeding complaint and to reject the null hypothesis at the .05 level (p-value $= .046$).

7.2. ANALYSIS OF PAIR-MATCHED DATA

The method presented in this section applies to cases where each subject or member of a group is observed twice (for example, before and after certain intervention), or matched pairs are measured for the same continuous characteristic. In the study reported in Example 7.2, blood pressure was measured from a group of women before and after each of them took an oral contraceptive. In Exercise 7.2, blood level of insulin was measured from dogs before and after some kind of nerve stimulation. In another exercise, we compared self-reported versus measured height. A popular application is an *epidemiological design* called a *pair-matched case–control study*. In case–control studies, cases of a specific disease are ascertained as they arise from population-based registers or lists of hospital admissions, and controls are sampled either as disease-free individuals from the population at risk or as hospitalized patients having a diagnosis other than the one under investigation. As a technique to control confounding factors, individual cases are matched, often one-to-one, to controls chosen to have similar values for confounding variables, such as age, sex, race, and so on.

Data from matched or before-and-after experiments should never be considered as coming from two independent samples. The procedure is to reduce the data to a one-sample by computing before-and-after (or case-and-control) difference for each subject or pairs of matched subjects. By doing this with paired observations, we get a set of differences, each of which is independent of the characteristics of the individual from which measurements were made. The analysis of pair-matched data with a continuous measurement can be seen as follows. What we really want to do is to compare the means, before versus after or cases versus controls, and the use of the sample of differences d's, one for each subject, helps to achieve that. With large sample size and assuming that the null hypothesis H_0 of *no difference* is true, the mean of the differences d's is distributed as *normal* with mean and variance given by

$$\mu_{\bar{d}} = 0$$

$$\sigma_{\bar{d}}^2 = \frac{\sigma_d^2}{n}$$

respectively. The extra needed parameter, the variance σ_d^2 has to be estimated from our data by the sample variance. In other words, the analysis of pair-matched data with a continuous measurement can be seen as a special case of the one-sample problem of Section 7.1 with $\mu_0 = 0$. Recall the form of the test statistic of the previous section, we have:

$$t = \frac{\bar{d} - 0}{s_d / \sqrt{n}}$$

and the rejection region is determined using the t distribution at $(n-1)$ degrees of freedom. This test is also referred to as the *one-sample t-test*, the same one-sample t-test as in the previous section.

Example 7.2

Trace metals in drinking water affect the flavor of the water, and unusually high concentration can pose a health hazard. The following table shows trace-metal concentrations (zinc, in mg/l) for both surface water and bottom water at six different river locations (the difference is bottom-surface).

Location	Bottom	Surface	Difference, d	d^2
1	.430	.415	.015	.000225
2	.266	.238	.028	.000784
3	.567	.390	.177	.030276
4	.531	.410	.121	.014641
5	.707	.605	.102	.010404
6	.716	.609	.107	.011449
Total			.550	.068832

The necessary summarized figures are:

$$\bar{d} = \frac{.550}{6}$$

$$= .0917$$

$$s_d = \sqrt{\frac{.068832 - (.550)^2/6}{5}}$$

$$= .061$$

$$SE(\bar{d}) = \frac{.061}{\sqrt{6}}$$

$$= .0249$$

$$t = \frac{.0917}{.0249}$$

$$= 3.68$$

Using the column corresponding to the upper tail area of .025 in Appendix C, we have a tabulated value of 2.571 for 5 degrees of freedom. Since

$$t = 3.68 > (\text{tabulated})2.571$$

we conclude that the null hypothesis of *no difference* should be rejected at the .05 level; there is enough evidence to support the hypothesis of *different* mean zinc concentrations (two-sided alternative, p-value $= .0143$).

Example 7.3

The systolic blood pressures of 12 women between the ages of 20 and 35 were measured before and after administration of a newly developed oral contraceptive; data are:

Subject	Before	After	After–Before Difference, d	d^2
1	122	127	5	25
2	126	128	2	4
3	132	140	8	64
4	120	119	−1	1
5	142	145	3	9
6	130	130	0	0
7	142	148	6	36
8	137	135	−2	4
9	128	129	1	1
10	132	137	5	25
11	128	128	0	0
12	129	133	4	16

Given the above data, we have the following summarized figures from the last column

$$n = 12$$

$$\sum d = 31$$

$$\sum d^2 = 185$$

These lead to:

$$\bar{d} = \text{Average after–before difference}$$

$$= 31/12$$

$$= 2.58 \text{ mmHg}$$

$$s^2 = \frac{185 - (31)^2/12}{11}$$

$$= 9.54$$

$$s = 3.09$$

$$\text{SE}(\bar{d}) = 3.09/\sqrt{12}$$

$$= .89$$

$$t = \frac{2.58}{.89}$$

$$= 2.90$$

Using the column corresponding to the upper tail area of .05 in Appendix C, we have a tabulated value of 1.796 for 11 degrees of freedom. Since

$$t = 2.90 > (\text{tabulated})\,1.796$$

we conclude that the null hypothesis of *no blood pressure change* should be rejected at the .05 level; there is enough evidence to support the hypothesis of *increase* systolic blood pressure (one-sided alternative, p-value $= .0072$).

Example 7.4

Data in epidemiologic studies are sometimes self-reported. Screening data from the hypertension detection and follow-up program in Minneapolis, Minnesota (1973–1974) provided an opportunity to evaluate the accuracy of self-reported height and weight. The following table gives the percent discrepancy between self-reported and measured height:

$$x = \frac{\text{Self-reported height} - \text{measured height}}{\text{Measured height}} \times 100\%$$

Education	Men			Women		
	n	Mean	Standard Deviation	n	Mean	Standard Deviation
≤High School	476	1.38	1.53	323	.66	1.53
≥College	192	1.04	1.31	62	.41	1.46

Let focus on the sample of men with high school education; investigations of other groups and the differences between them can be found in the exercises at the end of this chapter. An application of the one-sample t-test yields:

$$\bar{x} = 1.38$$

$$s = \frac{1.53}{\sqrt{476}}$$

$$= .07$$

$$t = \frac{1.38}{.07}$$

$$= 19.71$$

It can be easily seen that the difference between self-reported height and measured height is highly statistically significant ($p < .001$; comparing 19.71 versus the "cut-point" of 2.58 for large sample).

7.3. COMPARISON OF TWO MEANS

Perhaps one of the most common problems in statistical inference is the comparison of two population means using data from two independent samples; the sample sizes may or may not be equal. In this type of problem, we have two sets of continuous measurements, one of size n_1 and one of size n_2, and we consider the null hypothesis:

$$H_0 : \mu_1 = \mu_2$$

expressing the equality of the two population means.

To perform a test of significance for H_0, we proceed with the following steps:

(1) Decide whether a *one-sided* test or a *two-sided* test is appropriate.
(2) Choose a *level of significance* alpha (α), a common choice being .05.

(3) Calculate the *t-statistic*

$$t = \frac{\bar{x}_2 - \bar{x}_1}{\text{SE}(\bar{x}_2 - \bar{x}_1)}$$

where

$$\text{SE}(\bar{x}_2 - \bar{x}_1) = s_p \sqrt{\frac{1}{n_1} + \frac{1}{n_2}}$$

$$s_p^2 = \frac{(n_1 - 1)s_1^2 + (n_2 - 1)s_2^2}{n_1 + n_2 - 2}$$

s_p^2 is the weighted average of the two sample variances; subscript "p" is for "pooled".

(4) From the table for the standard normal distribution (Appendix C) with $(n_1 + n_2 - 2)$ degree of freedom and the choice of α, for example, $\alpha = .05$, the *rejection region* is determined by

(a) For a one-sided test,

$$t < (-\text{tabulated one-sided } t\text{-value}) \quad \text{for } H_A : \mu_2 < \mu_1$$
$$t > (+\text{tabulated one-sided } t\text{-value}) \quad \text{for } H_A : \mu_2 > \mu_1$$

(b) For a two-sided test or $H_A : \mu \neq \mu_0$

$$t < (-\text{tabulate two-sided } t\text{-value}) \quad \text{or} \quad t > (+\text{tabulated two-sided } t\text{-value})$$

This test is referred to as the *two-sample t-test*.

Example 7.5

In an attempt to assess the physical condition of joggers, a sample of $n_1 = 25$ joggers and a sample of $n_2 = 26$ nonjoggers were selected and their maximum volumes of oxygen uptake VO_2 were measured with the following results:

For 25 joggers: $\bar{x}_2 = 47.5$ ml/kg; $s_2 = 4.8$ ml/kg

For 26 non-joggers: $\bar{x}_1 = 37.5$ ml/kg; $s_1 = 5.1$ ml/kg

To proceed with the *two-sided, two-sample t-test*, we have

$$s_p = \sqrt{\frac{(25)(5.1)^2 + (24)(4.8)^2}{49}}$$

$$= 4.96$$

$$\text{SE}(\bar{x}_2 - \bar{x}_1) = (4.96)\sqrt{\frac{1}{25} + \frac{1}{26}}$$

$$= 1.39$$

It follows that:

$$t = \frac{47.5 - 37.5}{1.39}$$

$$= 7.19$$

indicating a significant difference between the joggers and the nonjoggers (at 49 degrees of freedom and $\alpha = .01$, the tabulated "t" value—with upper tail area of .025—is about 2.0 approximately; p-value <.001).

Example 7.6

Vision, or more specially visual acuity, depends on a number of factors. A study was undertaken in Australia to determine the effect of one of these factors: racial variation. Visual acuity of recognition as assessed in clinical practice has a defined normal value of 20/20 (or zero in log scale). The following summarized data on monocular visual acuity (expressed in log scale) were obtained from two groups:

(1) Australian males of Aboriginal origin

$$n_1 = 107; \quad \bar{x}_1 = -.26; \quad s_1 = .13$$

(2) Australian males of European origin

$$n_2 = 89; \quad \bar{x}_2 = -.20; \quad s_2 = .18$$

To proceed with a *two-sample t-test* we have:

$$s_p = \sqrt{\frac{(106)(.13)^2 + (88)(.18)^2}{194}}$$

$$= .155$$

$$SE(\bar{x}_2 - \bar{x}_1) = (.155)\sqrt{\frac{1}{107} + \frac{1}{89}}$$

$$= 0.022$$

It follows that,

$$t = \frac{(-.20) - (-.26)}{0.022}$$

$$= 2.73$$

The result indicates that the difference is statistically significant at the .01 level which corresponds to a two-sided cut-point of 2.58 for a large degree of freedom (p-value $= .006$).

This last example of the section involves a very important public health concern, the possible effects of environmental smoke (also referred to as second-hand smoke.

Example 7.7

The extend to which an infant's health is affected by parental smoking is an important public health concern. The following data give the urinary concentrations of cotinine (a metabolite of nicotine); measurements were taken both from a sample of infants who had been exposed to household smoke and from a sample of unexposed infants.

(1) Unexposed ($n = 7$): 8, 11, 12, 14, 20, 43, and 111
(2) Exposed ($n = 8$): 35, 56, 83, 92, 128, 150, 176, and 208

The descriptive statistics needed our two-sample t-test are:

(1) For unexposed infants:

$$n_1 = 7; \quad \bar{x}_1 = 31.29; \quad s_1 = 37.07$$

(2) For exposed infants:

$$n_2 = 8; \quad \bar{x}_2 = 116.0; \quad s_2 = 59.99$$

To proceed with a *two-sample t-test* we have:

$$s_p = \sqrt{\frac{(6)(37.07)^2 + (7)(59.99)^2}{13}}$$
$$= 50.72$$

$$SE(\bar{x}_2 - \bar{x}_1) = (50.72)\sqrt{\frac{1}{7} + \frac{1}{8}}$$
$$= 26.25$$

It follows that,

$$t = \frac{116.0 - 31.29}{26.25}$$
$$= 3.23$$

The result indicates that the difference is statistically significant at the .01 level which corresponds to a two-sided cut-point of 3.012 for 13 degrees of freedom (p-value $= .007$).

7.4. ONE-WAY ANALYSIS OF VARIANCE (ANOVA)

Suppose that the goal of a research project is to discover whether there are differences in the means of several independent groups. The problem is how we will measure the extent of differences among the means. If we had two groups then we would measure the difference by the distance between sample means and use the two-sample t-test. Here we have more than two groups; we could take all possible pairs of means and do many two-sample t-tests. What is the matter with this approach of doing many two-sample t-tests, one for each pair of samples? As the number of groups increases, so does the number of tests to perform; for example, we would have to do 45 tests if we have 10 groups to compare. Obviously, the amount of work is greater, but that should not be the critical problem—especially with technological aids such as the use of calculators and computers. So, what is the problem? The answer is that performing many tests increases the probability that one or more of the comparisons will result in a Type I error (i.e., a significant test result when the null hypothesis is true). This statement should make sense intuitively. For example, suppose the null hypothesis is true and we perform 100 tests—each has a .05 probability of resulting in a Type I error; then 5 of these 100 tests would be statistically significant as the results of Type I errors. Of course, we usually do not need to do that many tests; however, every time we do more than one, then the probability that at least one will result in a Type I error exceeds .05, indicating a falsely significant difference! What is needed is a different way to summarize the differences between several means and a method of *simultaneously* comparing these means in one step. This method is called ANOVA or One-way ANOVA, which is an abbreviation of "ANalysis Of VAriance". The method, and so does the name ANOVA, can be described as follows.

We have continuous measurements X's from k independent samples; the sample sizes may or may not be equal. We assume that these are samples from k normal distributions with a common variance but the means may or may not be the same. The case where we apply the two-sample t-test is a special case of this One-way ANOVA model with ($k = 2$). Data from the ith sample can be summarized into sample size, sample mean, and sample variance. And if we pool data together, the (grand) mean of this combined sample can be calculated from:

$$\bar{x} = \frac{\sum n_i \bar{x}_i}{\sum n_i}$$

In that combined sample of size $n = \sum n_i$, the variation in X is conventionally measured in terms of the deviations

$$x_{ij} - \bar{x}$$

where x_{ij} is the jth measurement from the ith sample; the total variation, denoted by SST, is the *sum of squared deviations*:

$$\text{SST} = \sum (x_{ij} - \bar{x})^2$$

For example, $\text{SST} = 0$ when all observations are the same; SST is the numerator of the sample variance of the combined sample, the greater SST the greater the variation among all X-values. The total variation in the combined sample can be decomposed into two components:

$$x_{ij} - \bar{x} = (x_{ij} - \bar{x}_i) + (\bar{x}_i - \bar{x})$$

(i) The first term reflects the variation *within* the ith sample; the sum:

$$\text{SSW} = \sum_{i,j} (x_{ij} - \bar{x}_i)^2$$
$$= \sum_i (n_i - 1)s_i^2$$

is called the *within sum of squares*; it is called "within" because we first calculating the degree of variation *in each group* then adding up.

(ii) The difference between the above two sums of squares,

$$\text{SSB} = \text{SST} - \text{SSW}$$
$$= \sum_{i,j} (\bar{x}_i - \bar{x})^2$$
$$= \sum_i n_i(\bar{x}_i - \bar{x})^2$$

is called the *between sum of squares*. SSB represents the variation or *differences between the sample means*, a measure very much similar to the numerator of a sample variance; the n_i's serve as *weights*.

Corresponding to the partitioning of the total sum of squares SST, there is partitioning of the associated degrees of freedom. We have $(n - 1)$ degrees of freedom associated with SST, the denominator of the variance of the combined sample; SSB has $(k - 1)$ degrees of freedom representing the differences between k groups, the remaining $(n - k)$ degrees of freedom are associated with SSW. These results lead to the usual presentation of the ANOVA process:

(i) The *within mean square* is obtain by dividing SSW by its degree of freedom which serves as an estimate of the common variance as stipulated by the One-way ANOVA *model*:

$$\text{MSW} = \frac{\text{SSW}}{n - k}$$

In fact, it can be seen that MSW is a natural extension of the pooled estimate s_p^2 as used in the two-sample t-test ($k = 2$). It is a measure of the average variation within the k samples.

(ii) The *between mean square* is obtained by dividing SSW by its degree of freedom which represents the *average variation* (or differences) between the k sample means:

$$MSB = \frac{SSB}{k-1}$$

(iii) The breakdowns of the total sum of squares and its associated degree of freedom are *displayed* in the form of an analysis of variance table (ANOVA table) as follows.

Source of Variation	SS	df	MS	F-Statistic	p-Value
Between samples	SSB	$k-1$	MSB	MSB/MSW	p
Within samples	SSW	$n-k$	MSW		
Total	SST	$n-1$			

The test statistic F for the above one-way analysis of variance compares MSB (the *average* variation—or differences—between the k sample means) and MSE (the *average* variation within the k samples), a value near 1 support the null hypothesis of *no differences* between the k population means. Decisions are made by referring the observed value of the test statistic F to the F-table in Appendix E with $(k-1, n-k)$ degrees of freedom; $(k-1)$ is the "numerator degree of freedom" and $(n-k)$ is the "denominator degree of freedom". In fact, when $(k=2)$, we have:

$$F = t^2$$

where "t" is the test statistic for comparing the two population means of Section 7.3. In other words, when $(k=2)$, the F-test is equivalent to the two-sided two-sample t-test. It is also obvious that the calculations are overwhelming; you will see how they are obtained by using *Excel* in Section 7.5.

Example 7.8

Vision, or more specially visual acuity, depends on a number of factors. A study was undertaken in Australia to determine the effect of one of these factors: racial variation. Visual acuity of recognition as assessed in clinical practice has a defined normal value of 20/20 (or zero in log scale). The following summarized the data on monocular visual acuity (expressed in log scale); part of this data set was given in Example 7.6:

Sample	Sample Size, n	Mean	Standard Deviation
Australian males of European origin	89	−.20	.18
Australian males of Aboriginal origin	107	−.26	.13
Australian females of European origin	63	−.13	.17
Australian females of Aboriginal origin	54	−.24	.18

To proceed with a One-way Analysis of Variance, we calculate the mean of the combined sample:

$$\bar{x} = \frac{(89)(-.20) + (107)(-.26) + (63)(-.13) + (54)(-.24)}{89 + 107 + 63 + 54}$$

$$= .213$$

Other figures needed are obtained as follows:

$$SSB = (89)(-.20 + .213)^2 + (107)(-.26 + .213)^2$$
$$+ (63)(-.13 + .213)^2 + (54)(-.24 + .213)^2$$
$$= .7248$$

$$MSB = \frac{.7248}{3}$$
$$= .2416$$

$$SSW = (88)(.18)^2 + (106)(.13)^2 + (62)(.17)^2 + (53)(.18)^2$$
$$= 8.1516$$

$$MSW = \frac{8.1516}{309}$$
$$= .0264$$

$$F = \frac{.2416}{.0264}$$
$$= 9.152$$

The results are summarized in the following ANOVA table:

Source of Variation	SS	df	MS	F-Statistic	p-Value
Between samples	.7248	3	.2426	9.152	<.0001
Within samples	8.1516	309	.0264		
Total	8.8764	312			

The resulting F-test indicates that the overall differences between the four population means is highly significant (p-value <.0001).

Example 7.9

A study was conducted to test the question as to whether cigarette smoking is associated with reduced serum–testosterone levels in men aged 35–45. The study involved the following four groups:

(1) Nonsmokers who had never smoked.

(2) Former smokers who had quit for at least 6 months prior to the study.

(3) Light smokers, defined as those who smoked 10 or fewer cigarettes per day.

(4) Heavy smokers, defined as those who smoked 30 or more cigarettes per day.

Each group consisted of 10 men and the following table shows raw data, where serum–testosterone levels were measured in μg/dl.

Nonsmokers	Former Smokers	Light Smokers	Heavy Smokers
.44	.46	.37	.44
.44	.50	.42	.25
.43	.51	.43	.40
.56	.58	.48	.27
.85	.85	.76	.34
.68	.72	.60	.62
.96	.93	.82	.47
.72	.86	.72	.70
.92	.76	.60	.60
.87	.65	.51	.54

An application of the One-way ANOVA method yields the following table:

Source of Variation	SS	df	MS	F-Statistic	p-Value
Between samples	.339	3	.113	3.798	.0183
Within samples	1.0711	36	.0298		
Total	1.4101	39			

The resulting F-test indicates that the overall differences between the four population means is statistically significant at the 5% level but not at the 1% level (p-value $= .0179$).

7.5. COMPUTATIONAL AIDS

The one-sample t-test and the two-sample t-test can also be implemented easily using Microsoft Excel. The first two steps are the same as in obtaining descriptive statistics:

(1) click the *paste function icon*, f*, and

(2) click *Statistical*.

Among functions available, choose TTEST. A box appears with four rows to be filled. The first two are for data in the two groups to be compared; in each you identify the range of cells, say B2:B23. The third box asking for "tails", enter "1" ("2") for one-sided (two-sided) alternative.

Enter the "type" of test on the last row, "1" ("2") for one-sample (two-sample) *t*-test.

If you follow the same two steps: (1) click the *paste function icon*, f*, and (2) click *Statistical*; among the functions available you would also see "FTEST". But that is *not* the *F*-test by the ANOVA procedure; that was the *F*-test used to compare two population variances, which we do not cover. To perform the One-way ANOVA, you follow a different path. The new first two steps are:

(1) Click "Tools" (near the top of the Window screen); among options available.
(2) Choose "Data Analysis"; a list of *Excel analysis tools* appear in a box (see picture below)

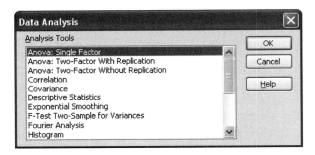

(3) Among the analysis tools available, click "Anova: Single Factor"—that is another name for One-way ANOVA.
(4) After selecting "Anova: Single Factor", a box appears with a blank "Input Range" to be filled; this is where you specify the location of your data on the spreadsheet—in the following figure, you see "A2:D11" where we keep the data of Example 7.9 (four groups—in columns A to D, each with 10 observations in rows 2–11).

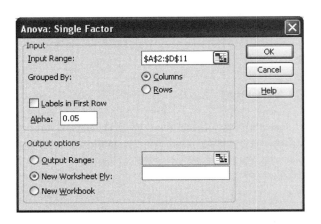

(5) After clicking "OK", you have all the results in the following picture consisting of:
  (a) Descriptive statistics: sample size (count), total (sum), mean (average), and variance for each of the four groups (called column).
  (b) The ANOVA table, the same table shown in Example 7.9. Computer output also includes an extra figure (in a column not shown) called "F crit"; this is the cut-point for the F statistic at the alpha level chosen (in a separate of the above figure—shown as ".05" but you can change to any figure). If your F statistic is greater than this cut-point, the Null hypothesis is rejected.

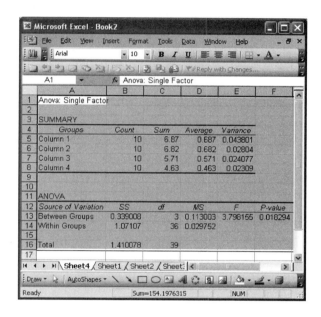

EXERCISES

7.1. The criterion for issuing a smog alert is established at greater than 7 ppm of a particular pollutant. Samples collected from ($n = 16$) stations in a certain city give a (sample) mean of 7.84 ppm with a standard deviation of $s = 2.01$ ppm. Do these findings indicate that the smog alert criterion has been exceeded? State clearly your null and alternative hypotheses, and your choice of the test size.

7.2. The purpose of an experiment is to investigate the effect of vagal nerve stimulation on insulin secretion. The subjects are mongrel dogs with varying body weights. The following table gives the amount of immunoreactive insulin in pancreatic venous plasma just before stimulation of the left vagus and the amount measured 5 min after stimulation for seven dogs.

	Immunoreactive Insulin (mU/ml)	
Dog	Before	After
1	350	480
2	200	130
3	240	250
4	290	310
5	90	280
6	370	1450
7	240	280

Test the null hypothesis that the stimulation of the vagus nerve has no effect on the blood level of immunoreactive insulin, that is

$$H_0 : \mu_{before} = \mu_{after}$$

State your alternative hypothesis, your choice of the test size, and draw appropriate conclusion.

7.3. In a study of saliva cotinine, seven subjects—all of whom had abstained from smoking for a week—were asked to smoke a single cigarette. The cotinine levels at 12 and 24 h after smoking are provided below:

	Cotinine Level (mmol/l)	
Subject	After 12 h	After 24 h
1	73	24
2	58	27
3	67	49
4	93	59
5	33	0
6	18	11
7	147	43

Test to compare the mean cotinine levels at 12 and 24 h after smoking; state clearly your null and alternative hypotheses, and your choice of the test size.

7.4. Dentists often make many people nervous. To see if such nervousness elevates blood pressure, systolic blood pressure of 60 subjects were measured in a dental setting then again in a medical setting. Data for 60 matched pairs (dental–medical) are summarized as follows.

$$Mean = 4.47$$

$$Standard\ deviation = 8.77$$

Test to compare the means blood pressure under two different settings; name the test and state clearly your null and alternative hypotheses, and your choice of the test size.

7.5. Ultrasounds were taken at the time of liver transplant and again 5–10 years later to determine the systolic blood pressure of the hepatic artery. Results for 21 transplants for 21 children are shown in the following table:

Child	After 5–10 years	At Transplant
1	46	35
2	40	40
3	50	58
4	50	71
5	41	33
6	70	79
7	35	20
8	40	19
9	56	56
10	30	26
11	30	44
12	60	90
13	43	43
14	45	42
15	40	55
16	50	60
17	66	62
18	45	26
19	40	60
20	35	27
21	25	31

Test to compare the means diastolic hepatic pressure; name the test and state clearly your null and alternative hypotheses, and your choice of the test size.

7.6. A study was conducted to investigate whether oat bran cereal helps to lower serum cholesterol in men with high cholesterol levels. Fourteen men were randomly placed on a diet, which included either oat bran or corn flakes; after 2 weeks, their low-density lipoprotein cholesterol levels were recorded. Each man was then switched to the alternative diet. After a second 2-week period, the LDL cholesterol level of each individual was again recorded. The data were:

Subject	LDL (mmol/l)	
	Corn Lakes	Oak Bran
1.00	4.61	3.84
2.00	6.42	5.57
3.00	5.40	5.85
4.00	4.54	4.84
5.00	3.98	3.68
6.00	3.82	2.96

(continued)

(Continued)

	LDL (mmol/l)	
Subject	Corn Lakes	Oak Bran
7.00	5.01	4.41
8.00	4.34	3.72
9.00	3.80	3.49
10.00	4.56	3.84
11.00	5.35	5.26
12.00	3.89	3.73
13.00	2.25	1.84
14.00	4.24	4.14

Test to compare the means LDL cholesterol level; name the test and state clearly your null and alternative hypotheses, and your choice of the test size.

7.7. Data in epidemiologic studies are sometimes self-reported. Screening data from the hypertension detection and follow-up program in Minneapolis, Minnesota (1973–1974) provided an opportunity to evaluate the accuracy of self-reported height and weight.

$$x = \frac{\text{Self-reported height} - \text{measured height}}{\text{Measured height}} \times 100\%$$

The following table gives the percent discrepancy between self-reported and measured height:

	Men			Women		
Education	n	Mean	Standard Deviation	n	Mean	Standard Deviation
≤High School	476	1.38	1.53	323	.66	1.53
≥College	192	1.04	1.31	62	.41	1.46

Example 7.4 was focused on the sample of men with high school education; using the same procedure, investigate the difference between self-reported height and measured height among:

(i) men with college education,
(ii) women with high school, and
(iii) women with college education.

In each case, name the test and state clearly your null and alternative hypotheses, and your choice of the test size. Also, compare the mean difference in the percentage discrepancy between

(a) men with different education levels,
(b) women with different education levels, and
(c) men versus women at each educational level.

In each case, name the test and state clearly your null and alternative hypotheses, and your choice of the test size.

7.8. A case–control study was undertaken to study the relationship between hypertension and obesity. Persons aged 30–49 years who were clearly nonhypertensive at their first multiple phase health checkup and became hypertensive by age 55 were sought and identified as cases. Controls were selected from among participants in a health plan, those who had the first checkup and no sign of hypertension in subsequent checkups. One control was matched to each case based on sex, race, year of birth, and year of entrance into the health plan. Data for 609 matched pairs are summarized as follows.

Variable	Paired Difference	
	Mean	Standard Deviation
Systolic blood pressure (mmHg)	6.8	13.86
Diastolic blood pressure (mmHg)	5.4	12.17
Body mass index (BMI, kg/m^2)	1.3	4.78

Compare the cases versus the controls using each measured characteristic; in each case, name the test and state clearly your null and alternative hypotheses, and your choice of the test size.

7.9. The Australian study of Example 6.13 also provided these data on monocular acuity (expressed in log scale) for two female groups of subjects (last two in the following table):

Sample	Sample size, n	Mean	Standard Deviation
Australian males of European origin	89	−.20	.18
Australian males of Aboriginal origin	107	−.26	.13
Australian females of European origin	63	−.13	.17
Australian females of Aboriginal origin	54	−.24	.18

Do these indicate a racial variation among women? Name your test and state clearly your null and alternative hypotheses, and your choice of the test size.

7.10. The ages (in days) at time of death for samples of 11 girls and 16 boys who died of sudden infant death syndrome are shown below:

Girls	{53, 56, 60, 60, 78, 87, 102, 117, 134, 160, 277}
Boys	{46, 52, 58, 59, 77, 78, 80, 81, 84, 103, 114, 115, 133, 134, 175, 175}

Do these indicate a gender difference? Name your test and state clearly your null and alternative hypotheses, and your choice of the test size.

7.11. An experimental study was conducted with 136 five-year-old children in four Quebec schools to investigate the impact of simulation games designed to teach children to obey certain traffic safety rules. The transfer of learning was measured by observing children's reactions to a quasi-real-life model of traffic risks. The scores on the transfer of learning for the control and attitude and behavior simulation game groups are summarized below:

Statistics	Control	Simulation Game
Sample size	30	33
Mean	7.9	10.1
Standard deviation	3.7	2.3

Test to investigate the impact of simulation games; name your test and state clearly your null and alternative hypotheses, and your choice of the test size.

7.12. In a trial to compare a stannous fluoride dentifrice (A) with a commercially available fluoride-free dentifrice (D), 270 children received A and 250 received D for a period of 3 years. The number "X" of DMFS increments (i.e., the number of new Decayed, Missing, and Filled Tooth Surfaces) was obtained for each child. Results were:

Statistics	Dentifrice A	Dentifrice D
Sample size	270	250
Mean	9.78	12.83
Standard deviation	7.51	8.31

Do the results provide strong enough evidence to suggest a real effect of fluoride in *reducing* the mean DMFS?

7.13. An experiment was conducted at the University of California at Berkeley to study the psychological environment effect on the anatomy of the brain. A group of 19 rats was randomly divided into two groups. Twelve animals in the treatment group lived together in a large cage, furnished with playthings, which were changed daily, while animals in the control group lived in isolation with no toys. After a month, the experimental animals were killed and dissected. The following table gives the cortex weights (the thinking part of the brain) in milligrams:

Treatment	{707, 740, 745, 652, 649, 676, 699, 696, 712, 708, 749, 690}
Control	{669, 650, 651, 627, 656, 642, 698}

Use the two-sample *t*-test to compare the means of two groups and draw appropriate conclusion.

7.14. Depression is one of the most commonly diagnosed conditions among hospitalized patients in mental institutions. The occurrence of depression was determined during the summer of 1979 in a multiethnic probability sample of 1000 adults in Los Angeles County, as part of a community survey of the epidemiology of depression and help-seeking behavior. The primary measure of depression was the CES-D scale developed by the Center for Epidemiologic Studies. On a scale of 0 to 60, a score of 16 or higher was classified as depression. The following table gives the average CES-D score for the two sexes.

Gender	n	CES-D Score Mean	Standard Deviation
Males	412	7.6	7.5
Females	588	10.4	10.3

Use a t-test to compare the males versus the females and draw appropriate conclusion.

7.15. A study was undertaken to study the relationship between exposure to polychlorinated biphenyls (PCBs) and reproduction among women occupationally exposed to PCBs during the manufacture of capacitors in upstate New York. Interviews were conducted in 1982 with women who had held jobs with direct exposure and women who had never held a direct-exposure job, in order to ascertain information on reproductive outcomes. Data are summarized in the following table.

Statistics	Direct Exposure ($n = 172$)	Indirect Exposure ($n = 184$)
Weight gain (lb)		
Mean	25.5	29.0
Standard deviation	14.0	14.7
Birth weight (g)		
Mean	3313	3417
Standard deviation	456	486
Gestational age (days)		
Mean	279.0	279.3
Standard deviation	17.0	13.5

Test to evaluate the effect of direct exposure (as compared to indirect exposure) using each measured characteristic; in each case, name the test and state clearly your null and alternative hypotheses, and your choice of the test size.

7.16. The following data are taken from a study that compares adolescents who have bulimia to healthy adolescents with similar body compositions and levels of physical activity. The following table provides measures of daily caloric intake for random samples of 23 bulimic adolescents and 15 healthy ones.

Group	Daily Calorie Intake (kcal/kg)
Bulimic Adolescents	15.9, 16.0, 16.5, 18.9, 18.4, 18.1, 30.9, 29.2, 17.0, 17.6, 28.7, 28.0, 25.6, 25.2, 25.1, 24.5, 18.9, 19.6, 21.5, 24.1, 23.6, 22.9, 21.6
Healthy Adolescents	30.6, 25.7, 25.3, 24.5, 20.7, 22.4, 23.1, 23.8, 40.8, 37.4, 37.1, 30.6, 33.2, 33.7, 36.6

Use the two-sample t-test to compare the two population means; state clearly your null and alternative hypotheses, and your choice of the test size.

7.17. College students were assigned to three study methods in an experiment to determine the effect of study technique on learning. The three methods are Read only, Read and underline, and Read and take notes; and the test scores are:

Technique	Test Score
Read only	15, 14, 16, 13, 11, 14
Read and underline	15, 14, 25, 10, 12, 14
Read and take notes	18, 18, 18, 16, 18, 20

Test to compare the three groups simultaneously; name your test and state clearly your null and alternative hypotheses, and your choice of the test size.

7.18. Four different brands of margarine were analyzed to determine the level of some unsaturated fatty acids (as percentage of fats). Results are:

Brand	Fatty Acids (%)
Brand A	13.5, 13.4, 14.1, 14.2
Brand B	13.2, 12.7, 12.6, 13.9
Brand C	16.8, 17.2, 16.4, 17.3, 18.0
Brand D	18.1, 17.2, 18.7, 18.4

Test to compare the four groups simultaneously; name your test and state clearly your null and alternative hypotheses, and your choice of the test size.

7.19. A study was done to determine if simplification of smoking literature improved patient comprehension. All subjects were administered a pretest. Subjects were then randomized into three groups. One group received no booklet, one group received one written at the 5th grade reading level, and the third received one written at the 10th grade reading level. After booklets were received, all subjects were administered a second test. The mean score differences (postscore minus prescore) are given below along with their standard deviations and sample sizes.

Test Group	Score Difference		
	n	Mean	Standard Deviation
No booklet	44	.25	2.28
Fifth grade level	44	1.57	2.54
Tenth grade level	41	.63	2.38

Test to compare the three groups simultaneously; name your test and state clearly your null and alternative hypotheses, and your choice of the test size.

7.20. A study was conducted to investigate the risk factors for peripheral arterial disease among persons 55–74 years of age. The following table provides data on LDL cholesterol levels (mmol/l) from four different sub-groups of subjects:

Patient Group	LDL Cholesterol (mmol/l)		
	n	Mean	Standard Deviation
No disease	1080	5.47	1.31
Major asymptotic disease	105	5.81	1.43
Minor asymptotic disease	240	5.77	1.24
Intermittent claudication	73	6.22	1.62

Test to compare the four groups simultaneously; name your test and state clearly your null and alternative hypotheses, and your choice of the test size.

7.21. A study was undertaken in order to clarify the relationship between heart disease and occupational carbon disulphide exposure along with another important factor, elevated diastolic blood pressure (DBP), in a data set obtained from a 10-year prospective follow-up of two cohorts of over 340 male industrial workers in Finland. Carbon disulphide is an industrial solvent, which is used to obtained from a 10-year prospective follow-up of two cohorts of over 340 male industrial workers in Finland. Carbon disulphide is an industrial solvent, which is used all over the world in the production of viscose rayon fibers. The following table gives the mean and standard deviation of serum cholesterol (mg/100 ml) among exposed and nonexposed cohorts, by diastolic blood pressure.

DBP (mmHg)	Exposed			Nonexposed		
	n	Mean	Standard Deviation	n	Mean	Standard Deviation
Below 95	205	220	50	271	221	42
95–100	92	227	57	53	236	46
Over 100	20	233	41	10	216	48

Test to compare simultaneously, separately for the exposed and nonexposed groups, the means serum cholesterol level at the three DBP levels using one-way ANOVA. Also, compare serum cholesterol levels between exposed and nonexposed cohorts at each level of DBP by using the two-sample t-tests. Draw your conclusions.

7.22. When a patient is diagnosed as having cancer of the prostate, an important question in deciding on treatment strategy for the patient is whether or not the cancer has spread to the neighboring lymph nodes. The question is so critical in prognosis and treatment that it is customary to operate on the patient (i.e., perform a laparotomy) for the sole purpose of examining the nodes and removing tissue samples to examine under the microscope for evidence of cancer. However, certain variables that can be measured without surgery are predictive of the nodal involvement; and the purpose of the study presented here was to examine the data for 53 prostate cancer patients receiving surgery, to determine which of five preoperative variables are predictive of nodal involvement. The following table presents the complete data set. For each of the 53 patients, there are two continuous independent variables, age at diagnosis and level of serum acid phosphatase (multiplied by 100; called "acid"), and three binary variables, X-ray reading, pathology reading (grade) of a biopsy of the tumor obtained by needle before surgery, and a rough measure of the size and location of the tumor (stage) obtained by palpation with the fingers via the rectum. For these three binary independent variables a value of one signifies a positive or more serious state and a zero denotes a negative or less serious finding. In addition, the sixth column presents the finding at surgery—the primary outcome of interest, which is binary, a value of one denoting nodal involvement, and a value of zero denoting no nodal involvement found at surgery. We investigate the effects of the three binary preoperative variables (X-ray, grade, and stage) on the outcome in Exercises 1.46 and 6.29. Descriptive statistics for the two continuous factors (age and acid phosphatase) were studied in Exercise 2.33. In this exercise we continue to focus on these continuous factors and their effects on the out come.

(a) Test to compare the group with nodal involvement and the group without in terms of Age and Acid phosphatase. Name your test and state clearly your null and alternative hypotheses, and your choice of the test size.

(b) Form four "Study Groups" as follows:
(1) those with nodal involvement but negative X-ray and negative grade, (2) those with nodal involvement but with either positive X-ray and/or positive grade, (3) those without nodal involvement, negative X-ray and negative grade, and (4) those without nodal involvement but with either positive X-ray and/or positive grade. Compare (simultaneously) the means of Age and Acid phosphatase of these four groups by the method of One-way ANOVA; state clearly your null and alternative hypotheses, and your choice of the test size.

Data

Case	X-Ray	Grade	Stage	Age	Acid	Nodes
1	0	1	1	64	40	0
2	0	0	1	63	40	0
3	1	0	0	65	46	0
4	0	1	0	67	47	0
5	0	0	0	66	48	0
6	0	1	1	65	48	0
7	0	0	0	60	49	0
8	0	0	0	51	49	0
8	0	0	0	66	50	0
10	0	0	0	58	50	0
11	0	1	0	56	50	0
12	0	0	1	61	50	0
13	0	1	1	64	50	0
14	0	0	0	56	52	0
15	0	0	0	67	52	0
16	1	0	0	49	55	0
17	0	1	1	52	55	0
18	0	0	0	68	56	0
19	0	1	1	66	59	0
20	1	0	0	60	62	0
21	0	0	0	61	62	0
22	1	1	1	59	63	0
23	0	0	0	51	65	0
24	0	1	1	53	66	0
25	0	0	0	58	71	0
26	0	0	0	63	75	0
27	0	0	1	53	76	0
28	0	0	0	60	78	0
29	0	0	0	52	83	0
30	0	0	1	67	95	0
31	0	0	0	56	98	0
32	0	0	1	61	102	0
33	0	0	0	64	187	0
34	1	0	1	58	48	1
35	0	0	1	65	49	1
36	1	1	1	57	51	1
37	0	1	0	50	56	1
38	1	1	0	67	67	1
39	0	0	1	67	67	1
40	0	1	1	57	67	1
41	0	1	1	45	70	1
42	0	0	1	46	70	1
43	1	0	1	51	72	1
44	1	1	1	60	76	1
45	1	1	1	56	78	1

(*continued*)

Data (*Continued*)

Case	X-Ray	Grade	Stage	Age	Acid	Nodes
46	1	1	1	50	81	1
47	0	0	0	56	82	1
48	0	0	1	63	82	1
49	1	1	1	65	84	1
50	1	0	1	64	89	1
51	0	1	0	59	99	1
52	1	1	1	68	126	1
53	1	0	0	61	136	1

Regression Analysis

Methods discussed in Chapters 6 and 7 are tests of significance; they provide analyses of data where a single measurement was made on each element of a sample, and the study may involve one or two, or several samples. If the measurement made is binary or categorical, we are often concerned with a comparison of proportions—the topics of Chapter 6. If the measurement made is continuous, we are often concerned with a comparison of means—the topics of Chapter 7. The main focus of both the chapters was the *difference* between populations or subpopulations. In many other studies, however, the purpose of the research is to assess *relationships* among a set of variables. For example, the sample consists of pairs of values, say a mother's weight and her newborn's weight measured from each of 50 sets of mother and baby, and the research objective is concerned with the *association* between these weights. Regression analysis is the technique for investigating relationships between variables; it can be used for both assessment of association and prediction. Consider, for example, an analysis of whether or not a woman's age is predictive of her systolic blood pressure. As another example, the research question could be whether or not a leukemia patient's white blood count is predictive of his survival time. Research designs may be classified as experimental or observational. *Regression analyses* are applicable to both types, yet the confidence one has in the results of a study can vary with the research type. In most cases, one variable is usually taken to be the *response* or *dependent variable*, which is the variable to be predicted from or explained by other variables. The other variables are called *predictors*, explanatory variable, or *independent variables*. The above examples, and others, show a wide range of applications in which the dependent variable is a continuous measurement. Such a variable is often assumed to be normally distributed, and a *model* is formulated to express the *mean* of this normal distribution as a function of potential independent variables under investigation. The dependent variable is denoted by Y and the study often involves a number of *risk factors* or *predictor variables*: $X_1, X_2, \ldots, X_k$ (it is the same as

Health and Numbers: A Problems-Based Introduction to Biostatistics, Third Edition, by Chap T. Le
Copyright © 2009 John Wiley & Sons, Inc.

in previous chapters, we use capital letters for variable names and lower case letters for their values).

8.1. SIMPLE REGRESSION ANALYSIS

In this section, we will discuss the basic ideas of *simple regression analysis* when only one predictor or independent variable is available for predicting the response of interest. In the interpretation of the primary parameter of the model, we will discuss both scales of measurement, discrete and continuous, even though in practical applications, the independent variable under investigation is often on a continuous scale.

8.1.1. The Simple Linear Regression Model

Choosing an appropriate model and analytical technique depends on the type of variable under investigation. In a variety of applications, the dependent variable of interest is a continuous variable that we can assume, may be after an appropriate transformation, to be normally distributed. The *regression model* describes the *mean* of that normally distributed dependent variable Y as a function of the value of the predictor or independent variable X, $X = x$. The model describes how possible values of Y are distributed give a fixed value "x" of X:

$$Y_i = \beta_0 + \beta_1 x_i + \varepsilon_i$$

where

(a) x_i is a given fixed value of the independent variable X, and Y_i is the (random) value of the response or dependent variable Y from the ith subject,

(b) β_0 and β_1 are the two fixed but unknown parameters; $(\beta_0 + \beta_1 x_i)$ is the mean of Y_i as stipulated by the model,

(c) ε_i is a random error term that is distributed as normal with mean zero and variance σ^2; σ^2 is also the variance of Y_i because $(\beta_0 + \beta_1 x_i)$ is fixed.

The above model is referred to as the *simple linear regression model*. It is simple because it contains only one independent variable. It is *linear* because the independent variable appears only in the first power; if we graph the mean of Y versus X, the graph is a *straight line* with *intercept* β_0 and *slope* β_1.

8.1.2. The Scatter Diagram

As mentioned above, and stipulated by the simple linear regression model, that if we graph the mean of Y versus X, the graph is a straight line. But that is the line for the means of Y; at each level of X, say $X = x$, the *observed value* of Y, $Y = y$, may exceed or fall short of its mean. Therefore, when we graph the observed value of Y versus x, the points do not fall perfectly on any line. This is an important characteristic for statistical relationships as pointed out in Chapter 2. If we let each pair of numbers (x, y) be represented by a dot in a diagram with the x's on the horizontal axis, we have a figure called *scatter diagram* as seen in later parts of Chapter 2 and again in the next few examples. The scatter diagram is a useful diagnostic tool for checking out the validity of features of the simple linear regression model. For example, if dots fall around a curve, not a straight line, then the *linearity* assumption may be violated. In addition, the model stipulates that, each level of X, $X = x$, the normal distribution for Y has constant variance not depending on the value of x. That would lead to a scatter diagram with dots spreading out—around the line—evenly across levels of X. Most of the times, an appropriate transformation, such as taking logarithm, of Y and/or X would improve and bring the data closer to fitting the model.

8.1.3. Meaning of Regression Parameters

The parameters β_0 and β_1 are called regression coefficients. The parameter β_0 is the intercept of the regression line. If the scope of the model include $X = 0$, β_0 gives the mean of Y when $X = 0$; when the scope of the model does not cover $X = 0$, β_0 does not have any particular meaning as a separate term in the regression model. As for the meaning of β_1, our more important parameter, it can be seen as follows.

We first consider the case of a binary independent variable with the conventional coding

$$x_i = \begin{cases} 0 & \text{if the patient is not exposed} \\ 1 & \text{if the patient is exposed} \end{cases}$$

Here, the term "exposed" may refer to a risk factor such as smoking, or a patient's characteristic such as race (white/nonwhite) or sex (male/female). It can be seen that,

(i) For a nonexposed subject, that is, $X = 0$,

$$\mu_y = \beta_0$$

(ii) For an exposed subject, that is, $X = 1$,

$$\mu_y = \beta_0 + \beta_1$$

Hence, β_1 represents the *increase* (or *decrease*, if β_1 is negative) in the mean of Y associated with the exposure. Similarly, we have for a continuous covariate X and any value x of X,

(i) When $X = x$,

$$\mu_y = \beta_0 + \beta_1 x$$

(ii) Whereas if $X = x + 1$,

$$\mu_y = \beta_0 + \beta_1(x + 1)$$

It can be seen that, by taking the difference, β_1 represents the *increase* (or *decrease*, if β_1 is negative) in the mean of Y associated with *one unit increase* in the value of X from $(X = x)$ to $(X = x + 1)$. For m units increase in the value of X, say $(X = x + m)$ versus $(X = x)$, the corresponding increase (or decrease) in the mean of Y is $m\beta_1$.

8.1.4. Estimation of Parameters

To find *good* estimates of the unknown parameters β_0 and β_1, statisticians use a method called *least squares method*, which is described as follows. For each subject or pair of values (x_i, y_i), we consider the *deviation* from the observed value y_i to its mean (or expected value) $(\beta_0 + \beta_1 x_i)$,

$$[y_i - (\beta_0 + \beta_1 x_i)]$$

According to the method of least squares, the good estimates of β_0 and β_1 are values b_0 and b_1 that minimize the *sum of squared deviations*:

$$S = \sum [y_i - (\beta_0 + \beta_1 x_i)]^2$$

The results are

$$b_1 = \frac{\sum xy - \frac{(\sum x)(\sum y)}{n}}{\sum x^2 - \frac{(\sum x)^2}{n}}$$

$$b_0 = \bar{y} - b_1 \bar{x}$$

The calculations are very tedious, and in Section 8.3 we will show you how to obtain these results by Excel. Given the estimates b_0 and b_1 obtained from the sample, we estimate the mean response by

$$\hat{y} = b_0 + b_1 x$$

This is our *predicted value* for (the mean of) Y at a given level/value of x.

Example 8.1

In the following table, the first two columns give the values for the birth weight (x, in ounces) and the increase in weight between 70th and 100th days of life, expressed as a percentage of the birth weight (y) for 12 infants.

Birth Weight x (oz)	Growth y (%)	x^2	y^2	xy
112	63	12544	3969	7056
111	66	12321	4356	7326
107	72	11449	5184	7704
119	52	14161	2704	6188
92	75	8464	5625	6900
80	118	6400	13924	9440
81	120	6561	14400	9720
84	114	7056	12996	9576
118	42	13924	1764	4956
106	72	11236	5184	7632
103	90	10609	8100	9270
94	91	8836	8281	8554
1207	975	123561	86487	94322

We first let each pair of numbers (x, y) be represented by a dot in a diagram with the x's on the horizontal axis, and we have the scatter diagram shown below. The dots do not fall perfectly on a straight line, but rather scatter around one, very typical for statistical relationships. However, a straight line seems to fit very well.

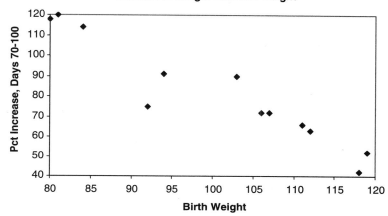

Increase in Weight Vs. Birth Weight

Generally, the 12 dots go from upper left to lower right indicating a negative association. We obtained, as shown in Example 2.11, a Pearson's correlation coefficient of $r = -.946$,

$$r = \frac{94,322 - \frac{(1207)(975)}{12}}{\sqrt{\left[123,561 - \frac{(1207)^2}{12}\right]\left[86,487 - \frac{(975)^2}{12}\right]}}$$

$$= -.946$$

Applying the formulas, we obtain the estimates for the slope and intercept as follows:

$$b_1 = \frac{\sum xy - \frac{(\sum x)(\sum y)}{n}}{\sum x^2 - \frac{(\sum x^2)}{n}}$$

$$= \frac{94,322 - \frac{(1207)(975)}{12}}{123,561 - \frac{(1207)^2}{12}}$$

$$= -1.74$$

$$b_0 = \bar{y} - b_1 \bar{x}$$

$$= \frac{975}{12} - (-1.74)\left(\frac{1207}{12}\right)$$

$$= 256.3$$

Similar to the coefficient of correlation r, the slope is positive for a positive association and negative for a negative association; in this example, both the slope (-1.74) and the coefficient of correlation $(-.946)$ are negative. The estimates of the slope and the intercept help us predict values of the dependent variable Y (the response) if we know the value of the independent variable X (the predictor)—even for the subject not included in the sample. For example, if the birth weight of some baby is 95 ounces, it is predicted that the increase between the 70th and 100th days of life would be

$$\hat{y} = b_0 + b_1 x$$
$$= 256.3 + (-1.74)(95)$$
$$= 90.1$$

Or the predicted growth is 90.1% of that baby's birth weight.

The graph of the regression line can also be imposed on the scatter diagram as shown below, and you will learn how to do this by Excel in Section 8.3.

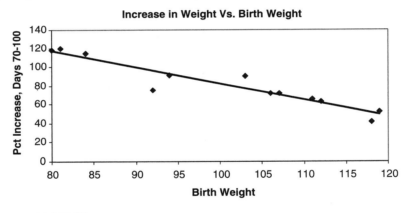

Increase in Weight Vs. Birth Weight

Example 8.2

In the following table, the first two columns give the values for age (x, in years) and systolic blood pressure (y, in mmHg) for 15 women. From the following table, we obtained, as shown in Example 2.12, a Pearson's correlation coefficient of $r = .566$ indicating a moderate positive association,

Age (x)	SBP (y)	x^2	y^2	xy
42	130	1764	16900	5460
46	115	2116	13225	5290

(Continued)

Age (x)	SBP (y)	x^2	y^2	xy
42	148	1764	21904	6216
71	100	5041	10000	7100
80	156	6400	24336	12480
74	162	5476	26244	11988
70	151	4900	22801	10570
80	156	6400	24336	12480
85	162	7225	26244	13770
72	158	5184	24964	11376
64	155	4096	24025	9920
81	160	6561	25600	12960
41	125	1681	15625	5125
61	150	3721	22500	9150
75	165	5625	27225	12375
984	2193	67954	325929	146260

We can also obtain the estimates for the slope and intercept as follows:

$$b_1 = \frac{\sum xy - \dfrac{(\sum x)(\sum y)}{n}}{\sum x^2 - \dfrac{(\sum x)^2}{n}}$$

$$= \frac{146{,}260 - \dfrac{(984)(2193)}{15}}{67{,}954 - \dfrac{(984)^2}{15}}$$

$$= .71$$

$$b_0 = \bar{y} - b_1 \bar{x}$$

$$= \frac{2{,}193}{15} - (.71)\left(\frac{984}{15}\right)$$

$$= 99.6$$

The estimates of the slope and the intercept help us predict values of the dependent variable Y if we know the value of the independent variable X (the predictor)—even for the subject not included in the sample. For example, for a 50-year-old woman, it is predicted that her systolic blood pressure would be about

$$\hat{y} = b_0 + b_1 x$$

$$= 256.3 + (-1.74)(95)$$

$$= 90.1$$

We can let each pair of numbers (x, y) be represented by a dot in a diagram with the x's on the horizontal axis, and we have the scatter diagram—as in Chapter 2. Again the dots do not fall perfectly on a straight line, but rather scatter around one, very typical for statistical relationships. In this example, a straight line still seems to fit too; however, the dots spread more and cluster less around the line, indicating a weaker association. The graph of the regression line can also be imposed on the scatter diagram as shown below. The positive Pearson's correlation coefficient ($r = .566$) confirms the positive slope (.51) and the direction of the line in the graph.

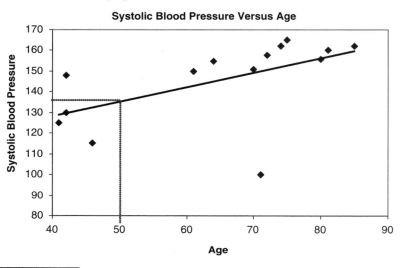

8.1.5. Testing for Independence

In addition to being able to *predict* the (mean) response at various levels of the independent variable, regression data can also be used to test for the independence between the two variables under investigation. Such a statistical test can be viewed or approached in two different ways: through the coefficient of correlation or through the slope; the coefficient of correlation r and the slope b_1 have the same numerator, and if one is zero so is the other.

(i) The correlation coefficient r measures the strength of the relationship between two variables. It is an estimate of an unknown population correlation coefficient ρ, the same way the sample mean is used as an estimate of some unknown population mean μ. We are usually interested in knowing whether we may conclude that $\rho \neq 0$, that is, that the two variables under investigation are really correlated. The test statistic is

$$t = r\sqrt{\frac{n-2}{1-r^2}}$$

The procedure is often performed as two-sided, that is,

$$H_A : \rho \neq 0$$

and it is a *t*-test with $(n-2)$ degrees of freedom, the same *t*-test as used in the comparisons of population means in Chapter 7.

(ii) The role of the slope β_1 can be seen as follows. Since the regression model describes the mean of the dependent variable Y as a function of the predictor or independent variable X,

$$\mu_y = \beta_0 + \beta_1 x$$

Y and X would be independent if $\beta_1 = 0$. The test for

$$H_0 : \beta_1 = 0$$

can be performed similar to the method for one-sample problems in Chapters 6 and 7 (Sections 6.1 and 7.1). In that process, the observed/estimated value b_1 is converted to standard unit: the number of standard errors away from the hypothesized value of zero. The formula for standard error of b_1 is rather complicated, and fortunately, the resulting test is *identical* to the above t-test. Whenever needed, for example in the computation of confidence intervals for the slope, we can always obtain the numerical value of its standard error from computer output.

When the above t-test for independence is significant, the value of X has a real effect on the distribution of Y. To be more precise, the square of the correlation coefficient, r^2, represents the proportion of the variability of Y accountable for by X. For example, a $r^2 = .25$ indicates that the total variation in Y is reduced by 25% by the use of information about X. In other words, if we have a sample of the same size, with all the n subjects having the same X-value, the variation in Y (say, measured by its variance) is 25% less than the variation of Y in the current sample. It is interesting to note that an $r = .5$ would give an impression of greater association between X and Y, but a 25% reduction in variation would not. The parameter r^2 is called the *coefficient of determination*, an index with a clear operational interpretation than the coefficient of correlation r.

Example 8.3

For the birth weight problem of Example 2.11 and Example 8.1, we have

$$n = 12,$$

$$r = -.946$$

$$t = (-.946)\sqrt{\frac{10}{1-(-.946)^2}}$$

$$= -9.23$$

At $\alpha = .05$ and 10 degrees of freedom, the tabulated (two-sided) t-coefficient is 2.228; this indicates that the null hypothesis of independence should be rejected, and the (computed) value $t = -9.23 < -2.228$. In this case, the birth weight (X) would account for

$$r^2 = .895$$

or 89.5% of the variation in growth rates between day 70 and day 100.

Example 8.4

For the blood pressure problem of Example 2.12 and Example 8.2, we have

$$n = 15,$$
$$r = .566$$

$$t = (.566)\sqrt{\frac{13}{1-(.566)^2}}$$

$$= 2.475$$

At $\alpha = .05$ and 13 degrees of freedom, the tabulated (two-sided) t-coefficient value is 2.16. Since the (computed) value $t > 2.16$, we have to conclude that the null hypothesis of independence should be rejected; the relationship between age and systolic blood pressure is real—not found by chance. However, a woman's age (X) would account for only

$$r^2 = .32$$

or 32% of the variation among systolic blood pressures.

8.1.6. Analysis of Variance Approach

The variation in Y is conventionally measured in terms of the deviations from observed values to the mean; the total variation, denoted by SST, is the sum of squared deviations:

$$\text{SST} = \sum (Y_i - \bar{Y})^2$$

For example, SST $= 0$ when all observations are the same; SST is the numerator of the sample variance of Y, the greater the SST the greater the variation among Y-values.

When we use the regression approach, the variation in Y is decomposed into two components:

$$(Y_i - \bar{Y}) = (Y_i - \hat{Y}_i) - (\hat{Y} - \bar{Y})$$

(i) The first term reflects the variation around the regression line measuring the deviation from each observed value to its predicted value, and the part than cannot be explained by the regression itself with the sum of squared deviations:

$$\text{SSE} = \sum (Y_i - \hat{Y}_i)^2$$

called the *error sum of squares*, and

(ii) the difference between the above two sums of squares,

$$\text{SSR} = \text{SST} - \text{SSE}$$
$$= \sum (\hat{Y}_i - \bar{Y})^2$$

is called the *regression sum of squares*. SSR may be considered a measure of the variation in Y associated with the regression line. In fact, we can express the *coefficient of determination* as

$$r^2 = \frac{SSR}{SST}$$

Corresponding to the partitioning of the total sum of squares SST, there is partitioning of the associated degrees of freedom (df). We have $(n-1)$ degrees of freedom associated with SST, the denominator of the sample variance of Y; SSR has one degree of freedom representing the slope, and the remaining $(n-2)$ are associated with SSE. These results lead to the usual presentation of regression analysis by most computer programs:

(i) The error mean square

$$MSE = \frac{SSE}{(n-2)}$$

serves as an estimate of the constant variance σ^2 as stipulated by the regression model.

(ii) The breakdowns of the total sum of squares and its associated degree of freedom are displayed in the form of an analysis of variance table (ANOVA table) as follows:

Source of Variation	SS	df	MS	F-statistic	p-value
Regression	SSR	1	MSE	$F = MSR/MSE$	p
Error	SSE	$n-2$	MSE		
Total	SST	$n-1$			

The test statistic F for the above analysis of variance approach compares MSR and MSE, and a value near 1 supports the null hypothesis of independence. In fact, we have

$$F = t^2$$

where t is the test statistic for testing whether or not the dependent variable Y and the independent variable X is correlated (i.e., $\rho = 0$); the F-test is equivalent to the two-sided t-test when referred to the F-table in Appendix E with $(1, n-2)$ degrees of freedom.

Example 8.5

For the birth weight problem of Examples 8.1 and 8.3, we have

Source of Variation	SS	df	MS	F-statistic	p-value
Regression	6508.43	1	6508.43	85.657	0.0001
Error	759.82	10	75.98		
Total	7268.25	11			

Example 8.6

For the blood pressure problem of Examples 8.2 and 8.4, we have

Source of Variation	SS	df	MS	F-statistic	p-value
Regression	16.91.20	1	1691.20	6.071	0.0285
Error	3621.20	13	278.55		
Total	5312.40	14			

8.2. MULTIPLE REGRESSION ANALYSIS

The effect of some factor on a dependent or response variable may be influenced by the presence of other factors because of redundancies or effect modifications, that is, interactions. Therefore, to provide a more comprehensive analysis, it may be desirable to consider a large number of factors and sort out which ones are most closely related to the dependent variable. In this section, we will discuss a *multivariate method* for this type of risk determination. This method, which is *multiple regression analysis*, involves a linear combination of the explanatory or independent variables, also called *covariates*; the variables must be quantitative with particular numerical values for each subject in the sample. A covariate or independent variable—such as a patient characteristic—may be dichotomous, polytomous, or continuous (categorical factors will be represented by dummy variables). Examples of dichotomous covariates are sex and presence or absence of certain comorbidity. Polytomous covariates include race and different grades of symptoms; these can be covered by the use of *dummy variables*. Continuous covariates include patient age, blood pressure, and so on. In many cases, data transformations (e.g., taking the logarithm) may be needed to satisfy the linearity assumption.

8.2.1. Regression Model with Several Independent Variables

Suppose we want to consider k independent variables simultaneously, and then the simple linear model of previous section can be easily generalized and expressed as

$$Y_i = \beta_0 + \beta_1 x_{1i} + \cdots + \beta_k x_{ki} + \varepsilon_i$$

$$= \beta_0 + \sum_{j=1}^{k} \beta_j x_{ji} + \varepsilon_i$$

where

(i) Y_i is the value of the response or dependent variable from the ith subject,

(ii) The quantities $\beta_0, \beta_1, \beta_2, \ldots, \beta_k$ represent unknown parameters; β_0 is the *intercept* and $\beta_1, \beta_2, \ldots, \beta_k$ are the *slopes*, one for each independent variables.

(iii) The x's are the values of the k independent variables $X_1, X_2, \ldots, X_k$ measured from the ith subject ($i = 1-n$), and

(iv) ε_i is a random error term which is distributed as normal with mean zero and variance σ^2, so that the mean of Y is

$$\mu_i = \beta_0 + \beta_1 x_{1i} + \cdots + \beta_k x_{ki}$$

$$= \beta_0 + \sum_{j=1}^{k} \beta_j x_{ji}$$

The above model is referred to as the *multiple linear regression model*. It is *multiple* because it contains several independent variables. It is still *linear* because the independent variables appear only in the first power; this feature is rather difficult to check because we do not have a scatter diagram to rely on as in the case of simple linear regression. In addition, the model can modified to include higher powers of independent variables as well as their various products as seen in subsequent sections.

8.2.2. Meaning of Regression Parameters

Similar to the univariate case of Section 8.1, the regression coefficient β_i represents

(i) The *increase* (or *decrease*, if β_i is negative) in the mean of Y associated with the exposure if X_i is binary (for example, $X_i = 1$ if exposed versus $X_i = 0$ if not exposed, where X represents an *exposure*) *assuming* that other independent variables are fixed, or

(ii) The *increase* (or *decrease*, if β_i is negative) in the mean of Y associated with *one unit increase* in the value of X_i if X_i is continuous (e.g., $X_i = x + 1$ versus $X_i = x$) *assuming* that other independent variables are fixed. For m units increase in the value of X_i ($X_i = x + m$) versus ($X_i = x$), the corresponding increase (or decrease) in the mean of Y is $m(\beta_i)$ *assuming* that other independent variables are fixed. In other words, β_i represents the *additional contribution* of X_i in the explanation of variation among values of Y. Of course, before such analyses are done, the problem and the data have to be examined carefully. If some of the variables are highly correlated, then one or fewer of the correlated factors are likely to be as good predictors as all of them; information from other similar studies also has to be incorporated so as to drop some of these correlated explanatory variables.

8.2.3. Effect Modifications

Consider the multiple regression model involving two independent variables:

$$Y_i = \beta_0 + \beta_1 x_{1i} + \beta_2 x_{2i} + \beta_3 x_{1i} x + \varepsilon_i$$

It can be seen that the meaning of β_1 and β_2 here is not the same as that given earlier because of the cross-product term $\beta_3 x_1 x_2$. Suppose, for simplicity, that both X_1 and X_2 are binary, then

(1) For $X_2 = 1$ or exposed, we have

$$\mu_i = \begin{cases} \beta_0 + \beta_1 + \beta_2 + \beta_3 & \text{if exposed to } X_1 \\ \beta_0 + \beta_2 & \text{if not exposed to } X_1 \end{cases}$$

so that the increase (or decrease) in the mean of Y due to an exposure to X_1 is $\beta_1 + \beta_3$, whereas

(2) For $X_2 = 0$ or unexposed, we have

$$\mu_i = \begin{cases} \beta_0 + \beta_1 + & \text{if exposed to } X_1 \\ \beta_0 & \text{if not exposed to } X_1 \end{cases}$$

so that the increase (or decrease) in the mean of Y due to an exposure to X_1 is β_1. In other words, the effect of X_1 depends on the level (presence or absence) of X_2 and vice versa. This phenomenon is called *effect modification*, that is, one factor modifies the effect of the other. The cross-product term $x_1 x_2$ is called an *interaction term*; the use of these products will help in the investigation of possible effect modifications. If $\beta_3 = 0$, the effect of two factors acting together (represented by $\beta_1 + \beta_3$) is equal to the combined effects of two factors acting separately. If $\beta_3 > 0$, we have a synergistic interaction; if $\beta_3 < 0$, we have an a antagonistic interaction.

8.2.4. Polynomial Regression

Consider the multiple regression model involving one independent variable

$$Y_i = \beta_0 + \beta_1 x_i + \beta_2 x_i^2 + \varepsilon_i$$

or it can be written as a multiple model

$$Y_i = \beta_0 + \beta_1 x_{1i} + \beta_2 x_{2i} + \varepsilon_i$$

with $(X_1 = X)$ and $(X_2 = X^2)$ where X is a continuous independent variable. The meaning of β_1 here is not the same as that given earlier because of the quadratic term $\beta_2 x_i^2$. We have, for example,

$$\mu_i = \begin{cases} \beta_0 + \beta_1 x + \beta_2 x^2 + \beta_3 & \text{when } X = x \\ \beta_0 + \beta_1(x+1) + \beta_2(x+1)^2 & \text{when } X = x+1 \end{cases}$$

So that the difference is

$$\beta_1 + \beta_2(2x+1)$$

a function of x.

Polynomial models with an independent variable presented in higher powers than the second are not often used. The second-order or quadratic model has two basic types of uses:

(i) When the true relationship is a second degree polynomial or when the true relationship is unknown but the second degree polynomial provides a better fit than a linear one, but

(ii) More often, a quadratic model is fitted for the purpose of establishing the linearity. The key item to look is whether $(\beta_2 = 0)$.

The use of polynomial models, however, is not without drawbacks. The most potential drawback is that X and X^2 are related—may be strongly, especially, if X is restricted to a narrow range; in this case, the standard errors are often very large.

8.2.5. Estimation of Parameters

To find good estimates of the $(k + 1)$ unknown parameters $\beta_0, \beta_1, \beta_2, \ldots, \beta_k$, statisticians use the same *method of least squares* that was described in the previous section. For each subject with data values $(y_i; x_{1i}, x_{2i}, \ldots, x_{ki})$, we consider the *deviation* from the observed value y_i to its mean (or expected value} $(\beta_0 + \beta_1 x_{1i} + \cdots + \beta_k x_{ki})$,

$$[y_i - (\beta_0 + \beta_1 x_{1i} + \cdots + \beta_k x_{ki})]$$

According to the method of least squares, the good estimates of $\beta_0, \beta_1, \beta_2, \ldots, \beta_k$ are values $b_0, b_1, b_2, \ldots, b_k$, which minimizes the *sum of squared deviations*

$$S = \sum [y_i - (\beta_0 + \beta_1 x_{1i} + \cdots + \beta_k x_{ki})]^2$$

The method is the same, but the results are much more difficult to obtain, and fortunately these results are provided by most standard computer programs, including Excel. In addition, computer output also provides standard errors for all estimates of regression coefficients.

8.2.6. Analysis of Variance Approach

Similar to the case of simple linear regression of Section 8.1.6, the variation in Y is also measured in terms of the deviations from observed values to the mean; the total variation, denoted by SST, is the sum of squared deviations:

$$\text{SST} = \sum (Y_i - \bar{Y})^2$$

The variation in Y is decomposed into two components:

$$(Y_i - \bar{Y}) = (Y_i - \hat{Y}_i) - (\hat{Y} - \bar{Y})$$

(i) The first term reflects the deviation from each observed value to its predicted value; the part than cannot be explained by the regression itself with the sum of squared deviations

$$\text{SSE} = \sum (Y_i - \hat{Y}_i)^2$$

called the *error sum of squares*, and

(ii) The difference between the above two sums of squares,

$$\text{SSR} = \text{SST} - \text{SSE}$$
$$= \sum (\hat{Y}_i - \bar{Y})^2$$

is called the *regression sum of squares*. SSR may be considered a measure of the variation in Y associated with the regression line. The coefficient of multiple determination is defined as

$$R^2 = \frac{\text{SSR}}{\text{SST}}$$

It measures the proportionate reduction of total variation in Y associated with the use of the set of independent variables. As for r^2 of the simple linear regression, we have

$$0 \leq R^2 \leq 1$$

and R^2 only assumes the value 0 when $\beta_0 = \beta_1 = \beta_2 = \ldots = \beta_k = 0$.

Corresponding to the partitioning of the total sum of squares SST, there is partitioning of the associated degrees of freedom (df). We have $(n - 1)$ degrees of freedom associated with SST, the denominator of the sample variance of Y; SSR has k degree of freedom representing the k independent variables, the remaining $(n - k - 1)$ are associated with SSE. These results lead to the usual presentation of regression analysis by most computer programs:

(i) The error mean square

$$\text{MSE} = \frac{\text{SSE}}{(n-k-1)}$$

serves as an estimate of the constant variance σ^2 as stipulated by the regression model, and

(ii) The breakdowns of the total sum of squares and its associated degree of freedom are displayed in the form of an analysis of variance table (ANOVA table) as follows:

Source of Variation	SS	df	MS	F-statistic	p-value
Regression	SSR	k	MSE	$F = \text{MSR/MSE}$	p
Error	SSE	$n - k - 1$	MSE		
Total	SST	$n - 1$			

8.2.7. Testing Hypotheses in Multiple Linear Regression

Once we have fit a multiple regression model and obtained estimates for the various parameters of interest, we want to answer questions about the contributions of various factors to the prediction of the binary response variable. The following are two such questions that we are interested in

(i) *An overall test*: Taken collectively, does the entire set of explanatory or independent variables contribute significantly to the prediction of the response? (or the explanation of variation among responses)

(ii) *Test for the value of a single factor*: Does the addition of one particular variable of interest add significantly to the prediction of response over and above that achieved by other independent variables?

Overall Regression Test

We now consider the first question stated above concerning an overall test for a model containing k factors. The null hypothesis for this test may be stated as: "All k independent variables *considered together* do not explain the variation in the responses." In other words, the null hypothesis is

$$H_0 : \beta_1 = \beta_2 = \cdots = \beta_k = 0$$

This *global* null hypothesis can tested using the "F statistic" in the above ANOVA table:

$$F = \frac{MSR}{MSE}$$

an F-test at $(k, n - k - 1)$ degrees of freedom; the test result (p-value) is contained in the last column of that ANOVA table.

Tests for Single Variables

Let us suppose that we now wish to test whether the addition of one particular independent variable of interest adds significantly to the prediction of the response over and above that achieved by other factors already present in the model. The null hypothesis for this test may be stated as: "Factor X_i does not have any value added to the prediction of the response *given* that other factors are already included in the model." In other words,

$$H_0 : \beta_i = 0$$

To test such a null hypothesis, one can use

$$t = \frac{\hat{\beta}}{SE(\hat{\beta})}$$

in a t-test with $(n - k - 1)$ degrees of freedom, where the quantity in the numerator is the estimated regression coefficient and the quantity in the denominator is the estimate of the standard error of that estimated regression coefficient, both are provided by Excel.

Example 8.7

Ultrasounds were taken at the time of liver transplant and again 5–10 years later to determine the systolic pressure of the hepatic artery. Results for 21 transplants for 21 children are shown in following table, and also available are sex ($1 =$ male, $2 =$ female) and age at the second measurement.

Child	After 5–10 yrs	At transplant	Sex	Age
1	46	35	1	16
2	40	40	1	19
3	50	58	1	19
4	50	71	0	23
5	41	33	0	16

(continued)

(*continued*)

Child	After 5–10 yrs	At transplant	Sex	Age
6	70	79	0	23
7	35	20	0	13
8	40	19	0	19
9	56	56	0	11
10	30	26	1	14
11	30	44	0	15
12	60	90	1	12
13	43	43	1	15
14	45	42	0	14
15	40	55	0	14
16	50	60	1	17
17	66	62	1	21
18	45	26	1	21
19	40	60	0	11
20	35	27	0	9
21	25	31	0	9

Using the second measurement of the systolic pressure of the hepatic artery as our dependent variable, the resulting ANOVA table is

ANOVA Table

Source of Variation	df	SS	MS	F	p-value
Regression	3	1810.93	603.64	12.158	0.00017
Residual	17	844.02	49.65		
Total	20	2654.95			

The result of the overall F-test ($p = 0.0002$) indicates that, taken collectively, three variables (systolic pressure at transplant, sex, and age) contribute significantly to the prediction of the dependent variable. The coefficient of multiple determination, obtained by Excel, is

$$R^2 = \frac{1810.93}{2654.95}$$

$$= .683$$

In other words, taken together the three independent variables (systolic pressure at transplant, sex, and age) account for 68.2% of variation in systolic blood pressure of the hepatic artery taken 5–10 years posttransplants.

In addition, we have:

	Coefficients	Standard Error	t Statistics	P-value
Intercept	11.384	6.517	1.747	0.0987
SBP at t transplant	0.381	0.082	4.631	0.0002
Sex	1.74	3.241	0.537	0.5982
Age	0.935	0.395	2.366	0.0301

The effects of pressure at transplant ($p = .0002$) and age ($p = 0301$) are significant at the 5% level whereas the effect of sex is not ($p = 0.5982$).

Example 8.8

There has been times the city of London experienced periods of dense fog. The following table shows such data for a 15-day very severe period that include the number of deaths in each day (y), the mean atmospheric smoke (X_1, in mg/m^3), and the mean atmospheric sulphur dioxide content (X_2, in parts/million):

Y	X_1	X_2
112	0.30	0.09
140	0.49	0.16
143	0.61	0.22
120	0.49	0.14
196	2.64	0.75
294	3.45	0.86
513	4.46	1.34
518	4.46	1.34
430	1.22	0.47
274	1.22	0.47
255	0.32	0.22
236	0.29	0.23
256	0.50	0.26
222	0.32	0.16
213	0.32	0.16

Using the number of deaths in each day as our dependent variable, the resulting ANOVA table is

ANOVA Table

Source of Variation	df	SS	MS	F	p-value
Regression	2	205,097.52	102,548.76	36.566	0.0001
Residual	12	33,654.20	2,804.52		
Total	14	238,751.73			

The result of the overall F-test ($p = 0.0001$) indicates that, taken collectively, the two independent variables contribute significantly to the prediction of the dependent variable. The coefficient of multiple determination, also obtained by Excel, is

$$R^2 = \frac{205,097.52}{238,751.73}$$

$$= .859$$

In other words, taken together the two independent variables (mean atmospheric smoke and mean atmospheric sulphur dioxide content) account for 85.9% of variation in the number of deaths in each day.

In addition, we have

	Coefficients	Standard Error	t Statistics	P-value
Smoke	−220.324	58.143	−3.789	0.0026
Sulfur	1051.816	212.596	4.947	0.0003

The effects of both factors, the mean atmospheric smoke and the mean atmospheric sulphur dioxide content, are significant even at the 1% level (both $p < 0.001$).

8.3. GRAPHICAL AND COMPUTATIONAL AIDS

Throughout several examples of this chapter, we show how to perform regression analysis, such as setting up ANOVA table and graphing the regression line. It has also been obvious that those needed formulas are very complicated, and the process is tedious and time-consuming. Fortunately, regression analysis can also be implemented easily using Microsoft's Excel; however, you need *Data Analysis*. "Data analysis" is an Excel add-in option that is available from the Excel installation CD; after installation, it is listed in your "Tools" menu (shown on top row—same place with other basic menus such as *File, Edit, View*, etc.).

ANOVA Table

The process is rather simple: (1) click the *Tools* and then (2) *Data Analysis*, and among functions available, choose *Regression*.

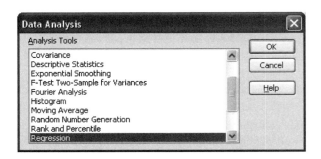

A box appears, use the cursor to fill in the ranges of Y and X's. The results include all items mentioned in this chapter, plus confidence intervals for regression coefficients. In the following figure, the data set (of Example 8.7) has one dependent variable (column B, rows 34–54) and three independent variables (columns C, D, and E—rows 34–54)

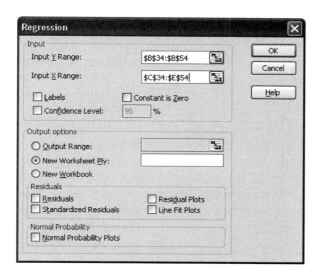

Regression Line

Step 1: Create a scatter diagram using *Chart Wizard* (see Sections 1.4 and 2.4).

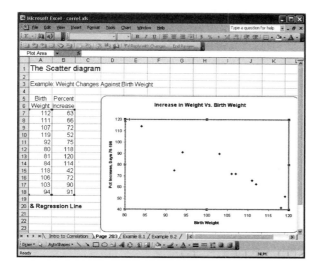

Step 2: (a) Click on the new Chart (scatter diagram) to make it active (at that point the menu on the top row has some minor changes), (b) Click on *Chart* (on the top row menu), (c) a box appears to let you choose "Type," and then select *Linear*.

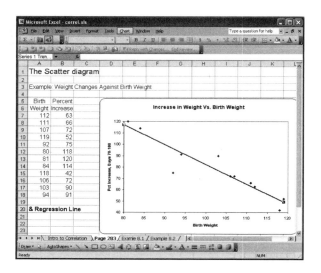

EXERCISES

8.1. Trace metals in drinking water affect the flavor of the water, and unusually high concentration can pose a health hazard. The following table shows trace metal concentrations (zinc, in mg/L) for both surface water and bottom water at six different river locations. Our aim is to see if surface water concentration (X) is predictive of bottom water concentration (Y).

Location	Bottom	Surface	Difference, d	d^2
1	0.430	0.415	0.015	0.000225
2	0.266	0.238	0.028	0.000784
3	0.567	0.390	0.177	0.030276
4	0.531	0.410	0.121	0.014641
5	0.707	0.605	0.102	0.010404
6	0.716	0.609	0.107	0.011449
Total			0.550	0.068832

(a) Draw a scatter diagram to show a possible association between the concentrations and check to see if a linear model is justified.

(b) Estimate the regression parameters, the bottom water concentration for location with a surface water concentration of .5 mg/L, and draw the regression line on the same graph with the scatter diagram.

(c) Test to see if the two concentrations are independent; state your hypotheses and your choice of the test size.

(d) Calculate the coefficient of determination and provide your interpretation.

8.2. In a study of saliva cotinine, seven subjects—all of whom had abstained from smoking for a week—were asked to smoke a single cigarette. The cotinine levels at 12 and 24 h after smoking are provided below:

Subject	Cotinine Level (mmol/L)	
	After 12 h	After 24 h
1	73	24
2	58	27
3	67	49
4	93	59
5	33	0
6	18	11
7	147	43

(a) Draw a scatter diagram to show a possible association between the cotinine levels (24 h measurement as the dependent variable) and check to see if a linear model is justified.

(b) Estimate the regression parameters, the 24 h measurement for a subject with a 12 h cotinine level of 60 mmol/L, and draw the regression line on the same graph with the scatter diagram.

(c) Test to see if the two cotinine levels are independent; state your hypotheses and your choice of the test size.

(d) Calculate the coefficient of determination and provide your interpretation.

8.3. The following data give the net food supply (X, number of calories per person per day) and the infant mortality rate (Y, number if infant deaths per 1000 live births) for certain selected countries before World War II:

Country	X	Y	Country	X	Y
Argentina	2730	98.8	Iceland	3160	42.4
Australia	3300	39.1	India	1970	161.6
Austria	2990	87.4	Ireland	3390	69.6
Belgium	3000	83.6	Italy	2510	102.7
Burma	1080	202.1	Japan	2180	60.6
Canada	3070	67.4	New Zealand	3260	32.2
Chile	2240	240.8	Netherlands	3010	37.4
Cuba	2610	116.8	Sweden	3210	43.3
Egypt	2450	162.9	England	3100	53.3
France	2880	66.1	USA	3150	53.2
Germany	2960	63.3	Uruguay	2380	94.1

(a) Draw a scatter diagram to show a possible association between the infant mortality rate (used as the dependent variable) and the net food supply and check to see if a linear model is justified.

(b) Estimate the regression parameters, the infant mortality rate for a country with a net food supply of 2900 calories per person per day, and draw the regression line on the same graph with the scatter diagram.

(c) Test to see if the two factors are independent; state your hypotheses and your choice of the test size.

(d) Calculate the coefficient of determination and provide your interpretation.

8.4. Refer to the data in previous Exercise 8.3, but in the context of a multiple regression problem with two independent variables: the net food supply ($X_1 = X$) and its square ($X_2 = X^2$).

(a) Taken collectively, do the two independent variables contribute significantly to the variation in the number of infant deaths?

(b) Calculate the coefficient of multiple determination and provide your interpretation.

(c) Fit the multiple regression model to obtain estimates of individual regression coefficients and their standard errors and draw your conclusion—especially the conditional contribution of the quadratic term.

8.5. The following are the heights (measured to the nearest 2 cm) and the weights (measured to the nearest kg) of 10 men and 10 women. Separately for each group, men and women,

(a) Draw a scatter diagram to show a possible association between the weight (used as the dependent variable) and the height and check to see if a linear model is justified.

(b) Estimate the regression parameters, the weight for a subject who is 160 cm (does the gender have an effect on this estimate?), and draw the regression line on the same graph with the scatter diagram.

(c) Test to see if the two factors are independent; state your hypotheses and your choice of the test size.

(d) Calculate the coefficient of determination and provide your interpretation.

(e) Is there evidence of an effect modification? (Compare the two coefficients of determination or coefficient of correlation—very informally)

Men

Height	162	168	174	176	180	180	182	184	186	186
Weight	65	65	84	63	75	76	82	65	80	81

Women

Height	152	156	158	160	162	162	164	164	166	166
Weight	52	50	47	48	52	55	55	56	60	60

8.6. Refer to the data in previous Exercise 8.5, but in the context of a multiple regression problem with three independent variables: height, gender, and product height by gender.

(a) Fit the multiple regression model to obtain estimates of individual regression coefficients and their standard errors. Draw your conclusion concerning the conditional contribution of each factor.

(b) Within the context of the multiple regression model in (a), does gender alter the effect of height on weight?

(c) Taken collectively, do the three independent variables contribute significantly to the variation in weights?

(d) Calculate the coefficient of multiple determination and provide your interpretation.

8.7. In an assay of heparin, a standard preparation is compared with a test preparation by observing the log clotting times (Y, in seconds) of blood containing different doses of heparin (X is log dose, replicate readings are made at each dose level):

Standard		Test		Log(Dose)
1.81	1.76	1.80	1.76	0.72
1.85	1.79	1.83	1.83	0.87
1.95	1.93	1.90	1.88	1.02
2.12	2.00	1.97	1.98	1.17
2.26	2.16	2.14	2.10	1.32

Separately for each preparation, standard and test,

(a) Draw a scatter diagram to show a possible association between the log clotting time (used as the dependent variable) and the log dose and check to see if a linear model is justified.

(b) Estimate the regression parameters, the log clotting time for a log dose of 1.0 (are estimates for different preparations different?), and draw the regression line on the same graph with the scatter diagram.

(c) Test to see if the two factors are independent; state your hypotheses and your choice of the test size.

(d) Calculate the coefficient of determination and provide your interpretation.

(e) Is there evidence of an effect modification? (Compare the two coefficients of determination or coefficient of correlation—very informally)

8.8. Refer to the data in previous Exercise 8.7, but in the context of a multiple regression problem with three independent variables: log dose, preparation, and product log dose by preparation.

(a) Fit the multiple regression model to obtain estimates of individual regression coefficients and their standard errors. Draw your conclusion concerning the conditional contribution of each factor.

(b) Within the context of the multiple regression model in (a), does preparation alter the effect of log dose on the log clotting time?

(c) Taken collectively, do the three independent variables contribute significantly to the variation in log clotting times?

(d) Calculate the coefficient of multiple determination and provide your interpretation.

8.9. Data are shown below for two groups of patients who died of acute myelogenous leukemia. Patients were classified into the two groups according to the presence or absence of a morphologic characteristic of white cells. Patients termed "AG positive" were identified by the presence of Auer rods and/or significant granulature of the leukemic cells in the bone marrow at diagnosis. For the AG negative patients, these factors were absent. Leukemia is a cancer characterized by an overproliferation of white blood cells; the higher the white blood count (WBC), the more severe the disease. Separately for each morphologic group, AG positive and AG negative,

(a) Draw a scatter diagram to show a possible association between the log survival time (take log yourself and use as the dependent variable) and the log WBC (take log yourself) and check to see if a linear model is justified.

(b) Estimate the regression parameters, the survival time for a patient with a WBC of 20,000 (are estimates for different groups different?), and draw the regression line on the same graph with the scatter diagram.

(c) Test to see if the two factors are independent; state your hypotheses and your choice of the test size.

(d) Calculate the coefficient of determination and provide your interpretation.

(e) Is there evidence of an effect modification? (Compare the two coefficients of determination or coefficient of correlation—very informally)

8.10. Refer to the data in Exercise 8.9, but in the context of a multiple regression problem with three independent variables: log WBC, morphologic characteristic (AG, represented by a binary indicator: 0 of AG negative and 1 if AG positive), and product log WBC by morphologic characteristic (AG).

(a) Fit the multiple regression model to obtain estimates of individual regression coefficients and their standard errors. Draw your conclusion concerning the conditional contribution of each factor.

(b) Within the context of the multiple regression model in (a), does the morphologic characteristic (AG) alter the effect of log WBC on log survival time?

(c) Taken collectively, do the three independent variables contribute significantly to the variation in log survival times?

(d) Calculate the coefficient of multiple determination and provide your interpretation.

AG-Positive, $n = 17$		AG-Negative, $n = 16$	
White Blood count (WBC)	Survival Time (weeks)	White Blood Count (WBC)	Survival Time (weeks)
2,300	65	4,400	56
750	156	3,000	65

(*Continued*)

AG-Positive, $n = 17$		AG-Negative, $n = 16$	
White Blood count (WBC)	Survival Time (weeks)	White Blood Count (WBC)	Survival Time (weeks)
4,300	100	4,000	17
2,600	134	1,500	7
6,000	16	9,000	16
10,500	108	5,300	22
10,000	121	10,000	3
17,000	4	19,000	4
5,400	39	27,000	2
7,000	143	28,000	3
9,400	56	31,000	8
32,000	26	26,000	4
35,000	22	21,000	3
100,000	1	79,000	30
100,000	1	100,000	4
52,000	5	100,000	43
100,000	65		

8.11. The purpose of this study was to examine the data for 44 physicians working for an emergency at a major hospital so as to determine which of a number of factors are related to the number of complaints (X) received during the previous year. In addition to the number of complaints, data available consist of the number of visits—which serves as the "size" for the observation unit, the physician—and four other factors under investigation. The following table presents the complete data set. For each of the 44 physicians, there are two continuous explanatory factors, the revenue (dollars per hour) and workload at the emergency service (hours), and two binary variables, sex (Female/Male) and residency training in emergency services ("Rcy," No/Yes). Divide the number of complaints by the number of visits and use this ratio (number of complaints per visit) as the *primary outcome* or dependent variable Y. Individually for each of the two continuous explanatory factors, the revenue (dollars per hour) and workload at the emergency service (hours),

(a) Draw a scatter diagram to show a possible association with the number of complaints per visit and check to see if a linear model is justified.

(b) Estimate the regression parameters, the number of complaints per visit for a physician having the (sample) mean level of the explanatory factor, and draw the regression line on the same graph with the scatter diagram.

(c) Test to see if the factor and the number of complaints per visit are independent; state your hypotheses and your choice of the test size.

(d) Calculate the coefficient of determination and provide your interpretation.

N-Visits	X	Rcy	Sex	Revenue	Hours	N-Visits	X	Rcy	Sex	Revenue	Hours
2014	2	Y	F	263.03	1287.25	3003	3	Y	F	280.52	1552.75
3091	3	N	M	334.94	1588.00	2178	2	N	M	237.31	1518.00
879	1	Y	M	206.42	705.25	2504	1	Y	F	218.7	1793.75
1780	1	N	M	226.32	1005.50	2211	1	N	F	250.01	1548.00
3646	11	N	M	288.91	1667.25	2338	6	Y	M	251.54	1446.00
2690	1	N	M	275.94	1517.75	3060	2	Y	M	270.52	1858.25
1864	2	Y	M	295.71	967.00	2302	1	N	M	247.31	1486.25
2782	6	N	M	224.91	1609.25	1486	1	Y	F	277.78	933.75
3071	9	N	F	249.32	1747.75	1863	1	Y	M	259.68	1168.25
1502	3	Y	M	269	906.25	1661	0	N	M	260.92	877.25
2438	2	N	F	225.61	1787.75	2008	2	N	M	240.22	1387.25
2278	2	N	M	212.43	1480.50	2138	2	N	M	217.49	1312.00
2458	5	N	M	211.05	1733.50	2556	5	N	M	250.31	1551.50
2269	2	N	F	213.23	1847.25	1451	3	Y	F	229.43	973.75
2431	7	N	M	257.3	1433.00	3328	3	Y	M	313.48	1638.25
3010	2	Y	M	326.49	1520.00	2927	8	N	M	293.47	1668.25
2234	5	Y	M	290.53	1404.75	2701	8	N	M	275.4	1652.75
2906	4	N	M	268.73	1608.50	2046	1	Y	M	289.56	1029.75
2043	2	Y	M	231.61	1220.00	2548	2	Y	M	305.67	1127.00
3022	7	N	M	241.04	1917.25	2592	1	N	M	252.35	1547.25
2123	5	N	F	238.65	1506.25	2741	1	Y	F	276.86	1499.25
1029	1	Y	F	287.76	589.00	3763	10	Y	M	308.84	1747.50

8.12. Refer to the data in Exercise 8.11 but consider all four explanatory factors and the product residency training-by-workload simultaneously.

(a) Fit the multiple regression model to obtain estimates of individual regression coefficients and their standard errors. Draw your conclusion concerning the conditional contribution of each factor.

(b) Within the context of the multiple regression model in (a), does the residency training alter the effect of workload on the number of complaints per visit?

(c) Taken collectively, do the five independent variables contribute significantly to the variation in log survival times?

(d) Calculate the coefficient of multiple determination and provide your interpretation.

Bibliography

Ahlquist, D. A., McGill, D. B., Schwartz, S. and Taylor, W. F. (1985). Fecal blood levels in health and disease: A study using HemoQuant. *New England Journal of Medicine* 314:1422.

Anderson, J. W., et al. (1990). Oat bran cereal lowers serum cholesterol total and LDL cholesterol in hypercholesterolemic men. *American Journal of Clinical Nutrition* 52:495–499.

Arsenault, P. S. (1980). Maternal and antenatal factors in the risk of sudden infant death syndrome. *American Journal of Epidemiology* 111:279–284.

Begg, C. B. and McNeil, B. (1988). Assessment of radiologic tests: Control of bias and other design considerations. *Radiology* 167:565–569.

Berkowitz, G. S. (1981). An epidemiologic study of pre-term delivery. *American Journal of Epidemiology* 113:81–92.

Blot, W. J., et al. (1978). Lung cancer after employment in shipyards during World War II. *New England Journal of Medicine* 299:620–624.

Brown, B. W. (1980). Prediction analyses for binary data. In: Biostatistics Casebook, edited by R.G. Miller, B. Efron, B. W. Brown, and L. E. Moses. : John Wiley and Sons, pp. 3–18.

Centers for Disease Control (1990). Summary of Notifiable Diseases: United States 1989 *Morbidity and Mortality Weekly Report* 38.

Cohen, J. (1960). A coefficient of agreement for nominal scale. *Educational and Psychological Measurements* 20:37–46.

Coren, S. (1989). Left-handedness and accident-related injury risk. *American Journal of Public Health* 79:1040–1041.

D'Angelo, L. J., Hierholzer, J. C., Holman, R. C. and Smith, J. D. (1981). Epidemic keratoconjunctivitis caused by adenovirus Type 8: Epidemiologic and laboratory aspects of a large outbreak. *American Journal of Epidemiology* 113:44–49.

Daniel, W. W. (1987) *Biostatistics: A Foundation for Analysis in The Health Sciences*, New York: John Wiley and Sons.

Dienstag, J. L. and Ryan, D. M. (1982). Occupational exposure to hepatitis B virus in hospital personnel: Infection or immunization. *American Journal of Epidemiology* 15:26–39.

Douglas, G. (1990). Drug therapy. *New England Journal of Medicine* 322:443–449.

Einarsson, K., et al. (1985). Influence of age on secretion of cholesterol and synthesis of bile acids by the liver. *New England Journal of Medicine* 313:277–282.

Engs, R. C. and Hanson, D. J. (1988). University students' drinking patterns and problems: Examining the effects of raising the purchase age. *Public Health Reports* 103:667–673.

Fiskens, E. J. M. and Kronshout, D. (1989). Cardiovascular risk factors and the 25 year incidence of diabetes mellitus in middle-aged men. *American Journal of Epidemiology* 130:1101–1108.

Fowkes, F. G. R., et al. (1992). Smoking, lipids, glucose intolerance, and blood pressure as risk factors for peripheral atherosclerosis compared with ischemic heart disease in the Edinburgh Artery Study. *American Journal of Epidemiology* 135:331–340.

Fox, A. J. and Collier, P. F. (1976). Low mortality rates in industrial cohort studies due to selection for work and survival in the industry. *British Journal of Preventive and Social Medicine* 30:225–230.

Freeman, D. H. (1980). *Applied Categorical Data Analysis*. New York: Marcel Dekker, Inc.

Freireich, E. J., et al. (1963). The effect of 6-mercaptopurine on the duration of steroid-induced remissions in acute leukemia: A model for evaluation of other potentially useful therapy. Blood 21:699–716.

Frerichs, R. R., et al. (1981). Prevalence of depression in Los Angeles County. *American Journal of Epidemiology* 113:691–699.

Fulwood, R., et al. (1986). Total serum cholesterol levels of adults 20–74 years of age: United States, 1976–1980. *Vital and Health Statistics, Series M*326.

Grady, W. R., et al. (1986). Contraceptives failure in the United States: Estimates from the 1982 National Survey of Family Growth. Family Planning Perspectives 18:200–209.

Graham, S., et al. (1988). Dietary epidemiology of cancer of the colon in western New York. *American Journal of Epidemiology*. 128: 490–503.

Gwirtsman, H. E., et al. (1989). Decreased caloric intake in normal weight patients with bulimia: Comparison with female volunteers. *American Journal of Clinical Nutrition* 49:86–92.

Helsing, K. J. and Szklo, M. (1981). Mortality after bereavement. *American Journal of Epidemiology* 114:41–52.

Herbst, A. L., Ulfelder, H. and Poskanzer, D.C. (1971). Adenocarcinoma of the vagina. *New England Journal of Medicine* 284:878–881.

Hiller, R. and Kahn, A. H. (1976). Blindness from glaucoma. *British Journal of Ophthalmology* 80: 62–69.

Hollows, F. C. and Graham, P. A. (1966) Intraocular pressure, glaucoma, and glaucoma suspects in a defined population. *British Journal of Ophthalmology* 50:570–586.

Hosmer, D. W. Jr., and Lemeshow, S. (1989). *Applied Logistic Regression*. New York: John Wiley and Sons.

Jackson, R., et al. (1992). Does recent alcohol consumption reduce the risk of acute myocardial infarction and coronary death in regular drinkers? *American Journal of Epidemiology* 136:819–824.

Kaplan, E. L. and Meier, P. (1958). Nonparametric estimation from incomplete observations. *Journal of the American Statistical Association* 53:457–481.

Kelsey, J. L., Livolsi, V. A., Holford, T. R., Fischer, D. B., Mostow, E. D., Schartz, P. E., O'Connor, T. and White, C. (1982). A case-control study of cancer of the endometrium. *American Journal of Epidemiology* 116:333–342.

Khabbaz, R., et al. (1990). Epidemiologic assessment of screening tests for antibody to human T lymphotropic virus type I. *American Journal of Public Health* 80:190–192.

Kleinbaum, D. G., Kupper, L. L. and Muller, K. E. (1988). *Applied Regression Analysis and Other Multivariate Methods*. Boston: PWS-Kent Publishing Company.

Kleinman, J. C. and Kopstein, A. (1981). Who is being screened for cervical cancer? *American Journal of Public Health* 71:73–76.

Klinhamer, P. J. J. M., et al. (1989). Intraobserver and interobserver variability in the quality assessment of cervical smears. *Acta Cytologica* 33: 215–218.

Knowler, W. C., et al. (1981). Diabetes incidence in Pima Indians: Contributions of obesity and parental diabetes. *American Journal of Epidemiology* 113: 144–156.

Koenig, J. Q., et al. (1990). Prior exposure to ozone potentiates subsequent response to sulfur dioxide in adolescent asthmatic subjects. *American Review of Respiratory Disease* 141:377–380.

Kono, S., et al. (1992). Prevalence of gallstone disease in relation to smoking, alcohol use, obesity, and glucose tolerance: A study of self-defense officials in Japan. *American Journal of Epidemiology*. 136:787–805.

Kushi, L. H., et al. (1988). The association of dietary fat with serum cholesterol in vegetarians: The effects of dietary assessment on the correlation coefficient. *American Journal of Epidemiology* 128:1054–1064.

Le, C. T. (1997). *Applied Survival Analysis*. New York: John Wiley and Sons.

Lee, M. (1989). Improving patient comprehension of literature on smoking. *American Journal of Public Health* 79:1411–1412.

Li, D. K., et al. (1990). Prior condom use and the risk of tubal pregnancy. American Journal of Public Health 80:964–966.

Mack, T. M., et al. (1976). Estrogens and endometrial cancer in a retirement community. *New England Journal of Medicine* 294:1262–1267.

Makuc, D., et al. (1989). National trends in the use of preventive health care by women. *American Journal of Public Health* 79:21–26.

Mantel, N. and Haenszel, W. (1959). Statistical aspects of the analysis of data from retrospective studies of disease. *Journal of the National Cancer Institute* 22:719–748.

Matinez, F. D., et al. (1992). Maternal age as a risk factor for wheezing lower respiratory illness in the first year of life. *American Journal of Epidemiology* 136:1258–1268.

May, D. (1974) Error rates in cervical cytological screening tests. *British Journal of Cancer* 29:106–113.

McCusker, J., et al. (1988). Association of electronic fetal monitoring during labor with caesarean section rate with neonatal morbidity and mortality. *American Journal of Public Health* 78:1170–1174.

Negri, E., et al. (1988). Risk factors for breast cancer: Pooled results from three Italian case-control studies. *American Journal of Epidemiology* 128:1207–1215.

Nischan, P., et al. (1988). Smoking and invasive cervical cancer risk: Results from a case-control study. *American Journal of Epidemiology* 128:74–77.

Nurminen, M., et al. (1982). Quantitated effects of carbon disulfide exposure, elevated blood pressure and aging on coronary mortality. *American Journal of Epidemiology* 115:107–118.

Ockene, J. (1990). The relationship of smoking cessation to coronary heart disease and lung cancer in the Multiple Risk Factor Intervention Trial. *American Journal of Public Health* 80:954–958.

Padian, N. S. (1990). Sexual histories of heterosexual couples with one HIV-infected partner. *American Journal of Public Health* 80:990–991.

Palta, M., et al. (1982). Comparison of self-reported and measured height and weight. *American Journal of Epidemiology* 115:223–230.

Pappas, G., et al. (1990). Hypertension prevalence and the status of awareness, treatment, and control in the Hispanic health and nutrition examination survey (HHANES). *American Journal of Public Health* 80:1431–1436.

Renaud, L. and Suissa, S. (1989). Evaluation of the efficacy of simulation games in traffic safety education of kindergarten children. *American Journal of Public Health* 79:307–309.

Renes, R., et al. (1981). Transmission of multiple drug-resistant tuberculosis: Report of a school and community outbreaks. *American Journal of Epidemiology* 113:423–435.

Rosenberg, L.,et al. (1981) Case-control studies on the acute effects of coffee upon the risk of myocardial infarction: Problems in the selection of a hospital control series. *American Journal of Epidemiology* 113:646–652.

Rossignol, A.M. (1989). Tea and premenstrual syndrome in the People's Republic of China. *American Journal of Public Health* 79:67–68.

Rousch, G. C., et al. (1982). Scrotal carcinoma in Connecticut metal workers: Sequel to a study of sinonasal cancer. *American Journal of Epidemiology* 116:76–85.

Salem-Schatz, S.,et al. (1990) Influence of clinical knowledge, organization context and practice style on transfusion decision making. *Journal of the American Medical Association* 25: 476–483.

Sandek, C.D., et al. (1989). A preliminary trial of the programmable implantable medication system for insulin delivery. *New England Journal of Medicine* 321:574–579.

Schwarts, B., et al. (1989). Olfactory function in chemical workers exposed to acrylate and methacrylate vapors. *American Journal of Public Health* 79:613–618.

Selby, J.V., et al. (1989). Precursors of essential hypertension: The role of body fat distribution. *American Journal of Epidemiology* 129:43–53.

Shapiro, S., et al. (1979). Oral contraceptive use in relation to myocardial infarction. *Lancet* 1:43–746.

Strader, C. H., et al. (1988). Vasectomy and the incidence of testicular cancer. *American Journal of Epidemiology* 128:56–63.

Strogatz, D. (1990). Use of medical care for chest pain differences between blacks and whites. *American Journal of Public Health* 80:290–293.

Taylor, H. (1981). Racial variations in vision. *American Journal of Epidemiology* 113:62–80.

Taylor, P. R., et al. (1989). The relationship of polychlorinated biphenyls to birth weight and gestational age in the offspring of occupationally exposed mothers. *American Journal of Epidemiology* 129:395–406.

Thompson, R. S., et al. (1989). A case-control study of the effectiveness of bicycle safety helmets. *New England Journal of Medicine* 320:1361–1367.

True, W. R., et al. (1988). Stress symptomology among Vietnam veterans. *American Journal of Epidemiology* 128:85–92.

Tuyns, A. J., et al. (1977). Esophageal cancer in Ille-et-Vilaine in relation to alcohol and tobacco consumption: Multiplicative risks. *Bulletin of Cancer* 64:45–60.

Umen, A. J. and Le, C. T. (1986). Prognostic factors, models, and related statistical problems in the survival of end-stage renal disease patients on hemodialysis. *Statistics in Medicine* 5:637–652.

Weinberg, G. B., et al. (1982). The relationship between the geographic distribution of lung cancer incidence and cigarette smoking in Allegheny County. Pennsylvania. *American Journal of Epidemiology* 115:40–58.

Whittemore, A. S., et al. (1988). Personal and environmental characteristics related to epithelial ovarian cancer. *American Journal of Epidemiology* 128:1228–1240.

Whittemore, A. S., et al. (1992). Characteristics relating to ovarian cancer risk: Collaborative analysis of 12 U. S. case-control studies. *American Journal of Epidemiology* 136:1184–1203.

Yassi, A., et al. (1991). An analysis of occupational blood level trends in Manitoba: 1979 through 1987. *American Journal of Public Health* 81:736–740.

Yen, S., Hsieh, C. and MacMahon, B. (1982) Consumption of alcohol and tobacco and other risk factors for pancreatitis. *American Journal of Epidemiology* 116:407–414.

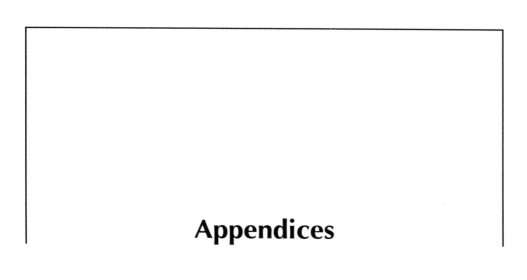

Appendices

Appendix A: Table of Random Numbers

63271	59986	71744	51102	15141	80714	58683	93108	13554	79945
88547	09896	95436	79115	08303	01041	20030	63754	08459	28364
55957	57243	83865	09911	19761	66535	40102	26646	60147	15704
46276	87453	44790	67122	45573	84358	21625	16999	13385	22782
55363	07449	34835	15290	76616	67191	12777	21861	68689	03263
69393	92785	49902	58447	42048	30378	87618	26933	40640	16281
13186	29431	88190	04588	38733	81290	89541	70290	40113	08243
17726	28652	56836	78351	47327	18518	92222	55201	27340	10493
36520	64465	05550	30157	82242	29520	69753	72602	23756	54935
81628	36100	39254	56835	37636	02421	98063	89641	64953	99337
84649	48968	75215	75498	49539	74240	03466	49292	36401	45525
63291	11618	12613	75055	43915	26488	41116	64531	56827	30825
70502	53225	03655	05915	37140	57051	48393	91322	25653	06543
06426	24771	59935	49801	11082	66762	94477	02494	88215	27191
20711	55609	29430	70165	45406	78484	31639	52009	18873	96927
41990	70538	77191	25860	55204	73417	83920	69468	74972	38712
72452	36618	76298	26678	89334	33938	95567	29380	75906	91807
37042	40318	57099	10528	09925	89773	41335	96244	29002	46453
53766	52875	15987	46962	67342	77592	57651	95508	80033	69828
90585	58955	53122	16025	84299	53310	67380	84249	25348	04332
32001	96293	37203	64516	51530	37069	40261	61374	05815	06714
62606	64324	46354	72157	67248	20135	49804	09226	64419	29457
10078	28073	85389	50324	14500	15562	64165	06125	71353	77669
91561	46145	24177	15294	10061	98124	75732	00815	83452	97355
13091	98112	53959	79607	52244	63303	10413	63839	74762	50289
73864	83014	72457	22682	03033	61714	88173	90835	00634	85169
66668	25467	48894	51043	02365	91726	09365	63167	95264	45643
84745	41042	29493	01836	09044	51926	43630	63470	76508	14194
48068	26805	94595	47907	13357	38412	33318	26098	82782	42851
54310	96175	97594	88616	42035	38093	36745	56702	40644	83514
14877	33095	10924	58013	61439	21882	42059	24177	58739	60170
78295	23179	02771	43464	59061	71411	05697	67194	30495	21157
67524	02865	39593	54278	04237	92441	26602	63835	38032	94770
58268	57219	68124	73455	83236	08710	04284	55005	84171	42596
97158	28672	50685	01181	24262	19427	52106	34308	73685	74246
04230	16831	69085	30802	65559	09205	71829	06489	85650	38707
94879	56606	30401	02602	57658	70091	54986	41394	60437	03195
71446	15232	66715	26385	91518	70566	02888	79941	39684	54315
32886	05644	79316	09819	00813	88407	17461	73925	53037	91904
62048	33711	25290	21526	02223	75947	66466	06232	10913	75336
84534	42351	21628	53669	81352	95152	08107	98814	72743	12849
84707	15885	84710	35866	06446	86311	32648	88141	73902	69981
19409	40868	64220	80861	13860	68493	52908	26374	63297	45052
57978	48015	25973	66777	45924	56144	24742	96702	88200	66162
57295	98298	11199	96510	75228	41600	47192	43267	35973	23152
94044	83785	93388	07833	38216	31413	70555	03023	54147	06647
30014	25879	71763	96679	90603	99396	74557	74224	18211	91637
07265	69563	64268	88802	72264	66540	01782	08396	19251	83613
84404	88642	30263	80310	11522	57810	27627	78376	36240	48952
21778	02085	27762	46097	43324	34354	09369	14966	10158	76089

Appendix B: Area Under the Standard Normal Curve

Entries in the table give the area under the curve between the zero and "z" standard deviations above the mean. For example, for $z = 1.25$ the area under the curve between the mean and z is .3944.

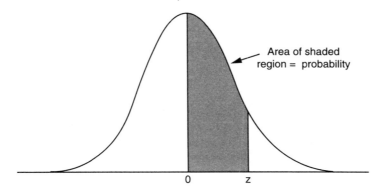

Area of shaded region = probability

z	.00	.01	.02	.03	.04	.05	.06	.07	.08	.09
.0	.0000	.0040	.0080	.0120	.0160	.0199	.0239	.0279	.0319	.0359
.1	.0398	.0438	.0478	.0517	.0557	.0596	.0636	.0675	.0714	.0753
.2	.0793	.0832	.0871	.0910	.0948	.0987	.1026	.1064	.1103	.1141
.3	.1179	.1217	.1255	.1293	.1331	.1368	.1406	.1443	.1480	.1517
.4	.1554	.1591	.1628	.1664	.1700	.1736	.1772	.1808	.1844	.1879
.5	.1915	.1950	.1985	.2019	.2054	.2088	.2123	.2157	.2190	.2224
.6	.2257	.2291	.2324	.2357	.2389	.2422	.2454	.2486	.2518	.2549
.7	.2580	.2612	.2642	.2673	.2704	.2734	.2764	.2794	.2823	.2852
.8	.2881	.2910	.2939	.2967	.2995	.3023	.3051	.3078	.3106	.3133
.9	.3159	.3186	.3212	.3238	.3264	.3289	.3315	.3340	.3365	.3389
1.0	.3413	.3438	.3461	.3485	.3508	.3531	.3665	.3577	.3599	.3621
1.1	.3643	.3554	.3686	.3708	.3729	.3749	.3770	.3790	.3810	.3830
1.2	.3849	.3869	.3888	.3907	.3925	.3944	.3962	.3980	.3997	.4015
1.3	.4032	.4049	.4066	.4082	.4099	.4115	.4131	.4147	.4162	.4177
1.4	.4192	.4207	.4222	.4236	.4251	.4265	.4279	.4292	.4306	.4319
1.5	.4332	.4345	.4357	.4370	.4382	.4394	.4406	.4418	.4429	.4441
1.6	.4452	.4463	.4474	.4484	.4495	.4505	.4515	.4525	.4535	.4545
1.7	.4554	.4564	.4573	.4582	.4591	.4599	.4608	.4616	.4625	.4633
1.8	.4641	.4649	.4656	.4664	.4671	.4678	.4686	.4693	.4699	.4706
1.9	.4713	.4719	.4726	.4732	.4738	.4744	.4750	.4756	.4761	.4767
2.0	.4772	.4778	.4783	.4788	.4793	.4798	.4803	.4808	.4812	.4817
2.1	.4821	.4826	.4830	.4834	.4838	.4842	.4846	.4850	.4854	.4857
2.2	.4861	.4864	.4868	.4871	.4875	.4878	.4881	.4884	.4887	.4890
2.3	.4893	.4896	.4898	.4901	.4904	.4906	.4909	.4911	.4913	.4916
2.4	.4918	.4920	.4922	.4925	.4927	.4929	.4931	.4932	.4934	.4936
2.5	.4938	.4940	.4941	.4943	.4945	.4946	.4948	.4949	.4951	.4942
2.6	.4953	.4955	.4956	.4957	.4959	.4960	.4961	.4962	.4963	.4964
2.7	.4965	.4966	.4967	.4968	.4969	.4970	.4971	.4972	.4973	.4974
2.8	.4974	.4975	.4976	.4977	.4977	.4978	.4979	.4979	.4980	.4981
2.9	.4981	.4982	.4982	.4983	.4984	.4984	.4985	.4985	.4986	.4986
3.0	.4986	.4987	.4987	.4988	.4988	.4989	.4989	.4989	.4990	.4990

Appendix C: Percentiles of the *t* Distributions

Entries in the table give t_α values, where α is the area or probability in the upper tail of the *t* distribution. For example, with 10 degrees of freedom and a .05 area in the upper tail, $t_{.05} = 1.812$.

df	.10	.05	.025	.01	.005
			Area in Upper Tail		
1	3.078	6.314	12.706	31.821	63.657
2	1.886	2.920	4.303	6.965	9.925
3	1.638	2.353	3.182	4.541	5.841
4	1.533	2.132	2.776	3.747	4.604
5	1.476	2.015	2.571	3.365	4.032
6	1.440	1.943	2.447	3.143	3.707
7	1.415	1.895	2.365	2.998	3.499
8	1.397	1.860	2.306	2.896	3.355
9	1.383	1.833	2.262	2.821	3.250
10	1.372	1.812	2.228	2.764	3.169
11	1.363	1.796	2.201	2.718	3.106
12	1.356	1.782	2.179	2.681	3.055
13	1.350	1.771	2.160	2.650	3.012
14	1.345	1.761	2.145	2.624	2.977
15	1.341	1.753	2.131	2.602	2.947
16	1.337	1.746	2.120	2.583	2.921
17	1.333	1.740	2.110	2.567	2.898
18	1.330	1.734	2.101	2.552	2.878
19	1.328	1.729	2.093	2.539	2.861
20	1.325	1.725	2.086	2.528	2.845
21	1.323	1.721	2.080	2.518	2.831
22	1.321	1.717	2.074	2.508	2.819
23	1.319	1.714	2.069	2.500	2.807
24	1.318	1.711	2.064	2.492	2.797
25	1.316	1.708	2.060	2.485	2.787
26	1.315	1.706	2.056	2.479	2.779
27	1.314	1.703	2.052	2.473	2.771
28	1.313	1.701	2.048	2.467	2.763
29	1.311	1.699	2.045	2.462	2.756
30	1.310	1.697	2.042	2.457	2.750
40	1.303	1.684	2.021	2.423	2.704
60	1.296	1.671	2.000	2.390	2.660
120	1.289	1.658	1.980	2.358	2.617
∞	1.282	1.645	1.960	2.326	2.576

Appendix D: Percentiles of Chi-square Distributions

Entries in the table give χ^2_α values, where α is the area or probability in the upper tail of the Chi-square distribution. For example, with 10 degrees of freedom and a .01 area in the upper tail, $\chi^2_\alpha = 23.2093$.

df	Area in Upper Tail	
	.05	.01
1	3.841	6.635
2	5.991	9.210
3	7.815	11.350
4	9.488	13.277
5	11.071	15.086
6	12.592	16.812
7	14.067	18.475
8	15.507	20.090
9	16.919	21.666
10	18.307	23.209
11	19.675	24.725
12	21.026	26.217
13	22.362	27.688
14	23.685	29.141
15	24.996	30.578
16	26.296	32.000
17	27.587	33.408
18	28.869	34.805
19	30.144	36.191
20	31.410	37.566
21	32.671	38.932
22	33.924	40.289
23	35.173	41.638
24	36.415	42.980
25	37.653	44.314
26	38.885	45.642
27	40.113	46.963
28	41.337	48.278
29	42.557	49.588
30	43.773	50.892
40	55.759	63.691
50	67.505	76.154
60	79.082	88.380
70	90.531	100.425
80	101.879	112.329
90	113.145	124.116
100	124.342	135.807

Appendix E: Percentiles of the *F* Distributions

Entries in the table give F_α values, where α is the area or probability in the upper tail of the *F* distribution. For example, with 3 numerator degrees of freedom, 20 denominator degrees of freedom, and a .01 area in the upper tail, $F_{.01} = 4.94$ at df = (3,20).

df	(2,.05)	(2,.01)	(3,.05)	(3,.01)	(4,.05)	(4,.01)	(5,.05)	(5,.01)
5	5.79	13.27	5.41	12.06	5.19	11.39	4.82	10.97
6	5.14	10.92	4.76	9.78	4.53	9.15	4.39	8.75
7	4.74	9.55	4.35	8.45	4.12	7.85	3.97	7.46
8	4.46	8.65	4.07	7.59	3.84	7.01	3.69	6.63
9	4.26	8.02	3.86	6.99	3.63	6.42	3.48	6.06
10	4.10	7.56	3.71	6.55	3.48	5.99	3.33	5.64
11	3.98	7.21	3.59	6.22	3.36	5.67	3.20	5.32
12	3.89	6.93	3.49	5.95	3.26	5.41	3.11	5.06
13	3.81	6.70	3.41	5.74	3.18	5.21	3.03	4.86
14	3.74	6.51	3.34	5.56	3.11	5.24	2.96	4.69
15	3.68	6.36	3.29	5.42	3.06	4.89	2.90	4.56
16	3.63	6.23	3.24	5.29	3.01	4.77	2.85	4.44
17	3.59	6.11	3.20	5.18	2.96	4.67	2.81	4.34
18	3.55	6.01	3.16	5.09	2.93	4.58	2.77	4.25
19	3.52	5.93	3.13	5.01	2.90	4.50	2.74	4.17
20	3.49	5.85	3.10	4.94	2.87	4.43	2.71	4.10
21	3.47	5.78	3.07	4.87	2.84	4.37	2.68	4.04
22	3.44	5.72	3.05	4.82	2.82	4.31	2.66	3.99
23	3.42	5.66	3.03	4.76	2.80	4.26	2.64	3.94
24	3.40	5.61	3.01	4.72	2.78	4.22	2.62	3.90
25	3.39	5.57	2.99	4.68	2.76	4.18	2.60	3.85
26	3.37	5.53	2.98	4.64	2.74	4.14	2.59	3.82
27	3.35	5.49	2.96	4.60	2.73	4.11	2.57	3.78
28	3.34	5.45	2.95	4.57	2.71	4.07	2.56	3.75
29	3.33	5.42	2.93	4.54	2.70	4.04	2.55	3.73
30	3.32	5.39	2.92	4.51	2.69	4.02	2.53	3.70
35	3.27	5.27	2.87	4.40	2.64	3.91	2.49	3.59
40	3.23	5.18	2.84	4.31	2.61	3.83	2.45	3.51
50	3.18	5.06	2.79	4.20	2.56	3.72	2.40	3.41
60	3.15	4.98	2.76	4.13	2.53	3.65	2.37	3.34
80	3.11	4.88	2.72	4.04	2.49	3.56	2.33	3.26
100	3.09	4.82	2.70	3.98	2.46	3.51	2.31	3.21
120	3.07	4.79	2.68	3.95	2.45	3.48	2.29	3.17
α	3.00	4.61	2.60	3.78	2.37	3.32	2.21	3.02

Numerator Degrees of Freedom, Area in Upper Tail

Answers to Selected Exercises

CHAPTER 1

1.1. For left-handed: $p = .517$; for right-handed: $p = .361$.

1.2. For factory workers: $x = 49$; for nursing students: $x = 73$.

1.3. For cases: $p = .775$; for controls: $p = .724$.

1.4. For Nursing home A: $p = .250$; for Nursing home B: $p = .025$.
     The proportion in Nursing home A where the "index" nurse worked is ten times higher than the proportion in Nursing home B.

1.5. (a) For high exposure level: $p = .488$; for low exposure level: $p = .111$; students in the high exposure group has a much higher proportion of cases, more than four times higher.

   (b) OR $= 7.66$; it supports the conclusion in (a) showing that high exposure is associated with higher odds, and so higher proportion, of positive cases.

1.6. (a) With EFM: $p = .126$; without EFM: $p = .077$; the EFM-exposed group has a higher proportion of caesarean deliveries.

   (b) OR $= 1.72$; it supports the conclusion in (a) showing that EFM exposure is associated with higher odds, and so higher proportion, of caesarean deliveries.

1.7. (a) With helmet: $p = .116$; without helmet: $p = .338$; the group without helmet protection has a higher proportion of head injuries.

   (b) OR $= .26$; it supports the conclusion in (a) showing that helmet protection is associated with reduced odds, and so lower proportion, of head injuries.

1.8. (a) Men: OR = .94 indicating a slightly lower risk of myocardial infarction.

Women: OR = .55 indicating a lower risk of myocardial infarction.

(b) The effect of drinking is stronger in women, reducing the risk: 45% versus 6%.

(c) Men: OR = .57 indicating a lower risk of coronary death.

Women: OR = .39 indicating a lower risk of coronary death.

(d) The effect of drinking is stronger in women, reducing the risk: 61% versus 43%.

1.9. (a) Zero or one partners: OR = 2.70.

Two or more partners: OR = 1.10.

(b) Both odds ratios indicate an elevated risk associated with smoking, but the effect on those with zero or one partners is clearer.

(c) Combined estimate of odds ratio: $OR_{MH} = 1.26$.

1.10. Chart is not available.

1.11. Chart is not available.

1.12. Chart is not available.

1.13. Chart is not available.

1.14. Chart is not available.

1.15. Sensitivity = .733; specificity = .972.

1.16. For Duponts EIA: sensitivity = .938; specificity = .988.

For cellular product's EIA: sensitivity = 1.0; specificity = .952.

1.17. (a) H. disease: 30.2%; cancer: 24.1%; C. disease: 8.2%; accidents: 4.0%; others: 33.4%.

(b) Population size: 3,525,297.

(c) Rates per 100,000: cancer: 235.4; C. disease: 80.3; accidents: 39.2; others: 325.5.

1.18. Chart is not available.

1.19. Odds ratio OR = 1.43.

1.20. (a) For nonsmokers: OR = 1.28.

(b) For smokers: OR = 1.61.

(c) The risk seems to be higher for smokers.

(d) Combined estimate: $OR_{MH} = 1.53$.

1.21. (a) Odds ratios associated with race (black versus white, nonpoor): 25–44: 1.07, 45–64: 2.00; 65 + : 1.54. Different ratios indicate possible effect modifications by age.

(b) Odds ratios associated with income (poor versus nonpoor, black): 25–44: 2.46, 45–64: 1.65; 65 + : 1.18. Different ratios indicate a possible effect modification by age.

(c) Odds ratios associated with race (black versus white) for 65 + years + poor:

1.18; for 65 + years + nonpoor: 1.54. The difference ($1.18 \neq 1.52$) indicates an effect modification by income.

1.22. (a)

Age Group	Odds Ratio
25–44	7.71
45–64	6.03
65 +	3.91

(b) The odds ratios decrease with increasing age.

(c) $OR_{MH} = 5.40$, but assumption may be wrong.

1.23. (a)

Weight Group	Odds Ratio
<57	5
57–75	2.75
>75	1.30

(b) The odds ratios decrease with increasing weight.

(c) $OR_{MH} = 2.78$, but assumption may be wrong.

1.24.

Age Group	Odds Ratio
Age at first live birth	
22–24	1.26
25–27	1.49
28 +	1.95
Age at menopause	
45–49	1.10
50 +	1.40

1.25. (a)

Factor	Level	No. of Men Surveyed Without Gallstone	No. of Men Surveyed With Gallstone
Smoking	Never	610	11
	Past	759	17
	Current	1309	33
Alcohol	Never	436	11
	Past	110	3
	Current	2132	47

(continued)

(Continued)

Factor	Level	No. of Men Surveyed	
		Without Gallstone	With Gallstone
BMI (kg/m²)	<22.5	706	13
	22.5–24.9	1271	30
	>24.9	701	18

(b)

Smoking	Status	Odds Ratio
	Past	1.24
	Current	1.4
Alcohol	Status	Odds Ratio
	Past	1.08
	Current	.87
BMI	Level	Odds Ratio
	22.5–24.9	1.41
	25.0+	1.39

1.26.

Duration	Year	Odds Ratio
	2–9	.94
	10–14	1.04
	15 or more	1.54
History	Status	Odds Ratio
	Yes; No drug	1.13
	Yes; drug	3.34

1.27.

Age (years)	Odds Ratio	
	Boys	Girls
21–25	.97	.80
26–30	.67	.81
Over 30	.43	.62

1.28. Sensitivity $= .650$; specificity $= .917$.

1.29. Number of new AIDS cases for 1987: 24,027; for 1986: 15,017
Number of cases of AIDS transmitted from mothers to newborns in 1988: 468.

1.30. Follow-up death rates:

Age (years)	Deaths/1000 months
21–30	3.95
31–40	5.05
41–50	11.72
51–60	9.8
61–70	10.19
Over 70	20.09

RR (70+ years versus 51–60 years) $= 2.05$.

1.31. Death rates for Georgia (per 100,000)
   (a) Crude rate for Georgia: 908.3.
   (b) Adjusted rate (U.S. as standard), Georgia: 1060.9
       versus adjusted rate for Alaska: 788.6
       versus adjusted rate for Florida: 770.6
   (c) Adjusted rate (Alaska as standard): 560.5
       versus crude rate for Alaska: 396.8

1.32. With Georgia as standard:
   Alaska $= 668.4$; Florida $= 658.5$ versus crude rate for Georgia of 908.3.

1.33. Chart is not available.

1.34. Charts are not available.

1.35. (a)

Group	Level	Proportion	Odds Ratio
Physicians	Frequent	.210	3.11
	Infrequent	.079	
Nurses	Frequent	.212	2.80
	Infrequent	.087	

   (b) Odds ratios are similar but larger for physicians.
   (c) $OR_{MH} = 2.93$.

1.36. Graphs are not available.

1.37. (a) For age

Group	Odds Ratio
14–17	2.09
18–19	1.96
20–24	1.69
25–29	1.02

Yes, the younger the mother, the higher the risk.

(b) For Socioeconomic level:

Group	Odds Ratio
Upper	.3
Upper-middle	.34
Middle	.56
Lower-middle	.71

Yes, the poorer the mother, the higher the risk.

1.38.

Group	Odds Ratio
Protestants	.5
Catholics	4.69
Others	.79

Yes, there is clear evidence of an effect modification (4.69 ≠ .50, .79).

1.39. See table in Exercise 1.24.

1.40.

Diets	Odds Ratio Males	Odds Ratio Females
Low fat, low fiber	1.15	1.72
High fat, high fiber	1.80	1.85
High fat, low fiber	1.81	2.20

Yes, there are evidences of effect modifications: for example:

(i) For males: high versus low fat, the odds ratio is 1.8 with high fiber and 1.57 with low fiber.

(ii) For females: high versus low fat, the odds ratio is 1.85 with high fiber and 1.28 with low fiber.

1.41.

Symptoms	Odds Ratio
Nightmares	3.72
Sleep problems	1.54
Troubled memories	3.46
Depression	1.46
Temper control problems	1.78
Life goal association	1.50
Omit feelings	1.39
Confusion	1.57

1.42. Graph is not available.

1.43. Choosing "never" as baseline, here are the odds ratios associated with being a resident (versus attending physician):

Action Level	Odds Ratio
Rarely	1.93
Occasionally	24.30
Frequent	33.80
Very frequent	5.20

1.44. Results are:

Factor	Odds Ratio
X-Ray	8.86
Stage	5.25
Grade	3.26

CHAPTER 2

2.1. Graphs are not available; median $= 193$.

2.2. Graphs are not available; median for 1979 is 47.6, for 1987 is 27.8.

2.3. Graphs are not available.

2.4. Graphs are not available.

2.5. Graphs are not available.

2.6. Graphs are not available.

2.7. Graphs are not available.

2.8. Graphs are not available; median from graph is 83, exact is 86.

2.9. Graphs are not available.

	Men	Women
Mean	84.71	88.51
Variance	573.68	760.90
Standard deviation	28.30	31.20

2.10. Graphs are not available.

		Mean	Variance	Standard Deviation	CV
2.11.		168.75	1372.75	37.05	
2.12.		3.05	.37	.61	
2.13.		112.78	208.07	14.42	
2.14.		100.58	196.08	14	
2.15.		.72	.26	.51	
2.16.	Age	65.6	243.11	15.19	
	SBP	146.2	379.46	19.48	
2.17.	Females	107.6	4373.5	66.1	
	Males	97.8	1635.9	40.4	
2.18.		.22	.44	.66	
2.19.	Treatment	651.9	31,394.30	177.2	
	Control	656.1	505.1	22.5	
2.20.		169	81.5	9	5%
2.21.		2.5	9.5	3.1	

2.22. Mean = 14.1; geometric mean = 10.3; median = 12.5.

2.23. Mean = 21.3; geometric mean = 10.6; median = 10.0.

2.24. Mean = 98.5; geometric mean = 93.4; median = 92.5.

2.25. Bulimic: mean = 22.1; variance = 21.0.
Healthy: mean = 29.7; variance = 42.1.
Bulimic group has smaller mean and smaller variance.

2.26. Drug A: mean $= 133.9$; variance $= 503.8$; standard deviation $= 130.0$.
Drug R: mean $= 267.4$; variance $= 4449.0$; standard deviation $= 253.0$.

2.27. (a) For survival time
AG Positive: mean $= 62.5$; variance $= 2954.3$; standard deviation $= 54.4$.
AG Negative: mean $= 17.9$; variance $= 412.2$; standard deviation $= 20.3$.
(b) For WBC:
AG Positive: 29,073.5; geometric mean $= 12,471.9$; median $= 10,000$.
AG Negative: 29,262.5; geometric mean $= 15,096.3$; median $= 20,000$.

2.28. $r = -.536$ for AG Positive and $r = .011$ for AG Negative.

2.29. Pearson's $r = .931$.

2.30. Graph is not available.
Pearson's $r = .514$ for men and $r = .718$ for women.

2.31. Graph is not available.
Pearson's $r = -.786$.

2.32. Graph is not available.
Pearson's $r = .940$ for Standard and $r = .956$ for Test.

2.33. Twenty patients with nodes, 33 patients without nodes:

Factor		Mean	Variance	Standard Deviation
Age	Without node	60.1	31.4	5.6
	With node	58.3	49.1	7.0
Acid	Without node	64.5	744.2	27.3
	With node	77.5	515.3	22.7

2.34. All patients: .054; with nodes: .273; without nodes: $-.016$.
Nodal involvement seems to change the strength of the relationship.

2.35. (a) 12 females, 32 males; 20 with residency, 24 without.

Factor		Mean	Standard Deviation
Gender	Females	.00116	.00083
	Males	.00139	.00091
Residency	Without	.00147	.00099
	With	.00116	.00071

(b) Between complaints and revenue: .031; between complaints and work load: .279.
(c) Graph is not available.

2.36. Between Y and X_1, $r = .756$; between Y and X_2, $r = .831$.

CHAPTER 3

3.1. Odds ratio = .62; Pr(Pap = yes) = .82, Pr(Pap = yes|black) = .75 ≠ .82.

3.2. Odds ratio = 5.99; Pr(second = present) = .65.
Pr(second = present|first = present) = .78 ≠ .65.

3.3. (a) .202; (b) .217; (c) .376; (d) .268.

3.4. Positive predictive value for Pop A: .991; for Pop B: .900.

3.5. (a) Sensitivity = .733, specificity = .972; (b) .016; (c) .301.

3.6. Results:

Prevalence	Positive Predictive Value
.2	.867
.4	.946
.6	.975
.7	.984
.8	.991
.9	.996

Yes:

$$\text{Prevalence} = \frac{(\text{PPV})(1-\text{specificity})}{(\text{PPV})(1-\text{specificity}) + (1-\text{PPV})(\text{sensitivity})}$$

$$= .113 \text{ if PPV} = .8$$

3.7. (a) .1056; (b) .7995.

3.8. (a) .9500; (b) .0790; (c) .6992.

3.9. (a) .9573; (b) .1056.

3.10. (a) 1.645; (b) 1.96; (c) .84.

3.11. $102.8 = 118.4 - (1.28)(12.17)$.

3.12.

20–24 years:	101.23	106.31	141.49	146.57
25–29 years:	104.34	109.00	141.20	145.86

For example, $123.9 - (1.645)(13.74) = 101.3$.

3.13. (a) 200 + days: .1587; 365 + days: almost 0; (b) .0228.

3.14. (a) .0808; (b) 82.4.

3.15. (a) 17.2; (b) 19.2%; (c) .0409.

3.16. (a) .5934; (b) .0475; (c) .0475.

3.17. (a) almost 0 ($z = 3.79$); (b) almost 0 ($z = -3.10$).

3.18. (a) .2266; (b) .0045; (c) .0014.

3.19. (a) .0985; (a) .0019.

3.20. Rate = 13.89 per 1000 live births; $z = 13.52$.

3.21. For t distribution, 20 df:

(a) Left of 2.086:.975; left of 2.845:.995.

(b) Right of 1.725:.05; right of 2.528:.01.

(c) Beyond ± 2.086:.05; beyond ± 2.845:.01.

3.22. For Chi-square distribution, 2 df:

   (a) Right of 5.991:.05; right of 9.210:.01.

   (b) Right of 6.348: between .01 and .05.

   (c) Between 5.991 and 9.210:.04.

3.23. For F distribution (2,30) df:

   (a) Right of 3.32:.05; right of 5.39:.01.

   (b) Right of 2.61: <.01.

   (c) Between 3.32 and 5.39:.04.

3.24. Kappa $= .399$, marginally good agreement.

3.25. Kappa $= .734$, good agreement—almost excellent.

CHAPTER 4

4.1. (Population) mean $= .5$; 6 possible samples with mean $= .5$.

4.2.
$$\Pr(\mu - 1 \leq \bar{x} \leq \mu + 1) = PR(-2.33 \leq Z \leq 2.33)$$
$$= .9802$$

		Pt Estimate	95% Confidence Interval	
4.3.	Left-handed		(.444,.590)	
	Right-handed		(.338,.384)	
4.4.	Students		(.320,.460)	
	Workers		(.667,.873)	
4.5.	In 1983		(.445,.393)	
	In 1987		(.355,.391)	
4.6.	High level		(.402,.574)	
	Low level		(.077,.145)	
4.7.	For Whites	25.3	(23.54,27.06)	
	For Blacks	38.6	(35.07,42.13)	No, n was used in CI
4.8.	Sensitivity		(.575,.891)	
	Specificity		(.964,.980)	
4.9.	Dupont's			Very small n's
	Sensitivity		(.820,1.0)	
	Specificity		(.971,1.0)	
	Cellular's			Very small n's too
	Sensitivity		Not available	
	Specificity		(.935,.990)	
4.10.	Physicians			
	Frequent		(.121,.299)	
	Infrequent		(.023,.135)	
	Nurses			
	Frequent		(.133,.136)	
	Infrequent		(.038,.136)	

4.11. (a) Proportion: (.067,.087); Odds ratio: (1.44,2.05).

4.12. (a) Proportion: (.302,.374); Odds ratio: (.15,.44).

4.13. Confidence intervals:

Event	Gender	95% Confidence Interval
Myocardial Infarction	Men	(.69,1.28)
	Women	(.30,.99)
Coronary Death	Men	(.39,.83)
	Women	(.12,1.25)

No clear evidence of effect modification; intervals are overlapped.

		Pt Estimate	95% Confidence Interval	
4.14.	Protestants		(.31,.84)	
	Catholics		(1.58,13.94)	
				Evidence of effect modification
	Others		(.41,1.51)	
4.15.	Proportion		(.141,.209)	
	Odds ratio		(1.06,1.93)	
4.16	Versus hospital controls	2.00	(.98,4.09)	
	Versus population controls	1.78	(.86,3.73)	
4.17.	Boys			
	<21 years	2.32	(.90,5.99)	
	21–25	2.24	(1.23,4.09)	
	26–30	1.55	(.87,2.77)	
	Girls			
	<21 years	1.62	(.62,4.25)	
	21–25	1.31	(.74,2.30)	
	26–30	1.31	(.76,2.29)	
4.18.	(a) Duration (years)			
	2–9	.94	(.74,1.20)	
	10–14	1.04	(.71,1.53)	
	15 or more	1.54	(1.17,2.02)	
	(b) Infertility			
	No drug use	1.13	(.83,1.53)	
	Drug use	3.34	(1.59,7.02)	
4.19.		3.05	(2.61,3.49)	
4.20.		112.78	(105.61,119.95)	
4.21.		100.58	(91.68,109.48)	
4.22.	Females		(63.2,152.0)	
	Males		(76.3,119.3)	

(Continued)

	Pt Estimate	95% Confidence Interval
4.23.	.36	(.12,.60)
4.24. Treatment		(653.3,676.9)
Control		(681.1,722.7)
4.25. Mean		(.63,4.57)
Coefficient correlation		(.764,.981)
4.26. Log scale		(1.88,2.84)
In weeks		(6.53,17.19)
4.27. Control	7.9	(6.58,9.22)
Simulation	10.1	(9.32,10.88)
4.28. (a)	25.0	(24.31,25.69)
(b) Large BMI likely leads to diabetes mellitus		
4.29. <95 Exp		(213.2,226.8)
Non-exp		(216.0,226.0)
95–100 Exp		(215.3,238.6)
Non-exp		(223.6,248.4)
100+ Exp		(215.0,251.0)
Non-exp		(186.2,245.8)
4.30.		(−.220,.320)
4.31.		(.545,.907)
4.32. Standard		(.760,.986)
Test		(.820,.990)
4.33. Smoke		(.398,.914)
Sulfur dioxide		(.555,.942)
4.34. Men		(−.171,.864)
Women		(.161,.928
4.35. AG Positive		(.341,.886)
AG Negative		(−.276,.666)

CHAPTER 5

5.1.

	Null Hypothesis	Alternative Hypothesis
(a)	$\mu = 30$	$\mu > 30$
(b)	$\mu = 11.5$	$\mu \neq 11.5$
(c)	Hypotheses are for population parameters	
(d)	$\mu = 31.5$	$\mu < 31.5$
(e)	$\mu = 16$	$\mu \neq 16$
(f)	Same answer as in (c)	

5.2. $H_0: \mu = 74.5$ and $H_A: \mu > 74.5$.

5.3. $H_0: \mu = 7250$ and $H_A: \mu < 7250$; one-sided.

5.4. $H_0: \pi = .38$ and $H_A: \pi > 38$; Type I error leads to unnecessary intervention and Type II error would mask a public health problem—opportunity is lost.

5.5. H_0: $\pi = .007$ and H_A: $\pi > .007$

Under H_0, the mean is $(1000)(.007) = 7$ and variance is $(1000)(.007)(.993) = (2.64)^2$.

$$z = \frac{20-7}{2.64}$$

$= 4.92$; p-value is almost zero because z is very large.

5.6. H_0: $\mu_d = 0$ and H_A: $\mu_d \neq 0$.

5.7. H_0: $\pi = 20.5/5000$ and H_A: $\pi > 20.5/5000$.

5.8. H_0: $\sigma = 20$ and H_A: $\sigma \neq 20$.

5.9. One-sided.

5.10. H_0: $\pi = .25$

Under H_0, the mean is $.25$ and variance is $(.25)(.75)/100 = (.043)^2$.

$$z = \frac{.18 - .25}{.043}$$

$= -1.63$; $\alpha = .052$

$$H_A : \pi = .15$$

Under H_0, the mean is $.25$ and variance is $(.15)(.85)/100 = (.036)^2$.

$$z = \frac{.18 - .15}{.036}$$

$= 0.83$; $\beta = .203$

5.11. Same null and alternative hypotheses as in Exercise 5.10.

Under H_0, the mean is $.25$ and variance is $(.25)(.75)/100 = (.043)^2$.

$$z = \frac{.22 - .25}{.043}$$

$= -.70$; $\alpha = .242$

Under H_0, the mean is $.25$ and variance is $(.15)(.85)/100 = (.036)^2$.

$$z = \frac{.22 - .15}{.036}$$

$= 1.94$; $\beta = .026$

The new change makes α larger and β smaller.

5.12.

$$p\text{-value} = \Pr(p < .18 \text{ or } p > .32)$$

$$= (2)\Pr\left(Z \geq \frac{.32 - .25}{.043}\right)$$

$$= .1032$$

CHAPTER 6

6.1. $z = -1.67$; p-value $= .095$.

6.2. $X^2 = 75.03$; p-value is almost zero.

6.3. $z = .66$ or $X^2 = .44$; p-value $= .5092$.

6.4. $z = 3.77$ or $X^2 = 14.23$; p-value $< .01$.

6.5. $z = 4.60$; p-value is almost zero.

6.6. H_0: consistent report for a couple, that is, man and woman agree
    $z = -.28$; p-value $= .7794$.

6.7. H_0: no effects of acrylate and methacrylate vapors on olfactory function
    $z = 2.33$; p-value $= .0198$.

6.8. $z = 4.11$ or $X^2 = 16.89$; p-value $= .0426$.

6.9. $z = 5.22$ or $X^2 = 27.22$; p-value $= .0223$.

6.10. $z = 7.44$ or $X^2 = 55.36$; p-value $= .0064$.

6.11. $X^2 = 44.49$; p-value $< .0001$.

6.12. $X^2 = 37.73$; p-value $< .0001$.

6.13. $X^2 = 37.95$; p-value $< .0001$.

6.14. $X^2 = 28.26$; p-value $< .0001$.

6.15. $X^2 = 5.58$; p-value $= .0182$.

6.16. For protestants: $X^2 = 7.205$; p-value $= .0073$.
    For catholics: $X^2 = 8.789$; p-value $= .0031$.
    For others: $X^2 = .502$; p-value $= .4786$.

6.17. $X^2 = 4.82$; p-value $= .0262$.

6.18. For physicians: $X^2 = 6.023$; p-value $= .0141$.
    For nurses: $X^2 = 7.156$; p-value $= .0075$.

6.19. For males

    Low fat, low fiber; $X^2 = .220$; p-value $= .6391$.
    High fat, high fiber; $X^2 = 3.635$; p-value $= .0566$.
    High fat, low fiber; $X^2 = 2.793$; p-value $= .0947$.

    For females

    Low fat, low fiber; $X^2 = 3.149$; p-value $= .0760$.
    High fat, high fiber; $X^2 = 4.010$; p-value $= .0452$.
    High fat, low fiber; $X^2 = 4.665$; p-value $= .0308$.

6.20. For smoking: $X^2 = .792$; p-value $= .3735$.
    For alcohol consumption: $X^2 = .1341$; p-value $= .7142$.
    For BMI: $X^2 = .7861$; p-value $= .3753$.

6.21. For nightmares: $X^2 = 95.56$; p-value $< .0001$.
    For sleep problems: $X^2 = 12.49$; p-value $= .0004$.
    For troubled memories: $X^2 = 97.18$; p-value $< .0001$.
    For depression: $X^2 = 14.36$; p-value $= .0002$.

For temper control problems: $X^2 = 21.97$; p-value $< .0001$.
For life goal association: $X^2 = 13.76$; p-value $= .0002$.
For omit feelings: $X^2 = 7.94$; p-value $= .0048$.
For confusion: $X^2 = 12.99$; p-value $= .0003$.

6.22. (i) Men

For myocardial infarction: $X^2 = .16$; p-value $= .6952$.
For coronary death: $X^2 = 8.47$; p-value $= .0036$.

(ii) Women

For myocardial infarction: $X^2 = 4.09$; p-value $= .0431$.
For coronary death: $X^2 = 2.62$; p-value $= .1055$.

6.23. (i) For myocardial infarction: $z = -1.31$; p-value $= .0951$.
(ii) For coronary death: $z = -3.28$; p-value $< .001$.

6.24. $z = 9.49$; p-value is almost zero
6.25. (a) For <57 kg: $X^2 = 19.186$; p-value $< .0001$.
For 57–75 kg: $X^2 = 18.081$; p-value $< .0001$.
For >75 kg: $X^2 = .382$; p-value $= .5365$.

(b) $z = 5.57$; p-value is almost zero but assumption might be wrong.
6.26. (a) For age:
Ages 14–17: $X^2 = 3.25$; p-value $= .0714$.
Ages 18–19: $X^2 = 3.63$; p-value $= .0567$.
Ages 21–24: $X^2 = 3.51$; p-value $= .0610$.
Ages 25–29: $X^2 = .01$; p-value is almost 1.0.

(b) Socio-economic level:
Upper: $X^2 = 10.02$; p-value $= .0015$.
Upper middle: $X^2 = 9.31$; p-value $= .0023$.
Middle: $X^2 = 4.02$; p-value $= .0450$.
Lower middle: $X^2 = 1.84$; p-value $= .1750$.

6.27. For boys: $X^2 = 9.46$; p-value $= .0021$.
For girls: $X^2 = 1.30$; p-value $= .2542$.

6.28. For duration (years): $X^2 = 1.28$; p-value $= .2579$.
For history of infertility: $X^2 = 3.45$; p-value $= .0633$.

6.29. For X-ray: $X^2 = 11.28$; p-value $= .0008$.
For grade: $X^2 = 4.07$; p-value $= .0437$.
For stage: $X^2 = 5.00$; p-value $= .0253$.

CHAPTER 7

7.1. $t = 1.68$; df $= 15$; p-value $= .0568$, one-sided.

7.2. $t = 1.33$; df $= 6$; p-value $= .2318$.

7.3. $t = 3.32$; df $= 6$; p-value$=.0160$.

7.4. $t = 3.95$; df $= 59$; p-value$=.0002$.

7.5. $t = .64$; df $= 20$; p-value $= .5294.20$.

7.6. $t = 3.29$; df $= 13$; p-value $= .0059$.

7.7. For men with college education: $t = 11.00$; p-value $< .0001$.

    For women with high school: $t = 7.75$; p-value $< .0001$.

    For women with college education: $t = 2.21$; p-value $= .0294$.

    Men with different education levels: $t = 2.70$; p-value $= .0081$.

    Women with different education levels: $t = 1.19$; p-value $= .2369.20$.

    High school: men versus women: $t = 6.53$; p-value $< .0001$.

    College: men versus women: $t = 3.20$; p-value $= .0018$.

7.8. SBP: $t = 12.11$; p-value $< .0001$.

    DBP: $t = 10.95$; p-value $< .0001$.

    BMI: $t = 6.71$; p-value $< .0001$.

7.9. $t = 3.40$; p-value $= .0010$.

7.10. $t = = .54$; df $= 25$; p-value $= .5940$.

7.11. $t = 2.86$; df $= 61$; p-value $= .0058$.

7.12. $t = 4.40$; p-value $< .0001$.

7.13. $t = 3.45$; df $= 17$; p-value $= .0031$.

7.14. $t = 4.71$; p-value $< .0001$.

7.15. Weight gain: $t = 2.30$; p-value $= .0235$.

    Birth weight: $t = 2.08$; p-value $= .0401$.

    Gestational age: $t \cong 0$; p-value is almost 1.0.

7.16. $t = 4.38$; df $= 35$; p-value $= .0001$.

7.17. An application of the One-way ANOVA yields:

Source of Variation	SS	df	MS	F Statistic	p-Value
Between samples	55.44	2	27.72	2.62	.1059
Within samples	158.83	15	10.59		
Total	214.28	17			

7.18. An application of the One-way ANOVA yields:

Source of Variation	SS	df	MS	F Statistic	p-Value
Between samples	74.803	3	24.934	76.23	.0001
Within samples	4.252	13	.327		
Total	79.055	16			

7.19. An application of the One-way ANOVA yields:

Source of Variation	SS	df	MS	F Statistic	p-Value
Between samples	40.526	2	20.263	3.509	0.0329
Within samples	527.526	126	5.744		
Total	568.052	128			

7.20. An application of the One-way ANOVA yields:

Source of Variation	SS	df	MS	F Statistic	p-Value
Between samples	57.184	3	19.061	37.026	<.0001
Within samples	769.113	1494	.515		
Total	826.297	1497			

7.21. An application of the One-way ANOVA yields:

For exposed group:

Source of Variation	SS	df	MS	F Statistic	p-Value
Between samples	5,310.03	2	2,655.016	.987	.3738
Within samples	845,028.000	314	2,691.172		
Total	850,338.032	316			

For non-exposed group:

Source of Variation	SS	df	MS	F Statistic	p-Value
Between samples	10,513.25	2	5,256.62	2.867	.06
Within samples	607,048.000	331	1,833.98		
Total	617,561.249	333			

7.22. (a) Age: $t = 1.037$; p-value $= .3337$.
    Acid: $t = -1.785$; p-value $= .0800$.
    (b) An application of the One-way ANOVA yields:

For age:

Source of Variation	SS	df	MS	F Statistic	p-Value
Between samples	49.710	3	16.570	0.4210	0.739
Within samples	1928.743	49	39.362		
Total	1978.453				

For acid:

Source of Variation	SS	df	MS	F Statistic	p-Value
Between samples	4797.380	3	1599.127	2.5357	0.068
Within samples	30901.490	49	630.643		
Total					

CHAPTER 8

8.1.
    (a) Graph is not available.
    (b) $b_0 = .0301$, $b_1 = 1.1386$, and $\hat{y} = .596$.
    (c) $t = 5.622$, df $= 4$, p-value $= .0049$.
    (d) $r^2 = .888$.

8.2.
    (a) Graph is not available.
    (b) $b_0 = 6.08$, $b_1 = .35$, and $\hat{y} = 27.08$.
    (c) $t = 2.173$, df $= 4$, p-value $= .082$.
    (d) $r^2 = .486$.

8.3.
    (a) Graph is not available.
    (b) $b_0 = 311.45$, $b_1 = -.08$, and $\hat{y} = 79.45$.
    (c) $t = -5.648$, df $= 20$, p-value $= .0001$.
    (d) $r^2 = .618$.

8.4.
    (a) $F = 16.2$, df $= (2,19)$, $p = .0001$.
    (b) $R^2 = .631$.
    (c) Results.

Factor	Regression Coefficient	Standard Error	t-Statistic	p-Value
X (food)	−.007	.091	−.082	.936
X^2	−.00001	.00001	−.811	.427

8.5. (1) For men:
 (a) Graph is not available.
 (b) $b_0 = -22.057$, $b_1 = -.538$, and $\hat{y} = 64.09$.
 (c) $t = -1.697$, df $= 5$, p-value $= .128$.
 (d) $r^2 = .265$.

(2) For women:
 (a) Graph is not available.
 (b) $b_0 = -61.624$, $b_1 = .715$, and $\hat{y} = 52.78$.
 (c) $t = 2.917$, df $= 5$, p-value $= .019$.
 (d) $r^2 = .516$.

8.6. (a) Results:

Factor	Regression Coefficient	Standard Error	t-Statistic	p-Value
Sex	-39.573	81.462	$-.486$	.634
Height	.361	.650	.555	.587
Sex-by-height	.177	.492	.360	.724

 (b) No (p-value $= .724$).
 (c) $F = 22.39$, df $= (3,16)$, $p = .0001$.
 (d) $R^2 = .808$.

8.7. (1) For Standard:
 (a) Graph is not available.
 (b) $b_0 = .292$, $b_1 = .362$, and $\hat{y} = 1.959$.
 (c) $t = 7.809$, df $= 5$, p-value $= .0001$.
 (d) $r^2 = .884$.

(2) For Test:
 (a) Graph is not available.
 (b) $b_0 = .283$, $b_1 = .280$, and $\hat{y} = 1.919$.
 (c) $t = 9.152$, df $= 5$, p-value $= .019$.
 (d) $r^2 = .913$.
 (e) No indication of effect modification.

8.8. (a) Results:

Factor	Regression Coefficient	Standard Error	t-Statistic	p-Value
Preparation	$-.009$	.005	-1.680	.112
Log dose	.443	.088	5.051	<.001
Preparation-by-Log dose	$-.081$	.056	-1.458	.164

 (b) No, very weak indication (p-value $= .164$).
 (c) $F = 46.23$, df $= (3,16)$, $p = .0001$.
 (d) $R^2 = .897$.

8.9. (1) For AG Positives:
    (a) Graph is not available.
    (b) $b_0 = .4810$, $b_1 = -.818$, and $\hat{y} = 19.58$.
    (c) $t = -3.821$, df $= 5$, p-value $= .002$.
    (d) $r^2 = .493$.

(2) For AG Negatives:
    (a) Graph is not available.
    (b) $b_0 = 1.903$, $b_1 = -.234$, and $\hat{y} = 9.06$.
    (c) $t = -.987$, df $= 5$, p-value $= .340$.
    (d) $r^2 = .065$.
    (e) Relationship is stronger and statistically significant for AG Positives but not so for AG Negatives.

8.10. (a) Results:

Factor	Regression Coefficient	Standard Error	t-Statistic	p-Value
AG status	2.847	1.343	2.119	.043
Log WBC	−.234	.243	−.961	.345
AG-by-Log WBC	−.583	.321	−1.817	.080

    (b) Rather strong indication (p-value $= .080$).
    (c) $F = 7.69$, df $= (3,29)$, $p = .0006$.
    (d) $R^2 = .443$.

8.11. (1) For revenue:
    (a) Graph is not available.
    (b) $b_0 = 1.113 \times 10^{-6}$, $b_1 = .829 \times 10^{-6}$, and $\hat{y} = 1.329$.
    (c) $t = -.198$, df $= 5$, p-value $= .884$.
    (d) $r^2 = .001$.

(2) For work load hours:
    (a) Graph is not available.
    (b) $b_0 = .260 \times 10^{-6}$, $b_1 = .754 \times 10^{-6}$, and $\hat{y} = 1.252$.
    (c) $t = 1.882$, df $= 5$, p-value $= .067$.
    (d) $r^2 = .078$.

8.12. (a) Results:

Factor	Regression Coefficient $\times 10^6$	Standard Error $\times 10^6$	t-Statistic	p-Value
Residency	3,176	1,393	2.279	.028
Sex	348	303.000	1.149	.258
Revenue	1.449	4.340	.334	.741
Work load hours	2.206	760	2.889	.006
Residency-by-hours	−2.264	.930	−2.436	.020

(b) Very strong indication (p-value $= .020$).

(c) $F = 2.14$, df $= (5,38)$, $p = .083$.

(d) $R^2 = .219$.

Index

Health and Numbers: A Problems-Based Introduction to Biostatistics, Third Edition, by Chap T. Le
Copyright © 2009 John Wiley & Sons, Inc.